Michael Y. Henein (Editor)

Heart Failure
in Clinical Practice

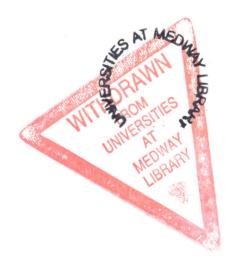

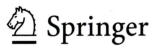 Springer

Prof. Michael Y. Henein
Department of Public Health and Clinical
Medicine, Umeå University, and
Umeå Heart Centre
Umeå, Sweden

ISBN: 978-1-84996-152-3   e-ISBN: 978-1-84996-153-0
DOI: 10.1007/978-1-84996-153-0
Springer Dordrecht Heidelberg London New York

A catalogue record for this book is available from the British Library

Library of Congress Control Number: 2010925793

Cover design: eStudio Calamar, Figueres/Berlin

Printed on acid-free paper

Springer is part of Springer Science+Business Media (www.springer.com)

Foreword

Heart failure is a complex clinical syndrome caused by a variety of etiologies: myocardial, valvular, and congenital. While the majority of its signs and symptoms are because of myocardial disease, one should not forget the less common cases which need the surgeon's intervention. In addition, the fast development of cardiac devices has set a platform for potential recovery of patients previously considered as end-stage heart failure. I strongly recommend this excellent and comprehensive book edited by Professor Michael Henein as a manual and guide for understanding and managing patients with heart failure.

Donald Ross

Preface

Over the years we have made considerable progress in the diagnosis and management of the syndrome of heart failure, the end-stage of most cardiac diseases. A Pharaonic diagnosis by means of observation of the signs of fluid retention has now been replaced by non-invasive cardiac function assessment, while tests for myocardial pathology and the assessment of intra-cardiac pressures aid in the diagnosis.

Similarly, management of heart failure patients has progressed from bed rest, until death, to a fully active exercise program. Thanks to the most recent pharmacological developments, even patients with very poor pump function can now enjoy near normal life without fluid retention. Furthermore, noninvasive cardiac imaging has allowed clinicians to identify patients in need of heart pump assistance and various devices are now available for temporary and long-term treatment strategies. While surgical devices aim at pressure off-loading of the ventricles for potential functional recovery, percutaneous devices aim at electrically optimizing and syncronizing ventricular function.

As a result of these improvements in diagnosis and patient management, clinical practice itself has had to change. Specialist clinics are now established worldwide and clinicians are sub-specializing in heart failure, as are nurses both in hospitals and community care.

While the outlook for heart failure patients is significantly improved, little has yet been achieved in prevention of the condition, and much remains to be done to delay disease progression and alleviate symptoms. This cannot be achieved without further high-quality research, particularly into the causes of heart failure itself and its progression from other less serious conditions. The more controversial issues mentioned in the chapters of this book, aim to stimulate clinicians to progress these ideas.

Michael Y. Henein

Contents

Contributors

Stefan D. Anker, MD, PhD
Department of Cardiology
Campus Vivdow Klinikum,
Charite
Universitatsmedizin Berlin
Berlin
Germany

**Constantinos Anagnostopoulos, MD,
FRCP, FRCR, FESC**
Department of Nuclear
Medicine and PET/CT
Barts and The London
School of Medicine and Dentistry
(QMUL)
London
UK

Diane Barker, MB ChB, MD
Cardiology
Liverpool Heart and Chest Hospital
Liverpool
UK

Resham Baruah, MD
National Heart and Lung Institute
Imperial College London
London
UK

Kurt Boman, MD, PhD
Department of Medicine
Public Health and Clinical Medicine
Skelleftea
Vasterbotten
Sweden

Lip Bun Tan, MBBChir, DPhil
Cardiology
Leeds General Infirmary
Leeds
UK

Margherita Calcagnino, MD
The Heart Hospital
London
UK

Andrew J.S. Coats, MD
University of East Anglia
Norwich Research Park
Norwich
Norfolk
UK

**Konstantinos Dimopoulos, MD, MSc,
PhD, FESC**
Adult Congenital Heart Centre
and Centre for Pulmonary Hypertension
Royal Brompton Hospital
London
UK

Wolfram Doehner, MD, PhD
Center for Stroke Research
Charité - Universitätsmedizin Berlin
Berlin
Germany

**Darryl P. Francis, Ma, MB,
BChir, MD, FRCP**
National Heart and Lung Institute
Imperial College London
London
UK

Jeffrey W.H. Fung, MD
Medicine and Therapeutics
Prince of Wales Hospital
The Chinese University of Hong Kong
Shatin
Hong Kong
China

Michael A. Gatzoulis, MD, PhD, FESC
Adult Congenital Heart Centre and Centre
for Pulmonary Hypertension
Royal Brompton Hospital
London
UK

**Georgios Giannakoulas, MD, PhD,
FESC**
Adult Congenital Heart Centre and Centre
for Pulmonary Hypertension
Royal Brompton Hospital
London
UK

Bengt Johansson, MD, PhD
Cardiology
Heart Centre
Umeå University Hospital
Umeå
Sweden

Nigel T. Lewis, MBChB
Cardiology
Leeds Teaching Hospitals NHS Trust
Leeds
UK

Wei Li, MD, PhD
Echocardiography Department
Royal Brompton & Harefield NHS Trust
London
UK

Per G. Lindqvist, PhD
Heart Centre
Public Health and Clincal Medicine
Umeå University Hospital
Umeå
Sweden

Krister Lindmark, MD, PhD
Department of Cardiology
Heart Center, Umeå University Hospital
Umeå
Sweden

Gregory Y.H. Lip, MD
Haemostasis Thrombosis & Vascular
Biology Unit
University of Birmingham Centre for
Cardiovascular Sciences
City Hospital
Birmingham
UK

**Robert J. MacFadyen, MD,
MRPharmS, FRCP**
University Department of Medicine
City Hospital
Birmingham
UK

Joseph F. Malouf, MD
Mayo Clinic
Internal Medicine
Rochester
Minnesota
USA

Cheuk-Man YU, MD
The Chinese University of Hong Kong
Shatin
Hong Kong
China

**William J. McKenna, BA, MD,
DSc, FRCP**
Institute of Cardiovascular Science
University College London
The Heart Hospital
London
UK

**Farouk Mookadam, MD,
FRCPC, FACC**
Mayo Clinic
Scottsdale
Arizona
USA

Stellan Mörner
Heart Centre
Public Health and Clincal Medicine
Umeå University Hospital
Umeå

Sherif E. Moustafa, MBBCh
Department of Cardiology
University of Alberta Hospital
Edmonton
Alberta
Canada

Andrew Owen, PhD, FESC
Department of Cardiology
Princess of Wales Hospital
Bridgend
Mid Glamorgan
Wales

Ashish Y. Patwala
Liverpool Heart and
Chest Hospital
Liverpool
UK

John Pepper, MA.MChir, FRCS
Royal Brompton Hospital
Department of Surgery
Sydney Street
London
UK

Eugenio Picano, MD
CNR, Institute of Clinical
Physiology
Pisa
Italy

**John E. Sanderson, MD, FRCP,
FACC, FHKAM**
Cardiovascular Medicine
University of Birmingham
Queen Elizabeth Hospital
Birmingham
UK

Stefan Soderberg, MD, PhD
Umeå University
Umeå
Sweden

James Stirrup, BSc MBBS MRCP
Department of Nuclear Medicine
Royal Brompton Hospital
London
UK

Lip-Bun Tan, MBBChir, DPhil
Cardiology
Leeds General Infirmary
Leeds
LS1 3EX
UK

Yu-ting Tan, MBBS
Cardiology
University of Birmingham
Edgbaston
Birmingham
UK

Lynne Williams, MD
University of Birmingham
Edgbaston
Birmingham
UK

Definition, Diagnosis, Epidemiology, Etiology and Pathophysiology of Heart Failure

1

Lip-Bun Tan, Nigel Lewis, and Diane Barker

Heart failure (HF) is the culmination of all preceding cardiovascular events and the successes and failures of attempted and administered interventions. It is the cumulative effects of all abnormalities in the heart, which culminate in the functional impairment of the cardiac pump. Once the patient reaches the stage of symptomatic HF, the prognosis becomes poor. The more severe the HF, the nearer the patient is to death, and therefore the less room for mistakes in managing these patients. For these reasons, attention to details such as accuracy of diagnoses, correct assessments of severity, profound understanding of the pathophysiological processes and institution of timely therapy are crucial, and it calls for no less than the most skilled of HF specialists if the patients were to stand any chance of successfully fighting against this lethal condition. This chapter intends to lay the foundations for rational approaches to therapy.

With multiple publications of guidelines by august national and international bodies, there is now a prevalent misconception that clinicians only need to follow these detailed guidelines, as they would follow a recipe book, and all will be well. In some quarters of clinical practitioners, it is deemed sufficient to follow guidelines and no longer necessary to comprehend such complex issues as definition, epidemiology, etiology and pathophysiology of HF, and these can be relegated to the ivory towers of academia. This could not be further from the truth. Managing HF demands the caring clinicians to not only judiciously adhere to published or local guidelines but also understand the bases upon which the guidelines were drafted, and be aware of their shortcomings, in order to exercise clinical judgment whenever necessary.

1.1
Definition of Heart Failure

Ambiguous or misleading definitions will lead to erroneous diagnosis and treatment. For example, patients with 'high output heart failure' (associated with pathologically low systemic vascular impedance) may be given the standard guideline approved HF therapy of

L.-B. Tan (✉)
Leeds General Infirmary, Leeds LS1 3EX, UK
e-mail: lbtan99@hotmail.com

M.Y. Henein (ed.), *Heart Failure in Clinical Practice*,
DOI: 10.1007/978-1-84996-153-0_1, © Springer-Verlag London Limited 2010

vasodilators, including angiotensin converting enzyme (ACE) inhibitors or negative inotropic and chronotropic agents such as beta-blockers, to the detriment of the individuals.
Or worse, the so-called 'failing' heart could have been removed and transplanted with a
donor heart, which was subsequently found to be inadequate to cope with the excessive
systemic vasodilation. Patients with hypertensive 'heart failure' may be given positive
inotropic agents, even though the systolic function is often unimpaired. Although in relative terms these hearts have 'failed' to support the requisite circulation, in absolute terms,
the hearts may be normal or even supernormal. The mistake stems from the misconception
that a normal heart is also expected to support an unphysiological circulation [either with
excessive cardiac output (CO) and/or blood pressure]. The term 'HF' should therefore not
be used to describe conditions of relative failure.

One not uncommon mistake with regard to defining HF is the confusion between definition and diagnosis. A definition should be universally applicable, not only to clinicians but
also to biochemists, engineers, geneticists, lay persons, pharmacologists or physiologists,
whereas a diagnosis only pertains to the clinical arena. Quite a number of the so-called 'definitions' are actually a guide to diagnosis, consisting of a list of clinical features, which if
present will help a clinician to arrive at a diagnosis of HF (e.g., ESC Guidelines on HF[1]).

HF implies the failure of the organ to function as it should. The historical milestone
definition of the function of the heart has been that attributed to William Harvey, the dis-
coverer of the circulation, who in 1628 stated:

> … that the *movement* of the blood is *constantly* in a circle, and is brought about by the *beat*
> of the heart … for the sake of nourishment …

Applying Newton's first Law of Motion to the cardiovascular system, we may infer that blood
cannot be constantly in motion in the circulation unless acted upon by the beat of the heart.
The entity that is provided by the beat of the heart to allow the continuous motion of blood is
hydraulic energy. Without the beat of the heart, blood in the circulation would come to a
standstill, because of the forces opposing flow, the frictional and separational forces. According
to the Law of Conservation of Energy, to maintain the circulation, the hydraulic energy lost in
the vasculature has to be replenished by the energy imparted by the heart. The function of the
heart, expressed in modern physiological terms, is therefore to provide adequate hydraulic
energy to maintain the circulation under physiological loading conditions. This definition
depicts the notion of energy dissipation in the vasculature, which has to be counterbalanced by
the work of the heart. In the circulation, the power (rate of work) of moving a volume of fluid
is the product of pressure and flow rate (power = energy or work per unit time = flow rate ×
pressure). Thus, the ability of the heart to generate energy and perform external work encom-
passes not only its ability to generate flow but also its ability to generate pressure. Pressure
generation is essential, unless the impedance to flow in the circulation is zero.

Taking the function of the heart as the sole pump responsible for maintaining the circulation, a modern definition of HF is therefore *the failure of the cardiac pump under physiological loading conditions to impart sufficient hydraulic energy output in order to
maintain a physiological circulation*. Implicit in the statement is the ability of the heart and
circulation to cope with all the usual physiological stresses such as severe exercise, desert
heat and altitude hypoxia. It is not expected that a normal human heart should be able to
cope with the circulation of a giraffe (such as encountered in severe hypertension) or of a
buffalo (such as during excessively high output states).

Defining HF correctly will lead to hierarchical categorization of our understanding of the pathophysiological processes in HF. This will avoid giving priority to treating secondary defects (such as vasoconstriction and neurohumoral activation) in HF at the expense of the primary defects (e.g., silent myocardial ischemia, pericardial effusion). A good definition will also lead to better conceptualization of the etiological processes of HF, and this will lead to a more rational approach to treatment. For example, treatment strategies can be divided into three: (1) definitive treatment such as reversing the pathological process(es) (as if turning the clock back). In clinical practice, it is only possible to approach such ideal interventions, such as replacement of valves, coronary bypass surgery, pericardiocentesis or regression of atherosclerosis; (2) palliative, in an attempt to alleviate distressing symptoms when nothing else can be done and (3) intermediate – i.e., buying time before the definitive treatment becomes indicated or available – including the use of diuretics, vasodilators and ACE inhibitors.

1.2
Diagnosis and Investigations

The clinical features that aid the diagnosis of the presence or absence of HF include the following (e.g., ESC Guidelines, 2008[1]):

- Symptoms typical of HF (breathlessness on exercise or at rest, fatigue, tiredness, ankle swelling).
- Signs typical of HF [tachycardia, hypotension, peripheral edema, hepatomegaly, venous congestion, ascites (Fig. 1.1), cool peripheries, tachypnea, pulmonary crackles or rales, pleural effusion, displaced apex beat/cardiomegaly, third heart sound, gallop rhythm, cardiac murmurs, oliguria/anuria].
- Objective evidence of functional or structural abnormality(ies) of the heart (radiographic or echocardiographic abnormality(ies), or via other imaging techniques, certain ECG abnormalities, raised natriuretic peptide concentration in the absence of renal failure).

The primary and most important duty of any clinician looking after any newly diagnosed HF patient is to identify whether there are any reversible or correctible lesions. Successful reversal or correction of these lesions may lift the patient out of the HF category altogether, or significantly ameliorate the severity of HF. HF should not be considered as an end-diagnosis without attempting to clarify the etiology. Therefore, the complete diagnostic process for a patient with suspected HF should include the following three steps:

1. The presence or absence of HF
2. The etiology of HF
3. The severity of HF

If any of these components is missing, then the diagnostic process is incomplete.

Objective tests are available to help clarify each of these diagnostic steps (Table 1.1). It is important to differentiate electrophysiological, structural and functional aspects of the

Fig. 1.1 An elderly heart
failure patient presenting
with ascites and prominent
superficial abdominal
venous congestion

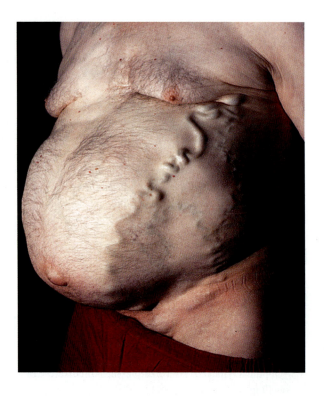

cardiac pump (Table 1.2). Patients with a low or high probability of HF based on the initial
assessments (Table 1.1) should undergo further evaluation to establish an alternative or
concomitant diagnosis. All patients with definite or probable HF should have an echocardiogram to identify cardiac structural abnormalities (e.g., cardiac chamber dimensions,
valve and other lesions). Other imaging techniques including cardiac magnetic resonance
(CMR) imaging may provide additional and more accurate assessment of cardiac structure, myocardial perfusion metabolism and resting ventricular systolic function. However,
the hallmark of patients with chronic HF is troublesome symptoms during exertion. True
function (i.e., what a patient can do) is better assessed when exertional symptoms occur,
through cardiopulmonary exercise testing, measuring their exercise capacity, peak oxygen
consumption (VO_2), peak CO and peak cardiac power output (CPO) (Table 1.2). From
these values, peak CPO has emerged as the strongest independent predictor of mortality in
HF patients.[2] This provides a direct grading of the functional severity of HF (Fig. 1.2).

1.2.1
Epidemiology of Heart Failure

The epidemiology of HF has been studied by many centers but the earliest and probably
the most comprehensive study has been conducted in Framingham.[3] Each of these epidemiological studies highlights various findings, but all of them show one common finding,

Table 1.1 Investigations to aid the diagnosis of heart failure

Investigations	HF likely if	HF unlikely if
ECG	Evidence of previous MI, significant arrhythmia, very low or wide QRS complexes	Entirely normal
CXR	Cardiomegaly, pulmonary congestion	Confounding pathology e.g., pneumonia (Fig. 1.2), COPD, pulmonary fibrosis, but may coexist with/exacerbate HF
BNP or N-BNP	• Elevation unexplained by renal impairment • Indirectly estimates severity of HF	Below laboratory range for normal subjects
Echocardiogram (or other imaging techniques, e.g., angiography, MRI, CT, scintigraphy)	• Nontrivial cardiac structural lesion(s) found as causative of pump dysfunction → establish etiology • Degree of compensatory changes/remodeling indirectly estimates severity	Normal cardiac structures & normal LV systolic and diastolic function
Cardiopulmonary Exercise testing	• Reduced cardiac reserve measured • Directly grades severity of HF • Abnormal Ex ECGs: ischemia, arrhythmia	Normal peak O_2 uptake or cardiac pumping reserve

Table 1.2 Assessing aspects of cardiac abnormalities

Electrical	Structural	Functional
Rate	LV dimensions, size	Exercise capacity
Rhythm	LVEF	Peak Ex VO2
Conduction	Regional walls	Peak CO, CPO
	Valvular lesions	Symptoms
	VSD, ASD	NYHA class
	Coronary lesions	Myocardial function
	Pericardium	

which is most relevant in clinical practice: that the incidence and prevalence of HF increases with age in all populations studied. A recent version of this relationship is shown in Fig. 1.3.[4] The median age at first diagnosis is usually over 70 years.[5] Symptomatic HF affects more than 900,000 people in the UK with a prevalence of 3% at 65–74 years, 7% at 75–84 years and over 12% above the age of 85 years (Fig. 1.3).[3] The incidence of HF is higher in men than in women in all age groups; however, because of higher life expectancy in women, there are more elderly women with HF than men. HF is increasingly causing a heavy burden on health resources, accounting for around 2% of the entire UK National

Fig. 1.2 CXR showing lobar pneumonia and pulmonary edema secondary to LV failure

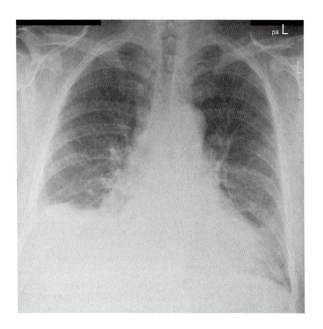

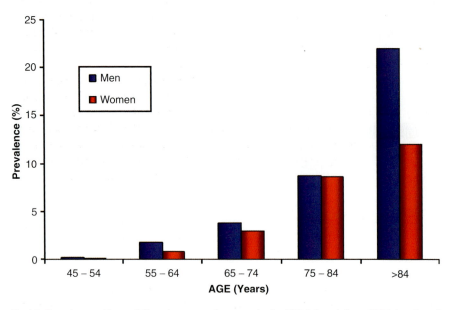

Fig. 1.3 Prevalence of heart failure in men and women in the UK (plotted from BHF data http://www.heartstats.org)

Health Service expenditure.[6] More than 80% of HF patients are 65 years and older, and they account for a disproportionate number of HF deaths and hospitalizations. Hypertension and coronary artery disease (CAD) account for the majority of cases of HF.[2]

1.2.2
Etiology

Although it is a common practice in most textbooks and review articles to provide a detailed listing of the frequencies of each etiology contributing to the population occurrences of HF, in actual clinical practice, such information is of peripheral importance. Whether an individual patient facing the clinician is more likely to have common conditions such as hypertension or ischemic heart disease causing his/her HF, or happens to be affected by a less common cardiomyopathy secondary to inflammatory or infiltrative disorders as the cause of HF is immaterial, because the history and clinical features are more likely to lead the clinician to the actual etiology. Thus, a first principle for the clinician is to treat each patient as a unique person and not merely as an epidemiological entity in population statistics. There is no substitute for good basic practice of taking careful medical history, physical examinations, investigations and interpreting the available information intelligently and wisely.

An important practical issue is what role etiology plays in the management of patients with HF. As an illustration, in one relatively small-scale epidemiological survey of the etiology of new cases of HF, the largest category of patients (34%) was classified as having unknown etiology.[7] As stated in the previous section, the HF diagnostic process is deemed incomplete if the cause of HF remains unknown. The causes of HF that are most important to diagnose are those which are amenable to surgical, interventional or pharmacological corrective treatment. For example, HF secondary to previously undetected cardiac tamponade or ruptured chordae tendinae can be readily corrected and the patient can be released from life-long treatment with diuretics and other HF drugs.

Generally, patients with HF are broadly classed into two groups: (1) cardiomyopathy secondary to ischemic heart disease and (2) cardiomyopathy due to nonischemic causes. Those with ischemic etiology tend to have a worse prognosis.[8] In the latter category, the two commonest underlying causes are hypertension and idiopathic dilated cardiomyopathy. Other not uncommon etiological causes are valvular diseases, arrhythmias (esp. atrial fibrillation) or conduction defects, and other structural defects. A significant proportion of patients with these etiologies can respond favourably to appropriate treatment.

Ischemic heart disease. The commonest cause of HF in the UK and Western world is ischemic heart disease. Ischemic heart disease often results in HF after a large myocardial infarction (MI), or multiple macro- and micro-infarctions. The presentation of HF may be acute or delayed. The most severe form of postinfarction HF is cardiogenic shock where the mortality rates are usually very high. Accurate diagnosis of this condition is urgent, and a reliable estimate of prognosis would help to triage the most effective treatment (Table 1.3).[9] Patients with substantial myocardial ischemia or hibernation would benefit from primary revascularization without delay, but those with substantial stunned myocardium would in time recover after appropriate and protracted circulatory support.[10]

Postinfarction patients with sizeable infarction will incur impaired pumping capacity of the left ventricle, resulting in clinical features of left ventricular failure. Typically the full thickness necrotic zone will undergo subsequent infarct expansion with attendant overall left ventricular chamber dilatation often referred to as adverse remodeling. The infarct expansion may be so large as to form an aneurysm, which further impairs pumping capacity

Table 1.3 Diagnosis and prognosis in cardiogenic shock

Clinical features aiding diagnosis of cardiogenic shock
Anuria, or oliguria with urine output <20 mL/h for consecutive hours
Cool moist skin of peripheries (fingers, toes, tip of nose)
Auscultatory or intra-arterial systolic blood pressure <90 mmHg
Obtunded mental state
Metabolic acidosis
Cardiac index <2 L/min
Not secondary to other causes of shock, e.g., hypovolemia, drug-induced (opiates, vasodilators, beta-blockers), arrhythmia, septicemia
Markers of grave prognosis in cardiogenic shock
Exhaustion of cardiac reserve despite inotropic stimulation[30]
Low cardiac power, esp <0.8 W[31]
Widespread Q waves with virtually absent R waves in all ECG leads
Protracted anuria despite normal serum creatinine
Echocardiographic global LVEF<10%
Systolic BP <60 mmHg and sinus tachycardia >100 beats/min

of the entire ventricle. The continual dilation of the left ventricular chamber progressively stretches the mitral valve ring leading to functional mitral regurgitation, thereby rendering the ventricle to function in the descending limb of Starling's curve.

With the advent of primary angioplasty and aggressive treatment of acute coronary syndrome, not all patients undergo completion of the infarct process during the acute phases, such that substantial noninfarcted myocardial territories end up being prone to ischemia, while others are either hibernating or stunned. Those with residual ischemia are more straightforward because they complain of angina usually during exertion but occasionally at rest. In such patients, the focus of the diagnostic process is to determine whether there is enough ischemic myocardium to benefit from anti-anginal medication or coronary revascularization. About a third of HF patients with ischemic heart disease have silent-ischemia myocardium, and their presenting complaint is often not angina but dyspnoea on exertion, just like patients with HF. Hence, amongst the HF patient with CAD, it is important to identify those with silent ischemia or hibernating myocardium, because coronary revascularization, via angioplasty or bypass surgery, may improve cardiac function so much as to obviate the need to continue with standard HF drugs. A small percentage of patients would have anginal symptoms or manifestations of silent ischemia due to coronary vasospasm. These may occur in coronary arterial segments with tight stenosis due to eccentric plaques, which are amenable to revascularization, or in apparently normal coronary arteries (Prinzmetal angina), which would respond to coronary vasodilatory drugs. Myocardial ischemia can sometimes present as tachyarrhythmia, especially during exertion but sometimes at rest, and the associated symptoms are dizziness, presyncope or syncope, exertional dyspnoea, or intermittent hyperventilation (often wrongly labeled as anxiety-related hyperventilatory syndrome). Prolonged Holter monitoring, especially those with facility for ST-segment monitoring, might unravel the underlying pathology. As a general rule, the hierarchy of seriousness of symptoms in ischemic HF patients is as follows (most serious first): syncope / presyncope > dyspnoea > angina, in terms of urgency of investigations and treatment.

Patients with substantial stunned myocardium may linger for some time with significant HF symptoms, but the prognosis is relatively good because once the stunning is resolved, the HF symptoms would abate. Patients with significant hibernating myocardium often masquerade as moderate-to-severe HF and are usually harder to diagnose, and treatment with escalating doses of HF medication (e.g., diuretics, ACE inhibitors) may be counterproductive. Referral to experts in this subspecialty may be required. The useful diagnostic steps to be considered and undertaken in HF patients with ischemic heart disease are those which will yield possibilities for therapeutic gains thereby alleviating the HF status, as shown in Table 1.4.

Nonischemic cardiomyopathies causing HF. Any intra-cardiac and extra-cardiac lesions affecting the heart, when severe enough as to significantly impair cardiac pump function, are liable to cause HF. Apart from ischemic heart disease, in the Western World, by far the two commonest causes are primary dilated cardiomyopathy and hypertensive HF. In some countries, valvular disorders secondary to rheumatic heart disease are still important etiologically,

Table 1.4 Ischemic heart disease and its sequelae as causes of heart failure

Treatable defects	Potential treatment options
Myocardial ischemia, esp. silent	Revascularization, anti-ischemia & preventative Rx
Ischemia due to coronary vasospasm	Coronary vasodilatory drugs
Arrhythmias	Anti-arrhythmic agents, ablation ICD
Conduction defects	Pacemaker, CRT
Excessive tachycardia/bradycardia	Drug or device Rx
Stunned myocardium	Supportive to promote recovery
Hibernating myocardium	Skill required in diagnosis, revascularization as appropriate, otherwise supportive
Structural abnormalities: e.g., acute mitral regurgitation due to ruptured papillary muscle(s), acute VSD, acute ventricular wall rupture resulting in tamponade	Acute surgical intervention
Adverse remodeling, LV aneurysm, functional mitral regurgitation	Surgical ventricular reconstruction, plication of mitral apparatus
Ventricular mechanical or electrical remodeling – resulting in eventual BBB and contractile dyssynchrony	CRT
End-stage HF	Cardiac transplantation, VAD, Palliative care

while Chagas disease features more in the South American continent. Other causes include the categories of congenital heart diseases, inflammatory heart diseases (e.g., myocarditis, sarcoid heart disease, eosinophilic heart disease), infiltrative cardiomyopathies (e.g., amyloid heart disease, haemachromatosis, tumours), pericardial diseases, hypertrophic cardiomyopathy, tachycardia-induced cardiomyopathy, toxic cardiomyopathies (e.g., secondary to chemotherapy), connective tissue disorders (e.g., systemic lupus erythematosus, scleroderma), neuroendocrine and metabolic disorders (e.g., diabetic cardiomyopathy, thyrotoxic heart diseases) and peripartum cardiomyopathy. Detailed diagnostic methods of each of these conditions are beyond the scope of this chapter, and readers are referred to major cardiology textbooks or reviews for details.

Of more relevance to clinical practice is early diagnosis, monitoring and managing of conditions, which are preventable, such as hypertensive heart disease and diabetic cardiomyopathy. Hypertension is one of the commonest causes of HF.[11] It causes pressure overload on the ventricle, leading to left ventricular hypertrophy. It was reported from the Framingham study that the presence of LVH on the ECG leads to a tenfold increase in risk of developing HF.[12] This can subsequently cause a hypertensive cardiomyopathy with LV systolic impairment. In addition, diastolic dysfunction is much more common in hypertensive patients. Similar considerations would also benefit diabetic patients. Although direct cardiomyopathic damages can occur, patients with diabetes and hypertension more commonly have cardiac complications via CAD. Good management needs to be directed at controlling the hypertension and diabetes as tightly as possible, but also attending closely to preventing atherosclerosis. Other reversible lesions to diagnose are any form of valvular diseases, arrhythmia, conduction defects including heart blocks or bundle branch blocks causing contractile dyssynchrony, pericardial effusion or constriction. Some of these lesions can be corrected through cardiological interventions. It may not be always straightforward to diagnose such conditions, and sometimes, very complex cases may need to be referred to the most able of cardiologists with HF specialist expertise.

Another helpful aspect about diagnosing and managing patients with nonischemic cardiomyopathies is to be aware of the relative prognosis of the various conditions.[13] Relative to idiopathic cardiomyopathy, patients with peripartum cardiomyoapthy and hypertensive cardiomyopathy tend to have better prognosis, whereas those with infiltrative cardiomypathy and secondary to anthracycline therapy or HIV infection have the worst prognosis.[12] In the latter cases, the importance of prevention cannot be over-emphasized.

1.3
Pathophysiology

Reading contemporary journals on topics about HF, one can be forgiven for inferring that a majority of papers cover subject areas in vascular, pulmonary, renal, skeletal muscular, and other pathology, and less on the heart itself. Be that as it may, in clinical practice however, it is always helpful to be reminded that the starting point of HF is in the heart. And therefore, the first duty of the clinician is to find whether there are any primary (Table 1.5) defects in the heart that can be corrected either to get the patient out of the HF category or to ameliorate its severity. Although the primary defects are being evaluated with a view to

Table 1.5 Cardiac defects categorized with reference to management strategies.

Defects	Treatment
Primary (= initiating cause of cardiac pump dysfunction)	
Ischemic/hibernating myocardium	Coronary revascularization
Pericardial effusion	Pericardiocentesis
Pericardial constriction	Pericardiectomy
Valvular disease	Valve repair/replacement
Valve stenosis	Valvotomy/valvuloplasty/valve replacement
Intra-cardiac shunts	Repair of shunts
Heart block, dyssynchrony	Pacemaker implantation, CRT
Rhythm disorder	Anti-arrhythmics, ablation, ICD
Secondary (as a consequence of pump failure and compensatory mechanisms)	
Fluid retention	Diuretics
Vasoconstriction	Vasodilators
Neurohumoral activation	ACEi, beta-blockers, ARB, Aldo receptor blockers
Rhythm/conduction disorder	Anti-arrhythmics, ICD, CRT
Peripheral organ hypoperfusion	Positive inotropes, vasodilators
Flow redistribution	Low-dose dopamine
Tertiary (as consequence of secondary defects or therapeutic attempts)	
Electrolyte imbalance	Judicious use of therapeutic agents & prevent/correct the abnormalities
Arrhythmia	
Myocardial toxicity	
Worse organ hypoperfusion	
Maldistribution of blood flow	

intervention if possible, the secondary and tertiary defects should also be considered and treated accordingly (Table 1.5).

Primary defects. When considering the pathophysiology of primary cardiac defects in HF, an important false avenue to avoid is the pursuance of measuring myocardial contractility, which was first proposed in 1962 and led to decades of a futile search for powerful positive inotropic agents.[14] By far the commonest primary defects amenable to correction are coronary artery stenoses, although the presence of morphological coronary lesions per se in the absence of any functional consequence does not provide any indication for intervention. Other identifiable structural defects (e.g., valvular disease, septal defects, pericardial effusion or constriction) causing functional impairments are worthy of consideration for corrective interventions. A key outcome of these primary cardiac defects is a loss of cardiac pumping reserve such that diminution in peak cardiac function first becomes noticeable

Fig. 1.4 Cardiac functional reserve showing clear reduction of the maximal levels and pumping reserve capacity with mild and moderate heart failure, but the resting level becoming manifest at the severe end of heart failure

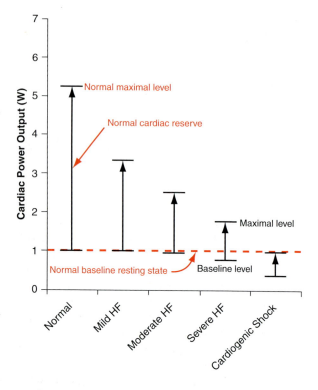

Fig. 1.5 A major loss of cardiac pumping capability and reserve is shown after a massive myocardial infarction (MI), and the ensuing progressive nature of functional deterioration which can be slowed by HF pharmacotherapy to improve the prognosis of HF patients as shown in clinical trials

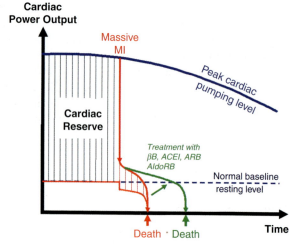

(Fig. 1.4). As the cardiac functional impairment progresses, then the resting cardiac function also becomes manifestly depressed (Fig. 1.4). Plotted against time, following a massive MI, cardiac reserve and peak performance are markedly reduced whereas the resting baseline cardiac performance is reduced to a smaller extent (Fig. 1.5).

Fig. 1.6 Vicious cycle of heart failure progression

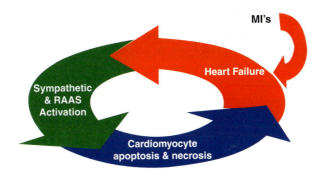

Secondary defects. Defects secondary to primary pump failure have attracted more research attention because of discoveries of beneficial pharmacological interventions since 1980s. The most important pathophysiological concept influencing the secondary defects of HF centers on the cardiovascular regulatory systems working together in order to maintain as normal an arterial pressure as possible. Following the onset of cardiac pumping failure, there is a tendency for the arterial pressure to fall, similar to the situation of hemorrhage.[15] This fall is detected by baroreceptors, which trigger compensatory mechanisms by systemic vasoconstriction, fluid retention and stimulation of cardiac performance, secondary to activation of the sympathetic, renin-angiotensin-aldosterone and vasopressin systems, which act together synergistically to restore BP towards normality. Unfortunately, it is well known that catecholamines, angiotensin and aldosterone are cardiotoxic. This in turn creates a vicious cycle whereby the compensatory mechanisms triggered by HF in turn worsen the HF, which will then require even higher levels of compensatory activation (Fig. 1.6). This pathophysiological vicious process can be arrested by inhibiting the activation of the sympathetic and RAA systems.

Tertiary defects. Iatrogenic complications, adverse reactions or side effects from therapeutic attempts can negate potential benefits of interventions, and if ignored can be detrimental. Clinical vigilance and close monitoring of the positive and negative effects of treatment are essential, especially when managing patients with unstable and severe HF.

1.3.1
Categories of Heart Failure

HF has been categorized in several ways:

1. *Acute vs. chronic HF* – this is the most important categorization in practice, because although they are both HF, the treatment is distinctly different. In acute decompensated HF, the patients are symptomatic at rest and exercise is out of the question, whereas those with chronic compensated HF are generally comfortable at rest but become symptomatic during exercise. Specific treatments for acute decompensated

HF (e.g., intravenous inotropes, dobutamine, milrinone, enoximone) are inappropriate for chronic ambulatory HF patients, and conversely therapy for chronic HF (e.g., ACE inhibitors, beta-blockers, angiotensin receptor blockers) may need to be temporarily stopped during acute exacerbation.

2. *Compensated vs. decompensated HF* – as above.
3. *Systolic vs. diastolic HF* – this is probably the most confusing and unhelpful categorization because in terms of cardiac muscle mechanics, systolic and diastolic dysfunction invariably coexist. It is more important to determine the severity and cause of HF in these patients to decide on how best to treat, than to worry about whether it is systolic or diastolic HF.
4. *Right-sided vs. left-sided HF* – because both right and left sides of the heart share a common pericardium and atrial and ventricular septa, there are always significant interactions between the two sides. Of practical importance are the questions whether the jugular various pressure (right-side filling pressure) can be used as an indirect indicator of the filling pressure for the left ventricle or not. Also whether the pulmonary system plays a major role in the etiology of HF or not.
5. *Low-output vs. high-output HF* – High-output HF is so rare nowadays that few will come across any case in a lifetime.
6. *Absolute vs. relative HF* – if a normal human heart is required to support a circulation with excessively high blood pressure (e.g., of a giraffe's circulation) or excessively large CO (e.g., of an elephant's circulation), there will be features typical of HF. This is relative HF, because the heart itself will function normally when connected to a normal physiological human circulation. The aim of treatment should not be stimulating the heart, but to lower its load. Absolute HF is when the heart itself is intrinsically failing and unable to maintain a normal physiological human circulation.

1.4
Comorbidity

Patients with HF have lower cardiac reserve to meet the greater circulatory demands required to cope with the stresses of extraordinary physiological states (exposure to very hot or cold weather) or disease states. For example, during septicemia, with toxic vasodilatation, much heightened circulation is necessary. The additional comorbid conditions render the HF patient even less able to cope with extra stresses. Comorbid conditions, which are associated with higher risks of hospitalizations and mortality, include chronic obstructive pulmonary disease (COPD), renal dysfunction, diabetes, depression and mental disorders (Table 1.6). With every additional comorbid condition, more drugs are added to an already substantial drug regimen for HF therapy. Inevitably, patients on multiple drugs ('poly-pharmacy') are more susceptible to drug interactions.[16] Consequentially, there is a higher rate of noncompliance with therapy in these patients.

Aging. Aging itself also produces profound effects on cardiovascular structure and function (Table 1.7) and predispose individuals to development of HF.[17–19] The aging male myocardium loses about 35% of its myocytes over the adult lifespan, whereas the female

Table 1.6 Prevalence of comorbidities in heart failure and their implications[32]

Condition	Prevalence (%)	Implications
Hypertension (HT)	27–55	LVH, HT cardiomyopathy, diastolic impairment
COPD/bronchiectasis	21–26	Diagnosis uncertain, increased dyspnoea
Anemia	15–50	Increased symptoms, worse prognosis
Diabetes (DM)	15–31	DM cardiomyopathy? More CAD/HT
Renal dysfunction	16	Exacerbated by diuretics and ACEi
Osteoarthritis	16	NSAIDS-fluid retention
CVA	5–18	Worse prognosis, more AF/HT/DM/CAD
Thyroid disease	14	High output HF, weight gain/loss, AF
Alzheimers/dementia	9–50	Worse prognosis, poor compliance
Depression	8–20	Worse prognosis, arrhythmias, poor compliance
Osteoporosis	5	Increased fracture risk, frailty
Asthma	5	Unable to use beta-blockers

ACEi angiotensin converting enzyme inhibitors; *CAD* coronary artery disease; *LVH* left ventricular hypertrophy; *NSAIDs* nonsteroidal anti-inflammatory drugs; *CVA* cerebrovascular accident; *AF* atrial fibrillation

Table 1.7 Effects of aging on the cardiovascular system

Effects of aging on the cardiovascular system
Cumulative attrition of cardiomyocytes (gender differences)
Compensatory myocyte hypertrophy, causing eccentric left ventricular hypertrophy, resulting in increased wall thickness with normal cavity size
Increased vascular hypertrophy and stiffness with increased impedance to LV ejection
Impaired endothelial dysfunction
Impaired LV diastolic filling
Impaired sinoatrial function and heart rate variability
Reduced peak oxygen consumption
Reduced peak cardiac power output in men, but not in women
Reduction in the aerobic enzyme activity of skeletal muscle, and thus a reduced peripheral oxygen extraction and ATP production capacity
Declining glomerular filtration rate

heart retains both its myocyte number and LV mass.[20] The cumulative effects of aging are a reduction in cardiovascular reserve, which impairs the heart's ability to respond to both physiological (exercise) and pathological stresses.[18, 19, 21] The prevalence of noncardiac comorbidity is well known to increase with age. The wide range of multiple conditions can contribute to the development and progression of HF and both limit therapy and alter responses to treatment (Table 1.6). Up to 86% of patients have two or more noncardiac comorbidities and 40% have ≥5 comorbidities, which accounts for 81% of the total HF inpatient hospital days.[22] Through passage of time, the older the patient, the greater the likelihood for the individual to have suffered one or more cardiac events culminating in the presentation of HF. Of all the age-groups, the elderly have the highest incidence and prevalence of HF (Fig. 1.1). Drug treatment in elderly patients is often complicated by polypharmacy and multiple comorbidity, greater risks of toxicity and adverse reactions secondary to multiorgan dysfunction (especially renal and hepatic), cognitive impairment, frailty and lack of social support. Since life expectancy is limited, the patients' perspectives on therapeutic objectives are often different, with less emphasis on mortality reduction or delaying death, and more on improving symptoms and quality of life.[23]

Respiratory disorders. COPD occurs in about 25% of HF patients.[12] Smoking is probably the common causal agent responsible for both. COPD and other comorbid lung diseases diminish pulmonary function and contribute to dyspnoea and impaired exercise tolerance. Often, it is difficult to distinguish whether cardiac or pulmonary disease is the limiting factor in the patient's symptom of dyspnoea. Reversible obstructive defects are seen in acute HF, as well as restrictive defects in chronic HF patients.

Renal impairment. Many patients with HF have renal dysfunction in the absence of intrinsic renal disease, which is usually progressive with longer durations of HF. This is generally as a consequence of reduced CO and hence decreased renal perfusion, accompanied by sodium and water retention.[24] Diuretics and ACE inhibitors can also contribute to worsening renal failure. Conversely, as a result of accelerated coronary atherosclerosis, hypertension and fluid retention, patients with primary renal disease are at high risk of HF. Renal function also declines with age, such that octogenarians often have a creatinine clearance of <50 mL/min.

Anemia becomes more common as HF progresses partly related to worsening of renal function and impairment in production of erythropoietin. Iron deficiency may also be a feature. HF-related anemia is associated with increased mortality and morbidity.[25] Elderly HF patients are at higher risk because of comorbid chronic illnesses such as renal dysfunction, reduced iron uptake and malabsorption and occult malignancy, and chronic blood loss associated with concomitant use of drugs such as NSAID's, steroids, aspirin, clopidogrel, warfarin.

Diabetes. Up to 30% of HF patients can have comorbidity of diabetes mellitus.[26] The suggestion of a diabetic cardiomyopathy has also been raised.[27] Diabetic hearts have been reported to show morphological changes, which include interstitial fibrosis, intramyocardial microangiopathy and myocyte hypertrophy.[25] Moreover, diabetics are known to have more coronary disease, hypertension, obesity and hyperlipidemia, which may partially explain a higher likelihood of developing HF.

1.5
Exacerbating and Precipitating Factors

HF is a chronic condition with a fluctuating course. There are a number of well known factors that precipitate or contribute to HF exacerbations. Cardiac-related precipitating and exacerbating factors include recurrence of MI or ischemia, arrhythmias (most commonly paroxysmal or persistent atrial fibrillation or flutter). Noncardiac factors include intercurrent infections esp. chest infection and sepsis, excess alcohol consumption, nonadherence with medication and fluid balance adjustments, injudicious salt intake, renal impairment, anemia, thyroid disease and adverse new pharmacotherapy (e.g., NSAIDs, dihydropyridines, thiazolidinediones).

In patients with severe HF, any systemic setback or other organ impairment may exacerbate the severity of HF and require hospital admissions. In winter, by far, the most common of any type is respiratory tract infection. Because fluid balance is a major issue in HF management, diuretics are still the main first-line therapy, and this invariably impacts on renal function. Close monitoring of serum electrolytes and creatinine is essential at all stages of HF management, to avoid arrhythmogenesis or worsening renal impairment. It is vital to protect renal function, because in a HF patient without adequate renal function, medical therapy is virtually impossible, because dialysis is not a realistic option.

1.6
Monitoring of Organ Dysfunction and HF Severity

In medical specialties, clinicians monitor organ function and dysfunction serially, such as serum creatinine and eGFR in renal medicine, peak flows and arterial pO_2 and pCO_2 in pulmonology, liver function tests in hepatology. In cardiology, left ventricular ejection fraction (LVEF) has been most often measured serially, but unfortunately it is not a measure of organ function. In the past two decades, it has emerged that the most representative measure of organ function is peak cardiac power output (CPO_{max}),[2] not dissimilar to peak brake horsepower used by engineers to grade car engines. Unfortunately, only very few centers in the world have expertise to measure this. Surrogate measures of CPO_{max} include peak exercise oxygen consumption, exercise duration or other indicators of exercise capacity and brain natriuretic peptide (BNP). BNP or, its more stable form, N-terminal pro-BNP, is a blood test that has been shown to (1) correlate significantly with the extent of cardiac dysfunction[28] and (2) be a powerful prognostic indicator for HF.[29] However, if doubt persists after undergoing available conventional investigations, measurement of CPO_{max} may provide the final answer about whether the patient has HF and how severe it is. To minimize margins of error in critical cases, we also use this test to determine how urgently a transplant candidate should receive a donor heart or a ventricular assist device as a bridge to transplant.

References

1. Task Force for Diagnosis and Treatment of Acute and Chronic Heart Failure 2008 of European Society of Cardiology; Dickstein K, Cohen-Solal A, Filippatos G, et al. ESC Guidelines for the diagnosis and treatment of acute and chronic heart failure 2008: the Task Force for the Diagnosis and Treatment of Acute and Chronic Heart Failure 2008 of the European Society of Cardiology. Developed in collaboration with the Heart Failure Association of the ESC (HFA) and endorsed by the European Society of Intensive Care Medicine (ESICM). *Eur Heart J.* 2008;29(19):2388-2442.

2. Cotter G, Williams SG, Vered Z, Tan LB. Role of cardiac power in heart failure. *Curr Opin Cardiol.* 2003;18:215-222.
3. Kannel WB, Belanger AJ. Epidemiology of heart failure. *Am Heart J.* 1991;121(3 pt 1):951-957.
4. http://www.heartstats.org. Accessed 21 Jan 2009.
5. Cowie MR, Wood DA, Coats AJS, et al. Incidence and aetiology of heart failure; a population-based study. *Eur Heart J.* 1999;20:421-428.
6. Stewart S, Jenkins A, Buchan S, McGuire A, Capewell S, McMurray JJ. The current cost of heart failure to the National Health Service in the UK. *Eur J Heart Fail.* 2002;4(3):361-371.
7. Cowie MR, Wood DA, Coats AJ, et al. Incidence and aetiology of heart failure; a population-based study. *Eur Heart J.* 1999;20(6):421-428.
8. Bart BA, Shaw LK, McCants CB Jr, et al. Clinical determinants of mortality in patients with angiographically diagnosed ischemic or nonischemic cardiomyopathy. *J Am Coll Cardiol.* 1997;30:1002-1008.
9. Williams SG, Tzeng B-H, Tan LB. Cardiogenic shock: physiological and biochemical concepts. In: David Hasdai, Peter B Berger, Alexander Battler, David R Holmes Jr, eds. *Cardiogenic Shock: Diagnosis and Treatment.* New Jersey: Humana; 2002:7-32.
10. Williams SG, Wright DJ, Tan LB. Management of cardiogenic shock complicating acute myocardial infarction: towards evidence based medical practice. *Heart.* 2000;83:621-626.
11. Kannel WB, Castelli WP, McNamara PM, McKee PA, Feinleib M. of blood pressure in the development of congestive heart failure. The Framingham study. *N Engl J Med.* 1972;287:781-787.
12. Levy D, Garrison RJ, Savage DD, Kannel WB, Castelli WP. Prognostic implications of echocardiographically determined left ventricular mass in the Framingham Heart Study. *N Engl J Med.* 1990;322:1561-1566.
13. Felker GM, Thompson RE, Hare JM, et al. Underlying causes and long-term survival in patients with initially unexplained cardiomyopathy. *N Engl J Med.* 2000;342(15):1077-1084.
14. Williams SG, Barker D, Goldspink DF, Tan LB. A reappraisal of concepts in heart failure: Central role of cardiac power reserve. *Arch Med Sci.* 2005;1:65-74.
15. Harris P. Evolution and the cardiac patient. *Cardiovasc Res.* 1983;17(7):437-445.
16. Lang CC, Mancini DM. Non-cardiac comorbidities in chronic heart failure. *Heart.* 2007; 93:665-671.
17. Rich MW. Epidemiology, pathophysiology, and etiology of congestive heart failure in older adults. *J Am Geriatr Soc.* 1997;45:968-974.
18. Wei JY. Age and the cardiovascular system. *N Engl J Med.* 1992;327:1735-1739.
19. Lakatta EG. Cardiovascular regulatory mechanisms in advanced age. *Physiol Rev.* 1993;73: 413-467.
20. Olivetti G, Melissari M, Capasso JM, Anversa P. Cardiomyopathy of the aging human heart. Myocyte loss and reactive cellular hypertrophy. *Circ Res.* 1991;68:1560-1568.
21. Fleg JL, O'Connor F, Gerstenblith G, et al. Impact of age on the cardiovascular response to dynamic upright exercise in healthy men and women. *J Appl Physiol.* 1995;78:890-900.
22. Braunstein JB, Anderson GF, Gerstenblith G, et al. Noncardiac comorbidity increases preventable hospitalizations and mortality among Medicare beneficiaries with chronic heart failure. *J Am Coll Cardiol.* 2003;42:1226-1233.
23. Tan LB, Murphy R. Shifts in mortality curves: saving or extending lives? *Lancet.* 1999; 354:1378-1381.
24. Rich MW. Heart failure in the oldest patients: the impact of comorbid conditions. *Am J Geriatr Cardiol.* 2005;14:134-141.
25. Horwich TB, Fonarow GC, Hamilton MA, MacLellan WR, Borenstein J. Anemia is associated with worse symptoms, greater impairment in functional capacity and a significant increase in mortality in patients with advanced heart failure. *J Am Coll Cardiol.* 2002;39:1780-1786.
26. Kannel WB, McGee DL. Diabetes and cardiovascular disease. The Framingham study. *JAMA.* 1979;241:2035-2038.

27. Rodrigues B, McNeill JH. The diabetic heart: metabolic causes for the development of a cardiomyopathy. *Cardiovasc Res*. 1992;26:913-922.
28. Williams SG, Ng LL, O'Brien R, Taylor S, Wright DJ, Tan LB. Is plasma N-BNP a good indicator of the functional reserve of failing hearts? The FRESH-BNP study. *Eur J Heart Fail*. 2004;6(7):891-900.
29. Latini R, Masson S, Wong M, et al. for the Val-HeFT Investigators. Incremental prognostic value of changes in B-type natriuretic peptide in heart failure with depressed ejection fraction. *Am J Med*. 2006;119:70.e23-70.e30.
30. Urban P, Stauffer JC, Bleed D, et al. A randomized evaluation of early revascularization to treat shock complicating acute myocardial infarction. The (Swiss) Multicenter Trial of Angioplasty for Shock-(S)MASH. *Eur Heart J*. 1999;20:1030-1038.
31. Fincke R, Hochman JS, Lowe AM, et al.; SHOCK Investigators. Cardiac power is the strongest hemodynamic correlate of mortality in cardiogenic shock: a report from the SHOCK trial registry. *J Am Coll Cardiol*. 2004;44(2):340-348.
32. Braunstein JB, Anderson GF, Gerstenblith G, et al. Noncardiac comorbidity increases preventable hospitalizations and mortality among medicare beneficiaries with chronic heart failure. *J Am Coll Cardiol*. 2003;42:1226-1233.

Inherited Myocardial Diseases

2

Margherita Calcagnino and William J. McKenna

2.1
Introduction

In the last classification of cardiomyopathies (CM) presented by the European Society of Cardiology, CM are defined as myocardial disorders in which the heart muscle is structurally and functionally abnormal, in the absence of sufficient coronary artery disease, hypertension, valvular disease, and congenital heart disease to cause the observed myocardial abnormality. CM are then grouped into specific morphological and functional phenotypes, and each phenotype is subclassified into familial and nonfamilial forms (Fig. 2.1).[1]

This chapter focuses on the clinical and practical management, with particular attention to heart failure (HF), of the main inherited CM including hypertrophic cardiomyopathy (HCM), dilated cardiomyopathy (DCM), and arrhythmogenic right ventricular cardiomyopathy (ARVC). All together, these account for ~10% of patients with HF,[2] the majority of whom are young.[3]

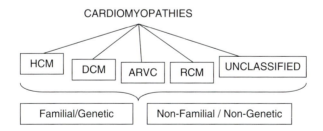

Fig. 2.1 Summary of proposed classification system. *HCM* hypertrophic cardiomyopathy; *DCM* dilated cardiomyopathy; *ARVC* arrhythmogenic right ventricular cardiomyopathy; *RCM* restrictive cardiomyopathy. (Modified from classification of the cardiomyopathies: a position statement from the European society of cardiology working group on myocardial and pericardial diseases[1])

M. Calcagnino (✉)
The Heart Hospital, London, UK
e-mail: marghecalcagnino@libero.it

M.Y. Henein (ed.), *Heart Failure in Clinical Practice*,
DOI: 10.1007/978-1-84996-153-0_2, © Springer-Verlag London Limited 2010

2.2
Hypertrophic Cardiomyopathy

2.2.1
Definition and General Features of the Disease

HCM is a genetically transmitted, phenotypically heterogeneous disease, which can affect individuals of all ages.

HCM has been defined by the presence of myocardial hypertrophy in the absence of loading conditions sufficient to account for the degree of hypertrophy.[4,5] A new genetic classification has emerged with the identification of mutations in sarcomeric protein genes in 50–70% patients with HCM.[6] However, this definition has important limitations in clinical practice, not least that genetic analysis is not available to most clinicians. Therefore, HCM is still a phenotypic diagnosis defined clinically by the presence of left ventricular hypertrophy (LVH) in the absence of a detectable cause.[7]

The myocardial hypertrophy most commonly affects the interventricular septum and is associated histologically with disorganization ("disarray") of cardiac myocytes and myofibrils, myocardial fibrosis, and small-vessel disease. Twenty-five percent of patients have resting left ventricular outflow tract obstruction (LVOTO).

HCM has a variable clinical course and outcome: many patients have little or no cardiovascular symptoms, whereas others have profound exercise limitation and recurrent arrhythmias.

The overall risk of disease-related complications such as endstage HF, sudden death (SD), and fatal stroke is quite low (roughly 1–2% per year), but the absolute risk in individuals varies as a function of age, underlying genetic abnormality, myocardial pathology, and other pathophysiological abnormalities, such as impaired peripheral vascular responses.[7]

2.2.2
Molecular Genetics

2.2.2.1
Inheritance Pattern and Sarcomeric Gene Mutations

The disease is usually inherited in an autosomal dominant fashion with variable clinical penetrance.

In adults, the majority of cases are familial, caused by mutations in cardiac sarcomeric protein genes. Recent studies suggest that in infants and children, approximately half of all cases of isolated cardiac hypertrophy are caused by a mutation of the same sarcomeric genes that are detected in adults with unexplained LVH.[8] Inherited disorders of metabolism and neuromuscular diseases can also be involved.

Approximately 50–70% of patients present mutations in one of the genes that encode different components of the cardiac sarcomere (Fig. 2.2). These components are

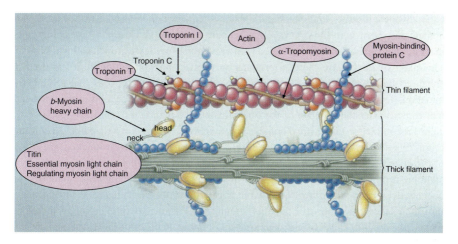

Fig. 2.2 Structure of the cardiac sarcomere. (From Nabel EG. Cardiovascular disease. NEngl J Med 2003: 349:60-72)

represented by β-myosin heavy chain (chromosome 14), cardiac troponin T (chromosome 1), cardiac troponin I (chromosome 19), α-tropomyosin (chromosome 15), cardiac myo-sin-binding protein C (chromosome 11), the essential and regulatory myosin light chains (chromosome 3 and 12, respectively), and cardiac actin (chromosome 15).[9,10] Mutations in three other sarcomeric protein genes (titin, Troponin C, and α-cardiac myosin heavy chain) have been reported.[5,7,9,11]

Some adult patients, like many children, might have non-sarcomeric disease such as Anderson–Fabry disease,[12] Noonan syndrome, mitochondrial disease,[13] and a phenotype that include HCM, Wolff–Parkinson–White syndrome, and premature conduction disease, associated with mutations in the gene encoding the γ-subunit of AMP-kinase, an important regulator of cellular energy homoeostasis.[14,15] Human muscle LIM protein,[16] LAMP-2 (Danon disease),[17] and phospholamban promoter[18] represent other non-sarcomeric gene mutations that might result in HCM phenocopies.

2.2.2.2
Pathophysiology of Sarcomeric Protein Gene Mutations

There are various ways in which mutations in genes encoding sarcomere proteins might interfere with sarcomere function.[19-42]

Allele inactivation can result in haploinsufficiency (a reduced amount of functional protein), or produce a mutant protein that has a novel function or that interferes with nor-mal protein function (dominant negative). Most but not all mutations appear to cause a dominant negative interference with the normal function of the wild-type protein rather than haploinsufficiency. There seems to be a dose–response, with a correlation between the levels of mutant sarcomere protein expressed and myocyte dysfunction.[24] Animal models of mutated sarcomeric protein genes mimic some aspects of human disease, including

LVH, myocyte disarray, and interstitial fibrosis.[22] However, the mechanisms for the development of hypertrophy and disarray remain poorly understood. Current evidence suggests that sarcomere mutations are associated with activation of myocyte growth pathways.[9,15,28,43] The effect of sarcomeric mutated proteins on cardiac function varies from impaired to enhanced contractility.[14,27,44] The energy depletion hypothesis proposes that sarcomeric mutations lead to inefficient ATP utilisation[45] and consequent increased energy demand that compromises the capacity of the cardiomyocyte to maintain free energy levels sufficient for contraction and critical homeostatic functions, such as Ca^{2+} reuptake. According to this hypothesis, chronic energy depletion with ensuing myocyte dysfunction, elevation of cytosolic Ca^{2+} and AMP-activated protein kinase activation, results in hypertrophy.[45] In addition, recent data show that β-myosin mutations cause highly variable (increased or decreased) calcium sensitivity from fiber to fiber, with ensuing imbalances in force generation. Imbalances in contractile function among individual muscle cells might therefore represent a primary cause for the development of myocyte disarray, LVH, and myocardial dysfunction.[46] Potential modifiers of disease expression include genetically determined variation in the renin-aldosterone-angiotensin system,[47-50] rare examples of homozygotes and compound heterozygotes.[33,51]

2.2.3
Pathophysiology of the Disease

1. Diastolic dysfunction

Almost all patients with HCM have impaired diastolic function, which has been attributed to abnormalities in both the active component of the dissociation of actin and myosin in the early filling phase, and the passive properties of the ventricle that affect compliance.[52-55] Enhanced LV stiffness provokes prolonged isovolumic relaxation, delayed peak filling, reduced relative volume during the rapid filling period, increased dependence on atrial contribution to filling and regional heterogeneity in the timing, rate and degree of LV relaxation, and diastolic filling.[5,56] Some patients have a flat LV pressure–volume relation, with a similar response to offloading to that seen in patients with constrictive pericarditis, which suggests the presence of increased external constraint to LV filling.[55]

The causes of diastolic dysfunction in HCM include myocyte hypertrophy, myocyte and myofibrillar disarray, abnormal chamber geometry, abnormal intracellular calcium metabolism and myocardial ischemia. Collagen turnover is increased (synthesis prevails over degradation), and there is evidence for abnormal inhibition of matrix metalloproteinases.[57-59]

Abnormal diastolic function represents one of the main causes of symptoms of congestive cardiac failure in HCM. Slow relaxation and elevated end-diastolic pressures are observed in the majority of cases.[52,60-68] In a minority of patients, elevation of filling pressures, biatrial dilation, and signs of right HF may predominate, even in the absence of substantial myocardial hypertrophy,[69,70] presenting a "restrictive" hemodynamic phenotype.

One of the problems linked to diastolic dysfunction is that it is complex to quantitate with noninvasive tools, especially because of its dependence on changes in preload and afterload conditions. Moreover, so far there are no effective pharmacological treatments to modify the underlying pathophysiology of diastolic dysfunction.

2. Systolic dysfunction

Conventional measurements of ejection fraction (EF) are "normal" in the majority of patients with HCM. M-mode assessment of short-axis LV dimensions have shown a low prevalence of systolic impairment (<3%).[52,60-62,71,72] Recently, tissue Doppler and strain imaging have demonstrated a much higher prevalence of abnormal systolic function, with reduced longitudinal shortening, delayed regional longitudinal contraction, and paradoxical systolic lenghthening,[73-77] but only a minority of patients evolve to gross systolic dysfunction and LV dilation.

Studies suggest that up to 50% of patients with HCM show global and regional systolic dysfunction during exercise[78,79] and that the presence of reduced systolic performance during pharmacologic stress is related to future deterioration of LV performance.[80]

Many patients have systemic markers of abnormal systolic performance (natriuretic peptides, cytokines, etc.)[81-85] that correlate with symptom class, exercise limitation, and diastolic function.

A reduced EF is associated with greater likelihood of LV enlargement, greater wall thinning, deterioration in functional class, cardiac transplantation, and death.[71,72,86,87] Left atrial (LA) size, LV end-diastolic dimension, end-diastolic pressure, and reduced exercise capacity at the initial evaluation represent the principal predictors of HF death. Depressed cardiac function may contribute to the high prevalence of atrial fibrillation (AF) in patients who die from HF.[71]

3. Left ventricular outflow tract obstruction

About 25% of HCM patients have a resting pressure gradient in the outflow tract of the LV caused by systolic anterior motion (SAM) of the mitral valve (MV) leaflets.[5,60-63,88-90] Occasionally (around 5% of cases),[5] gradients are caused by muscular apposition in the mid-cavity region.[91-93] By convention, LVOTO is defined by a pressure gradient greater than or equal to 30 mmHg,[61,63,94,95] but probably clinically significant (moderate to severe) obstruction should be considered only when the gradient is more than 50 mmHg.[91] Some patients without outflow obstruction at rest develop gradients during physiologic and pharmacologic interventions that diminish LV end-diastolic volume or augment LV contractility.

Geometric factors including primary abnormalities of the mitral apparatus, including anomalous anterior and inward or central displacement of the papillary muscles, leaflet elongation, and anteriorly positioned MV leaflet coaptation, play a role in causing LVOTO[96-98]; the outflow tract narrowing due to septal hypertrophy and the Venturi effect are also important.[5,99-104]

One of the most frequent consequences of SAM and abnormal mitral leaflet coaptation is mitral regurgitation,[60,99] which occurs in almost all patients with obstructive HCM. The regurgitant jet is usually posteriorly directed; central or anterior jets should raise the suspicion of intrinsic MV disease.

LVOTO represents an independent predictor of disease progression and death due to HF and stroke.

4. Myocardial ischemia

During pacing and pharmacologic stress, patients with HCM exhibit metabolic evidence for myocardial ischemia, and most of them have reduced coronary flow reserve.[105-114] Different pathophysiologic mechanisms have been suggested as causes of myocardial ischemia: small vessel disease, reduced capillary density, epicardial coronary compression, and increased oxygen demand (caused by myocardial hypertrophy and myocyte disarray). Myocardial ischemia may contribute to chest pain and breathlessness in many individuals, but there are limited data to suggest that ischemia is a common trigger for fatal ventricular arrhythmia or an important contributor to long-term morbidity and mortality.[112-114]

2.2.4
Clinical Profile

2.2.4.1
Epidemiology and Age at Presentation

The majority of studies suggest that HCM has a prevalence of approximately 1 in 500 adults.[1,5,7] The frequency of unexplained LVH in children remains unknown, but an annual incidence of LVH between 0.3 and 0.5 per 100,000 has been reported from medical centers in the United States and Australia.[115-117]

Ventricular hypertrophy usually develops during periods of rapid somatic growth, typically during adolescence.[118] De novo myocardial hypertrophy may occur in later decades, but is uncommon and appears to be associated with MYBPC3 mutations.[119,120] HF accounts for an increasing proportion of HCM-related deaths with advancing age.[71,87]

2.2.4.2
Symptoms

Most patients with HCM are asymptomatic or have mild symptoms. Often the diagnosis is made incidentally or during family screening. Breathlessness and chest pain during exertion are the commonest symptoms, with a characteristic day-to-day variation in the activity needed to cause symptoms.[76,82,87,88,106,109,111,112,114,120-127] Chest pain can occur at rest and is frequently precipitated by meals.[123] Fifteen to twenty-five percent of patients complain of syncope or presyncope, which can arise during exertion or at rest.[128] The underlying mechanisms for these symptoms include diastolic and systolic dysfunction, LVOTO, AF, bradyarrhythmias, and abnormal peripheral vascular responses during exercise. Alcohol exacerbation of LVOTO has been reported as a cause of syncope.[129]

Increase in breathlessness and fatigue are the prevailing symptoms of HF in HCM patients. These appear to be caused in large measure by diastolic dysfunction, with impaired filling due to abnormal relaxation and increased chamber stiffness, leading in turn to elevated LA and LV end diastolic pressures, reduced cardiac output, pulmonary congestion, and impaired exercise performance with reduced oxygen consumption at peak exercise.[5]

Additional disabling causes of HF symptoms are LVOTO, which causes elevated LV pressures and concomitant mitral regurgitation,[5] and transient myocardial ischemia. Palpitations are common and usually related to supraventricular tachyarrhythmias; AF with rapid ventricular response may cause acute decompensation and even syncope.

Paroxysmal nocturnal dyspnea, orthopnea, and ankle swelling are less common but can be present in a context of apparently mild disease.

Advanced HF symptoms with severe breathlessness at rest, cold periphery, and cachexia are rare.

2.2.4.3
Clinical Examination

Physical examination of the cardiovascular system in patients with familial HCM often reveals little information, but an accurate inspection can be useful to identify particular phenotypes of the disease, linked to congenital malformations and syndromes (e.g., facial dysmorphology in Noonan syndrome).

Patients with dynamic LVOTO have a systolic murmur at the left sternal edge, not radiating to the neck or axilla. The murmur characteristically increases with maneuvers that decrease afterload or venous return (standing or Valsalva maneuver), and decreases with interventions that increase afterload and venous return (squatting). Most patients with LVOTO also have mitral regurgitation, suggested by the presence of a longer, pansystolic murmur radiating to the axilla; severe regurgitation is sometimes associated with a mid diastolic rumble. In patients who develop HF, typical signs include tachycardia, tachypnoea, pulmonary rales, pleural effusion, raised jugular venous pressure, peripheral edema, and other fluid overload features.

2.2.5
Investigations

2.2.5.1
Electrocardiography

The detection of an abnormal electrocardiogram is very common in patients with HCM. The most frequent changes include LA enlargement, repolarization abnormalities, and pathologic Q waves, most commonly in the infero-lateral leads.[130-133] Voltage criteria for LVH in isolation do not suggest HCM in normal young adults. Giant negative T waves in the mid-praecordial leads are characteristic of hypertrophy predominantly in the distal

LV.[134] Many patients have a short PR interval with a slurred QRS upstroke, not usually associated with Wolff–Parkinson–White syndrome.[14,133,135] During ambulatory monitoring, the most frequent arrhythmias recorded are premature ventricular complexes (88%), supraventricular tachyarrhythmias such as AF and flutter (30–40%) and nonsustained ventricular tachycardia (25–30%).[136-141]

In patients with HCM, symptomatic palpitation is usually provoked by supraventricular arrhythmias/paroxysmal AF, whereas sustained ventricular tachycardia (SVT) is rare, except in patients with apical LV aneurysms.[140] Nonsustained VT (NSVT) is associated with severity of hypertrophy and symptom class, but is itself rarely symptomatic. Supraventricular arrhythmias are more common in patients with LVOTO.[142]

2.2.5.2
Echocardiography

Diagnostic criteria for HCM in adults are based on the detection of unexplained LVH on echocardiography.[4,5] Generally, a diastolic wall thickness greater than two standard deviations from the mean corrected for age, sex, and height (typically ≥15 mm in any myocardial segment) is sufficient to make the diagnosis of HCM in an adult. Most patients have a disproportionate increase in the thickness of the interventricular septum; a few have concentric, apical, and other patterns.[63,91,94,95,143] Right ventricular hypertrophy occurs in >1/3 of patients with HCM and is diagnosed when at least two right ventricular wall measurements exceed two standard deviations from the mean recorded in normal individuals.

The most common echocardiographic abnormalities[52,95,99,144] include asymmetric septal hypertrophy (ASH), SAM of the MV, a small ventricular cavity, septal immobility, and premature closure of the aortic valve. It is possible to score the severity of hypertrophy in several ways.[91,145,146]

LVOTO magnitude is usually measured by continuous wave Doppler.[61,94,95,143,147] This outflow gradient is typically dynamic: for this reason, many laboratories perform provocation maneuvres and, increasingly, upright exercise in symptomatic patients to detect inducible gradients.

Diastolic abnormalities are frequent, in particular, in symptomatic patients, but the use of conventional pulsed-wave Doppler to assess diastolic function in HCM has a number of limitations, and importantly mitral flow velocity curves cannot be used reliably to determine filling pressure.[148] Tissue Doppler imaging (TDI) of mitral annular motion measured from the apical window has been proposed as a load-independent parameter of diastolic function.[77] Moreover, TDI and strain imaging echocardiography may detect subclinical systolic and diastolic dysfunction when conventional echocardiography is normal.[73-77]

Conventional echocardiographic indices of global LV systolic function are normal at rest in most patients, but regional function (particularly in the interventricular septum) and stroke volume during exercise is reduced in some.[79]

In a minority of patients (~3.5%),[3,149] myocardial thinning and progressive systolic impairment also arise, representing the pattern of the "end-stage" phase of the disease, with LV remodeling and systolic dysfunction.

2.2.5.3
Exercise Testing

Disease severity is objectively assessed by exercise testing with simultaneous respiratory gas analysis. HCM patients usually have some reduction in peak oxygen consumption compared with healthy controls,[150,151] even when asymptomatic.

Up to 25% of patients have an abnormal blood pressure response during upright exercise: systolic blood pressure fails to rise by more than 20–25 mmHg from baseline values or falls.[152-154] Abnormal vasodilatation in nonexercising muscles, thought to be triggered by inappropriate firing of LV baroreceptors, explains the mechanism underlying this response in the majority of cases.[155] In a minority of patients, abnormal exercise blood pressure response is secondary to exercise induced LVOT, mitral regurgitation, or ischemia.[156]

2.2.5.4
Cardiac Magnetic Resonance Imaging

A potentially important role of Cardiac Magnetic Resonance in HCM is to assess myocardial tissue characteristics in vivo, with gadolinium contrast agents. Up to 80% of patients with HCM have patchy areas of late enhancement (LE)[157-163]: correlation with histologic data indicates that LE is caused by myocardial interstitial replacement.[157] The extent of LE correlates with wall thickness and regional function and is associated with progressive remodeling of the LV and risk markers for SCD.[157]

2.2.6
Principles of Clinical Management

The treatment of HCM patients may be complex and can change during the course of the disease.[5,164,165] The aims of management are to improve symptoms and prevent disease-related complications. There are a few basic principles of management, which can have an effect on quality of life and prognosis. It is important to define and treat the mechanisms underlying symptoms, to assess the risks of AF, stroke, SCD, and to evaluate the familial involvement.

2.2.6.1
Symptomatic Treatment in HCM

A key goal of treatment in HCM is the alleviation of symptoms related to HF.[5] Symptoms related to diastolic dysfunction should be treated with drugs which enables heart rate (HR) control with a consequent prolongation of diastole and relaxation and an increase in passive ventricular filling. These effects are also useful to treat chest pain.

β-Blockers can be effective by decreasing HR, lessening LV contractility, and reducing myocardial oxygen demand,[164-170] but paradoxically may reduce exercise capacity by inducing chronotropic incompetence as well as causing the recognized β-Blocker side effects (e.g., fatigue or impotence).

Sustained release Verapamil, in doses up to 480 mg/day, may be useful in controlling HR and relieving chest pain.[54,171-176] Its principal actions are to improve ventricular relaxation and filling, to relieve myocardial ischemia, and to decrease LV contractility. However, aside from the mild side effect of constipation, Verapamil can occasionally cause hemodynamic deterioration and even death in patients with severe disabling symptoms, elevated pulmonary arterial pressure, and severe LVOTO.[167] Current practice is to use β-Blockers before Verapamil,[142] but no data suggest the superiority of one drug over the other. Diltiazem may have beneficial effects[177] on symptoms and LV function and provides a useful alternative to Verapamil when side effects are problematic.

In some patients with refractory chest pain, sometimes, nitrates can be useful (in the absence of LVOTO), but they should be used with caution to avoid excessive reductions in preload and afterload.

Symptoms related to LVOTO are usually treated with the negative inotropic agent Disopyramide (type I-A antiarrhythmic), generally in addition to β-blockers. Doses of 300–600 mg/day can decrease resting obstruction and mitral regurgitant volume.[169,178-181] Its anti-cholinergic side effects include dry mouth and eyes, constipation, difficulty in micturition, and accelerated atrioventricular nodal conduction that increases ventricular rate during AF. Coadministration of β-blockers can minimize the last problem. There is no evidence for an adverse effect on prognosis in HCM patients caused by its proarrhythmic effects;[180] however, the QT interval should be monitored and coadministration of other antiarrhythmics avoided.

Various options are available to patients with obstructive HCM who are unable to tolerate drugs, or whose symptoms persist despite treatment. Septal myectomy, in which a trough of muscle is removed from the interventricular septum via a transaortic approach, is the gold standard.[182-186] The most promising alternative to surgery is percutaneous alcohol septal ablation.[187-201] Dual chamber pacing provides an alternative, which may be effective in elderly patients with mild LV hypertrophy.[202-210]

2.2.6.2
Advanced Heart Failure

When systolic dysfunction arises, it may be necessary to decrease or discontinue β-blockers or calcium antagonists and to introduce diuretics judiciously. Severe HF symptoms are rare and arise in a relatively small, but important subgroup of patients with nonobstructive HCM who develop ventricular dilatation, systolic impairment and severe HF, usually associated with LV remodeling, demonstrable as wall thinning and chamber enlargement.

The prevalence of this unique HCM subset has been reported to occur in approximately 3.5% of patients[3,149,211] and has been variously known as the "dilated," "end-stage," or "burnt-out" phase.[5] This evolution of HCM represents an increasingly recognized complication, with a high incidence of adverse outcomes (including SCD), requiring defibrillator implantation and, ultimately, cardiac transplantation.

The *sine qua non* of end-stage phase of HCM is a functional abnormality characterized by an LVEF <50% at rest, reflecting global systolic dysfunction: this often precedes other evidence of remodeling, as well as severe symptoms.[3] Patterns of LV remodeling are generally nonuniform and variable. Studies suggest that only about 50% of patients have evidence of complete remodeling with the triad of LV wall thickness regression, cavity dilatation, and reduced EF; more than one third of the advanced HF patients show a nondilated or persistently hypertrophied LV or both.[3]

The relative infrequency with which advanced HF occurs underscores the importance of clinical suspicion. The transition from a hypertrophied and nondilated state to one of systolic dysfunction appears to evolve gradually and is often associated with development of AF.[3] If recognized, this permits changes in management strategies, including transition of standard HCM medical therapy to drugs for systolic pump failure. Similarly, patients with severe restrictive physiology may develop severe congestive features slowly over decades.

A family history of HCM with advanced HF helps identify at risk individuals.[3]

The clinical course of advanced HF is variable, but generally unfavorable, with heart transplantation the only definitive treatment for unrelenting progressive HF, unresponsive to medical management.[3] The overall annual mortality rate of 11% per year is in sharp contrast to 1% per year for the overall HCM population.[3,5] After recognition of advanced HF, patients experience a generally precipitous and aggressive course. Therefore, definitive management strategies may be required.

Mechanisms responsible for transformation of typical HCM to advanced HF are unresolved. Intuitively, the expanded collagen matrix in HCM would appear to offer a structural framework for substantial ventricular stiffness and consequently, a measure of protection from the advanced HF.[212] This raises the alternative possibility of a unique molecular or genetic susceptibility to advanced HF.[213]

In advanced HF drug treatment strategies differ substantially from those approaches in patients with typical LVH, nondilated chambers, and preserved systolic function.

Conventional HF therapy is indicated in patients with systolic impairment,[7] with ACE inhibitors (ACE-Is) or angiotensin-II receptor blockers (ARBs), diuretics, digitalis, β-blockers, spironolactone, and anticoagulation.[5] There is no evidence, however, that β-blockers, ACE-Is or ARBs prevent or convey a survival benefit to congestive HF and ventricular systolic dysfunction of advanced HCM (in contrast with the experience in DCM).

Treatment of patients with restrictive disease is more difficult, but β-blockers, diuretics, and Spironolactone, in particular, can help.[7]

In potential transplant candidates, prophylactic implantable cardioverter defibrillator (ICD) requires consideration when systolic dysfunction is severe, to protect against lethal ventricular tachyarrhythmias while they await donor hearts.[214-216]

Recent data suggest that biventricular pacing may be beneficial in some patients with advanced HCM.[217,218] Symptomatic improvement was associated with reverse remodeling of the LA and LV.

Ultimately, patients with end-stage HF represent the primary subgroup of HCM for whom heart transplantation, which is the only definitive treatment option, is considered.[219]

2.2.6.3
Management of Supraventricular Arrhythmia

AF in patients with HCM is associated with a high risk of thromboembolism and when the heart rate is not controlled can cause sudden and sometimes severe deterioration in symptoms and exercise capacity.[139,220,221] Restoration of sinus rhythm either with drugs or electrical cardioversion usually results in a rapid improvement in symptoms. If this is unsuccessful, control of the ventricular rate with β-blockers, calcium antagonists, or both is almost effective as the restoration of the sinus rhythm.[139] Patients with persistent or permanent AF should be anticoagulated. Anticoagulation should also be considered in those who have frequent paroxysms of AF and enlarged LA. Amiodarone is effective in preventing AF and subsequent thromboembolism.[139]

2.2.6.4
Sudden Cardiac Death

SCD occurs with a frequency of up to 1% per year in adults with HCM.[86,126,145,164,165,216,222-225] Its incidence has declined as a consequence of evolving diagnostic criteria, family screening, and modern treatment protocols.

The mechanism of SCD is thought to be ventricular arrhythmia in most patients, although bradyarrhythmias and thromboembolism might account for some cases. There are other potential triggers including atrial arrhythmia, myocardial ischemia, and exercise.[139,220,221,226,227]

Many clinical features have been suggested as useful predictors of SCD; of these, the most widely advocated are family history of premature SCD, unexplained syncope, flat or hypotensive blood pressure response during upright exercise, NSVT during 24–48 h ECG monitoring and severe hypertrophy (≥30 mm).[126,145,153,154,216,222-225,228-231]

The presence of multiple clinical risk factors substantially increases the risk of sudden death. It is recommended that patients with multiple risk factors should be considered for ICD therapy.[5,214,232-234]

The treatment of patients with only one risk factor is more complex because other factors such as age and clinical context need to be considered. In view of these data, ICD should be regarded as the best current treatment for patients with a history of cardiac arrest or sustained ventricular arrhythmia and in those with a high risk clinical profile including advanced HF.

2.2.6.5
Family Screening

First-degree relatives should undergo 12-lead ECG and two-dimensional echocardiographic studies annually during puberty and adolescence.[5] Delayed adult-onset LVH is rare, but possible, so it is reasonable to recommend that adult relatives with normal echocardiograms at or beyond age 18 have subsequent clinical studies performed about every 5 years, particularly if symptoms develop or there is an adverse family history.[5] Screening in children (younger than age 12) is not usually performed systematically, unless the child has a high-risk family history or is involved in particularly intense competitive sports programs.[5]

Asymptomatic affected patients identified through family screening are usually evaluated on approximately a 12- to 18-month basis.[5]

The most definitive method for confirming the clinical diagnosis of HCM is the identification of a disease-causing mutant gene. To date, however, there are logistical problems applying mutation analysis into clinical practice.[5] Once a disease-causing mutation is defined in a proband, an accurate definition of genetic status in all family members is both efficient and inexpensive.

Efforts to identify early markers of disease expression in adolescents who are known to carry disease-causing genes have focused on echocardiographic Doppler indices of impaired relaxation, which may be abnormal in the absence of LVH. The earliest changes are, however, usually seen in the 12-lead ECG tracing: pathologic Q waves, left axis deviation, and inferolateral T wave inversion.[5]

Family evaluation should include genetic counseling regarding the risk of developing HCM and its complications.

2.3
Dilated Cardiomyopathy

2.3.1
Definition and General Features of the Disease

DCM is characterized by the presence of LV dilatation and systolic dysfunction in the absence of coronary artery disease or abnormal loading conditions (valve disease, hypertension) sufficient to cause global systolic impairment.[1] Diastolic abnormalities and/or right ventricular (RV) dilation and dysfunction may be present, but are not necessary for the diagnosis.[1]

The prevalence of DCM in the general population varies with age and geography[1]; in adults, it is estimated to be 1:2,500.[6,235] DCM is the third most common cause of HF and the most frequent cause of heart transplantation.[6]

At least 25% of DCM patients have evidence for familial DCM.[1] Nonfamilial forms of DCM can occur following myocarditis (toxic/infective/immune), can be associated with Kawasaki disease, Churg–Strauss syndrome, pregnancy, as well as endocrine or nutritional disorders or be alcohol or tachycardia induced.[1] The most common causes of myocarditis are viral, including the enteroviruses, adenoviruses, and parvovirus B19.[236]

Both familial and nonfamilial forms have the same clinical features including progressive HF and a decline in LV contractile function, ventricular and supraventricular arrhythmias, conduction system abnormalities, thromboembolism, and sudden or HF-related death.[1,6,237,238]

With improvements in the treatment of HF, including the general availability of cardiac transplantation and better medical treatment, clinical outcome following the onset of symptoms has substantially improved.[235]

2.3.2
Clinical Genetics

Autosomal dominant inheritance is the predominant pattern of transmission of familial DCM (approximately 90%),[239,240] caused by mutations in sarcomeric, cytoskeletal, protein/ Z-band, and nuclear membrane genes.[1] The genetic and clinical heterogeneity suggests causation by a single gene, with multiple other genetic and environmental factors altering its expressivity.[241]

X-linked forms (XLCM) are reported to account for approximately 5–10% of familial DCM[239]; these result from mutations in the dystrophin gene (associated to Duchenne and Becker dystrophies)[242] or from mutations in the G4.5/Tafazzin gene (associated to Barth syndrome).[243] Inherited metabolic disorders (e.g., haemochromatosis),[1] autosomal recessive, and mitochondrial inheritance are less common.[239]

Familial DCM demonstrates incomplete age-dependent penetrance.[241,244,245] Among individuals carrying a particular gene mutation, there may be wide variability in phenotypic effects and severity, both within and between families. Within the same family, the disease may range from subtle clinical symptoms and/or mild arrhythmias to SCD or DCM leading to HF and/or cardiac transplantation.

2.3.3
Molecular Genetics

To date, the genes that are involved in causing familial DCM appear to encode two major subgroups of proteins, cytoskeletal and sarcomeric proteins.[246-249] The cytoskeletal proteins indentified include dystrophin,[250-252] desmin,[253] lamin A/C (LMNA),[254,255] δ-sarcoglycan,[256] β-sarcoglycan,[257] and metavinculin.[258]

In the case of sarcomere-encoding genes, some of the genes identified for HCM, including β-myosin heavy chain, cardiac troponin T, cardiac myosin-binding protein C, cardiac actin, and α-tropomyosin, appear to be culprits.[259-264]

A new group of sarcomeric genes, encoding Z-disk proteins,[265] have also been identified; those include cypher/ZASP,[266] muscle LIM protein (MLP),[267,268] α-actinin-2,[267] myopallidin,[269] and telethonin (Tcap).[270] In addition, mutations in phospholamban,[271,272] in SCN5A (the principal Na⁺-channel α-subunit expressed in human heart)[273-275] and in G4.5/ Tafazzin,[243] have also been reported (Table 2.1).

2.3.4
Molecular Pathophysiology

Metabolic and mechanosensory abnormalities, disturbed calcium homeostasis, force generation, and transmission defects[276-279] are the main mechanisms involved in disease causation, leading to poor systolic function and compensatory chamber dilatation. The altered hemodynamic parameters of decreased stroke volume and increased chamber pressures trigger the recognized neurohumoral changes of HF and produce ventricular remodeling with eccentric hypertrophy and cavity dilation. Insidious progression is the rule in inherited DCM.

Table 2.1 Familial dilated cardiomyopathy: genes, proteins, and phenotypes (Modified from Cecil Medicine XXIII edition)[308]

Gene	Protein sarcomeric	Phenotype
MYH7	β-Myosin heavy chain	DCM
MYBPC3	Cardiac myosin binding protein C	DCM
TNNT2	Cardiac troponin T	DCM
TNNI3	Cardiac troponin I	DCM
TPM1	α-Tropomyosin	DCM
ACTC	α-Cardiac actin	DCM
TNNC1	Cardiac troponin C	DCM
MYH6	α-Myosin heavy chain	DCM
Sarcomere and Z-disc related		
TTN	Titin	DCM
CRP3	Muscle LIM protein	DCM
VCL	Metavinculin	DCM
LDB3	Cypher/ZASP	DCM, noncompaction
Intermediate filaments		
DES	Desmin	DCM
LMNA	Lamin A/C	DCM, conduction defect, muscular dystrophy
Cytoskeletal		
DMD	Dystrophin	DCM
SGCD	δ-Sarcoglycan	DCM
Ion channel and ion-channel related		
PLN	Phospholamban	DCM
SCN5A	Na⁺-channel α-subunit	DCM, atrial and ventricular arrhythmia
Mitochondrial		
G4.5	Tafazzin	DCM, myopathy (Barth's syndrome)

DCM dilated cardiomyopathy; *ZASP* Z-band alternatively spliced

In the case of cytoskeletal mutations, defects of force transmission are considered to result in the DCM phenotype, while sarcomeric-induced DCM has been speculated to result from defects of force generation.[259-261,276-279]

Mutations in the sarcomere may produce HCM or DCM. In the latter case, abnormalities in force generation or transmission are thought to contribute to the development of this phenotype. In addition to mutations in the thin filament protein actin, mutations in the thick filament protein encoding gene β-myosin heavy chain has been shown to cause DCM in children and adults. Mutations in this gene are thought to perturb the actin–myosin interaction and force generation or alter cross-bridge movement during contraction. Mutations in cardiac troponin T, a thin filament protein, have been speculated to disrupt calcium-sensitive troponin C binding.[280] Mutations in phospholamban have also been identified, which further support calcium handling as a potentially important mechanism in the development of DCM. Interestingly, studies suggest that homozygous mutations cause DCM and HF, while heterozygoes cause cardiac hypertrophy.[261] Recessive mutation in troponin I is thought to impair the interaction with troponin T,[263] while α-tropomyosin mutations have also been identified and were predicted to alter the surface charge of the protein leading to impaired interaction with actin.[261-264]

The Z disc represents a recent area of interest for evaluation at the molecular level. Mutations in MLP have been identified[268]; these have been suggested to result in defects in the interaction with telethonin. In mouse models,[268] MLP acts as a stretch sensor, which when mutated may cause disease. Mohapatra et al.[267] identified abnormalities in the T-tubule system and Z disc architecture, which correlates with the histopathology seen in MLP-knockout mice.[268,281] This was further supported by the finding of reduced expression of MLP in chronic human HF.[281,282] In addition, mutations in α-actinin-2, which is involved in crosslinking actin filaments and shares a common actin-binding domain with dystrophin, were also identified in familial DCM with disruption in binding to MLP.

Mutations have also been identified in the Z-band alternatively spliced PDZ-motif protein ZASP, the human homolog of the mouse cypher gene, which when disrupted leads to DCM[283]; this protein, which interacts with α-actinin-2, disrupts the actin cytoskeleton when mutated. Furthermore, mutations of titin (the giant sarcomeric cytoskeletal protein that contributes to the maintenance of the sarcomere organization and myofibrillar elasticity) have a role in the pathophysiology of DCM, interacting with these proteins at the Z-disc/I band transition zone.[284]

Interestingly, evidence exists that suggests that viral myocarditis and familial DCM have similar mechanisms of disease based on the proteins targeted.[285] In particular, studies show that the enteroviral protease 2A directly cleaves dystrophin in the hinge 3 region, leading to functional dystrophin impairment.[286] These findings suggest that in human myocarditis a focal disruption of dystrophin protein may contribute to the pathogenesis of human enterovirus-induced DCM.[285] These data are supported by the observation that such defects are reversible with successful LV assist device treatment.[287,288]

2.3.5
Clinical Genotype: Phenotype Correlations

2.3.5.1
Lamin A/C

The lamins are located in the nuclear envelope at the nucleoplasmic side of the inner nuclear membrane; lamin A and C are expressed both in heart and skeletal muscle.

Mutations in LMNA gene were initially reported to cause the autosomal dominant form of Emery–Dreifuss muscular dystrophy,[289] which has skeletal myopathy associated with DCM and conduction system disease. It has also been found to cause a form of autosomal dominant limb girdle muscular dystrophy (LGMD1B), which is also associated with conduction system disease.[289] Multiple mutations have been identified in patients with DCM and conduction system disease which, in some cases, had mildly elevated CK. The mechanisms responsible for the differential development of DCM, conduction system abnormalities, and skeletal myopathy are not yet elucidated.[254]

Lamin A/C mutations are associated with several distinct phenotypes. The disease frequently present with premature sinoatrial and atrioventricular node dysfunction, which progress to heart block commonly requiring pacemakers, associated with late-onset DCM; AF and other supraventricular arrhythmias are also frequent. Severe early DCM, unexpected SCD, or isolated premature cardiac death are also observed,[244,245,290-295] indicating that some patients affected by familial DCM associated with LMNA mutations may have a particularly adverse prognosis.

2.3.5.2
X-Linked DCM

Two X-linked forms of DCM have been well characterized: XLCM, which presents in adolescence and young adults, and Barth syndrome, which is most frequently identified in childhood.[296]

XLCM occur in males with rapid progression from HF to cardiac transplantation or to death due to ventricular arrhytmias; these patients are distinguished by elevated serum creatine kinase muscle isoforms (CK-MM), a sign of underlying skeletal muscle disease.[297] Female carriers tend to develop mild to moderate DCM in the fifth decade and the disease is slowly progressive.[296] Towbin et al.[298] identified the disease causing gene, Dystrophin, which is responsible for the clinical abnormalities of the disease; protein analysis by immunoblotting demonstrated severe reduction or absence of dystrophin protein in the heart of these patients.[298] Dystrophin is a cytoskeletal protein, which provides structural support to the myocyte by creating a lattice-like network to the sarcolemma, and it plays an important role in linking the sarcomeric contractile apparatus to the sarcolemma and extracellular matrix.[297,299,300] Furthermore, dystrophin is involved in cell signaling, interacting with nitric oxide synthase.[301]

Dystrophin gene mutations also cause Duchenne and Becker muscular dystrophy. These skeletal myopathies present early in life (adolescence) and the vast majority of patients develop DCM before the 25th birthday. In most patients, CK-MM is elevated; immunohistochemical analysis demonstrates reduced levels (or absence) of dystrophin; female carriers develop disease late in life, similar to that seen in XLCM. Murine models of dystrophin deficiency have abnormalities of muscle physiology based on membrane structural support anomalies, which are worsened by mechanical stress.[302,303] In addition, mutations in dystrophin secondarily affect proteins, which interact with dystrophin, causing impaired function of the myocytes of the heart and skeletal muscles.[304] Mechanical stress appears to play a significant role in the age-dependent dysfunction of these muscles.[302]

Barth syndrome is a disorder that presents in male infants as HF associated with cyclic neutropenia and 3-methylglutaconic aciduria; in some cases, these infants succumb early from HF, SCD, or sepsis due to leukocyte dysfunction.[305] Mitochondrial dysfunction and abnormalities in cardiolipin have also been documented.[305,306] The responsible gene of this syndrome is G4.5/Tafazzin, which encodes a protein called tafazzin, whose gene product is an acyltransferase. Mutations in G4.5 result in a wide clinical spectrum, which includes apparent classic DCM, hypertrophic DCM, endocardial fibroelastosis, and left ventricular noncompaction.[246,305]

2.3.6
Pathophysiology of Heart Failure in DCM

The initial manifestations of hemodynamic dysfunction in DCM are secondary to dilatation and systolic impairment that lead to a reduction in stroke volume and a rise in ventricular filling pressures. These changes have downstream effects on cardiovascular reflexes and systemic organ perfusion and function, which in turn stimulate a variety of interdependent compensatory responses. This constellation of responses (involving cardiovascular system, neurohormonal systems, and alterations in renal physiology) leads to the characteristic pathophysiology of the HF syndrome.

1. Systolic dysfunction

In the normal shaped ventricle, stroke volume increases over a wide range of end-diastolic volumes (the Frank–Starling effect). In the dilated DCM failing heart with depressed contractility, there is relatively little increment in systolic function with further increases in LV volume; in this case, the LV function curve is shifted downward and flattened. In the clinical setting, depressed stroke volume despite elevated ventricular filling pressures characterizes systolic dysfunction. The resulting symptoms are those of exercise intolerance, pulmonary or systemic congestion and, later, organ dysfunction. The clinical assessment of systolic function is pragmatic: the most practical measure is the LVEF by echocardiography, which, however, reflects a single point on the ventricular function curve.

2. Diastolic dysfunction

The relevance of impaired diastolic function in the pathogenesis of HF in DCM is increasingly appreciated.[307] In the LV with diastolic dysfunction, filling pressures rise because the compliance is reduced, with resulting LA hypertension and pulmonary congestion. Cardiac output may be reduced if ventricular filling is impaired. These abnormalities are exaggerated by activity, resulting in exertional dyspnoea and exercise intolerance. Diastolic dysfunction is difficult to quantitate, especially because of its dependence on changes in preload and afterload conditions.

3. Neurohormonal activation

The role of neurohormonal activation in HF is well recognized, thanks to the increasing understanding of its pathophysiology and with evidence that blockade of some of these responses can have a profound effect on outcomes.[308] The number of systems that are known to be activated in HF continues to grow. Sympathetic nervous system, renin-angiotensin-aldosterone system, and cytokine activation are the main ones involved. The sustained activation of these systems leads to secondary damage within the ventricle, with worsening LV remodeling and subsequent cardiac decompensation. ACE-Is, ARBs, and β-blockers attenuate and may reverse this adverse remodeling process, preventing LV dilation, geometric distortion, and deterioration in contractile function.

2.3.7
Clinical Profile

Familial DCM can be divided into presymptomatic and symptomatic stages and may manifest clinically at any age (most commonly in the third or fourth decade, or in child-hood)[6] and usually is identified when associated with severe limiting symptoms and disability.

HF, manifesting with acute decompensation triggered by an unrelated problem (such as anemia, thyrotoxicosis, or infection), is often the initial presentation of DCM. Presentation with an embolic event from the LV or LA, or with a sustained arrhythmia is less common. The classic presentation with a gradual decrease in exercise capacity may be appreciated only in retrospect.[308]

HF symptoms relating to raised filling pressures and pulmonary congestion (breathless-ness at rest, orthopnea, nocturnal cough, paroxysmal nocturnal dyspnea, peripheral edema) often precede manifestations of inadequate tissue perfusion due to low cardiac output[308] (early-onset fatigue, inability to tolerate physical exertion). Diaphoresis, hepatic pain and cachexia occur late in the course of the disease.

Patients may experience palpitation, related to supraventricular or ventricular arrhyth-mias, with symptoms of impaired consciousness (e.g., dizziness, syncope).

Common physical examination findings related to HF include sinus tachycardia, gallop rhythm, rales, jugular venous distention, pallor, cool extremities, hepatomegaly and a mur-mur consistent with mitral regurgitation. Peripheral edema, ascites, pleural and pericardial effusion, signs of hypoperfusion and renal dysfunction are late findings.[2]

2.3.8
Investigations

2.3.8.1
Electrocardiography

The ECG changes of early disease are not specific and may include left axis deviation and T wave abnormalities.[2,309] With progressive and advanced disease, conduction abnormalities may develop: PR prolongation, QRS widening, left bundle branch block (LBBB). The development of progressive conduction disease in association with LV dysfunction should raise suspicion of myotonic dystrophy, or disease caused by a mutation in lamin A/C.[254,310,311] Other intraventricu-lar conduction delays or loss of anterior or inferior forces are also common.

2.3.8.2
Chest X-Ray

Chest X-ray is useful to detect cardiomegaly, pulmonary congestion, and pleural fluid accumulation; it can also demonstrate the presence of coexistent pulmonary disease or infection contributing to dyspnoea.[2]

2.3.8.3
Laboratory Tests

Recommended tests include the following: a full blood count; renal, thyroid, and hepatic function; iron and transferrin levels to exclude hemochromatosis; creatine kinase levels to detect subclinical skeletal myopathy.[308]

Natriuretic peptides and neurohormonal markers are useful to determine whether HF is an active issue.[2,312,313] In cases of acute decompensated HF, the B-type natriuretic peptide (BNP) tends to be significantly elevated.[312,313] Novel approaches including the development of molecular biomarkers (derived from endomyocardial biopsy samples) for individual risk assessment in new-onset HF are on the near horizon.[314]

2.3.8.4
Echocardiography

Usually diagnosis of DCM (both familial and non familial forms) is made with two-dimensional echocardiography with findings of ventricular chamber enlargement and systolic dysfunction with normal LV wall thickness.[308] Mitral regurgitation is often present.

Common echocardiographic abnormalities are reduced LVEF (<45–50%), global LV dysfunction, increased end-diastolic (>55–60 mm) and end-systolic diameter (>45 mm), reduced fractional shortening (<25%), increased LA size (>45 mm), abnormalities of the early and late diastolic filling patterns at mitral diastolic flow profile, increased tricuspid regurgitation peak velocity (>3 m/s), reduced aortic outflow velocity time integral (<15 cm) and dilated inferior vena cava.[2]

Recently, new noninvasive imaging approaches such as measures of myocardial performance index (MPI), strain, sphericity, and tissue characterization using backscatter methods have been developed and used in an attempt to determine early-onset abnormalities consistent with early diagnosis.[315,316] The detection of early disease provides the opportunity to intervene and attenuate or prevent disease progression.

Patients should have a two-dimensional echocardiogram (with measurement of chamber dimensions and calculated indices of systolic function) to provide structural and functional characterization of their disease at initial evaluation and serially to assess treatment effect and disease progression.

2.3.8.5
Exercise Testing

Exercise testing is useful for the objective evaluation of exercise capacity and exertional symptoms, such as dyspnoea and fatigue. The 6-minute walk test is a reproducible and simple tool to assess submaximal functional capacity.

A maximal exercise test (preferably with metabolic gas exchange measurements) provides a reproducible measurement of maximal exercise capacity and should be done as a baseline and for serial assessment to monitor disease progression and the effect of treatment and to provide functional characterization of the disease.

2.3.8.6
Cardiac Magnetic Resonance Imaging

CMR is an accurate, reproducible technique for the assessment of LV and RV volumes and global function,[2] but is generally less practical for serial evaluation.

Furthermore, late gadolinium-enhanced CMR, having the ability to assess myocardial tissue characteristics in vivo, may be very helpful in DCM patients both for risk stratification and for differential diagnosis. This technique provides evidence of inflammation, infiltration, and scarring and allows identification of diverse ethiologies of DCM in patients with previous infarction, myocarditis, pericarditis, or infiltrative and storage diseases.[2] Studies report that in DCM, midwall fibrosis determined by CMR is a predictor of mortality, cardiovascular hospitalization, ventricular tachycardia, and SCD.[317-319] The role of CMR in DCM risk stratification may have value in determining the need for device therapy. In addition, the detection of cardiac scarring seems to have also the potential to identify non-responders to CRT.[320]

2.3.8.7
Holter ECG

Ambulatory ECG monitoring is important to assess patients with symptoms suggestive of an arrhythmia (palpitation, presyncope, or syncope) and in monitoring HR control in patients with AF.[2] Episodes of symptomatic or asymptomatic NSVT are frequent in decompensated DCM patients and are associated with poor prognosis.

2.3.9
Principles of Clinical Management

Treatment aims to minimize symptoms and prevent the development of complications and disease progression. In the absence of a specific underlying cause or aggravating factors, treatment is as described for the various stages of HF.

Supportive therapy includes sodium and fluid restriction, avoidance of alcohol and other toxins. Regular, moderate daily activity is desirable to sustain mobility, avoid deconditioning, and maintain physical and psychological well-being. It is also important to monitor patients' weight; weight reduction should be considered in obese subjects.[2]

Titration to the target dose (or to the maximum tolerated dose) of neurohormonal inhibitors such ACE-Is, β-blockers, ARBs, or aldosterone antagonists is strongly recommended. As demonstrated in several randomized trials, these drugs have a beneficial impact on mortality.[2] Optimal treatment with ACE-Is improves ventricular function, reduces hospitalizations for worsening HF and increases survival, as well as treatment with β-blockers. ACE-Is side-effects occur in a minority of patients and include a dry cough, rash, metallic taste, and rarely swelling of the tongue. Also, β-blockers may provoke side-effects in a minority of patients, including worsening fatigue, impotence, and cold hands. β-blockers should be reduced or temporarily suspended during episodes of acute HF.

ARBs or aldosterone antagonists should be considered in patients with severe symptomatic HF and advanced functional class, in the absence of hyperkalemia and significant renal dysfunction.[2] ARBs are also recommended as an alternative in patients intolerant to ACE-Is.[2]

Studies suggest[321-323] that in symptomatic patients intolerant to both ACE-Is and ARBs, the combination of hydralazine and isosorbide dinitrate may be used as an alternative; the same combination should also be considered in patients with persistent symptoms despite optimal treatment.

Digoxin is useful for initial HR control in decompensated patients with rapid AF, prior to initiation of a β-blocker. This drug may have a role in improving ventricular function and patient well-being also in patients in sinus rhythm, but has no effect on survival.[2]

Diuretics (loop diuretics, thiazides) should usually be used in combination with ACE-Is/ARBs in patients with HF and clinical signs or symptoms of congestion.[2]

AF in patients with DCM is associated with a high risk of thromboembolism and can cause severe deterioration of HF. Restoration of sinus rhythm either with drugs (Amiodarone) or electrical cardioversion usually results in a substantial improvement in symptoms. If this is unsuccessful, another option is the control of the ventricular rate with digoxin or β-blockers. Patients with episodes of AF or with echocardiographic evidence of a LA or LV mural thrombosis should be anticoagulated.

ICD therapy for primary prevention is indicated for DCM patients with an LVEF ≤35%, in functional class NYHA II or III, receiving optimal medical therapy, and with an expectation of survival with good functional status for >1 year.[2] Secondary prevention with ICD therapy is recommended for survivors of ventricular fibrillation and also for patients with documented haemodynamically unstable VT or VT with syncope, a LVEF ≤40%, on optimal medical therapy, who have a reasonable expectation of survival with good functional status for >1 year.[2]

Patients in NYHA class III–IV who are symptomatic despite optimal medical therapy and who have an important reduction of systolic function (LVEF ≤35%) and QRS prolongation (QRS width ≥120 ms) require management for advanced HF with cardiac resynchronization therapy, to syncronize interventricular and intraventricular contraction.[2] Moreover, in DCM, biventricular (instead of mono or bicameral) devices are preferred for patients with conventional indications for permanent pacing.[2]

Cardiac transplantation should be considered in patients with end-stage HF, severe symptoms, no serious comorbidity, requiring inotropes, mechanical ventilatory, and mechanical device support (i.e., balloon counterpulsation), with no alternative treatment options.[2] However, so far, waiting times for organs remains a significant limitation. To overcome this, left ventricular assist devices (LVADs) have been used as a "bridge to transplant" and show promise. Dystrophin is often reduced or absent in hearts of patients with both familial and nonfamilial DCM: studies suggest that the reduction of mechanical stress by use of LVADs results in reverse remodeling of dystrophin and of the heart itself.[287,288]

Although improved outcomes have been achieved, the ultimate outcome for these patients remains problematic. For these reasons, further studies on genetic-based therapies such as gene therapy,[324] stem cell therapy[325], and targeted treatments, such as the use of membrane sealants[326] and exon skipping, are under evaluation.

2.3.9.1
Family Screening

Familial evaluation of first-degree relatives of individuals with familial DCM is important at the time of diagnosis and serially thereafter. The detection and treatment of DCM is possible before the onset of advanced symptomatic disease.

A thorough family history should be taken on every individual with DCM[327,328] and a distinction should be made between a family history that is negative for cardiovascular disease and one that is inconclusive. The primary aim of pedigree analysis is to diagnose familial DCM and to identify at-risk family members to initiate early treatment and risk evaluation.[239]

Clinical screening of relatives of patients with familial DCM by physical examination, 12-lead ECG and two-dimensional echocardiogram is warranted, because a significant proportion of patients may not be detected without formal screening and once detected may assist in identifying more distant family members who are at risk.[239] Familial DCM gene carriers often do not manifest symptoms of HF or arrhythmias until late in the disease process and even if they have cardiovascular abnormalities detected by ECG or echocardiogram, they may be asymptomatic. Unfortunately, no ECG abnormalities are specific to familial DCM. It has been suggested that LV enlargement may be the single most useful criterion in identifying those with preclinical disease.[329,330]

The detection of early disease in a family member may lead to earlier interventions that may slow disease progression. Treatment with ACE-Is or β-blockers has been suggested,[327,331] but the efficacy of such therapy remains to be proven.

So far, the potential role of lifestyle modifications for subjects with preclinical disease is unknown, but avoidance of alcohol and illicit drugs should be encouraged.[239] The contribution of environmental factors to the pathogenesis of disease remains to be established.

Precise algorithms to determine the interval of evaluation remain to be determined; adults with normal screening who have a first-degree relative with familial DCM should have a repeat echocardiogram and ECG every 3–5 years.[327,332] More frequent evaluation of those with abnormalities or unexplained symptoms appears appropriate.

Genetic counseling is also important to lend support to families and to give explanations about the uncertainty and anxiety surrounding the significance of clinical and genetic evaluation. Genetic testing is not yet commonly available, but its emergence will provide new opportunities for presymptomatic diagnosis.[239]

2.4
Arrhythmogenic Right Ventricular Cardiomyopathy

2.4.1
Definition and General Features of the Disease

ARVC is an inherited heart muscle disease[333,334] defined by the presence of RV dysfunction (global or regional), with or without LV disease, in the presence of histological evidence for the disease and/or electrocardiographic abnormalities.[1,335]

ARVC is characterized by the loss of myocytes with replacement by fibro-adipose tissue, with a predilection for the RV.[336] Forms of ARVC affecting primarily the LV are increasingly recognized.

Clinical manifestations of the disease include ventricular arrhythmias, congestive HF and SCD, which may be the first presentation of the disease; patients have a propensity for reentry ventricular arrhythmias most commonly arising from diseased portions of the RV. Indeed, ARVC has been reported as a common cause of SCD in the young, including athletes.

ARVC has an estimated prevalence of 1:1,000–1:5,000.[1] This probably represents an underestimation and takes into account only the most severe spectrum of the disease.

2.4.2 Clinical Genetics

The prevalence of familial ARVC is usually cited as around 30–50%[337-339]; the disease has an autosomal dominant inheritance pattern and incomplete penetrance, although recessive forms are described, often in association with cutaneous disorders.[1]

2.4.3
Molecular Genetics and Genotype: Phenotype Correlations

ARVC is caused by mutations in desmosomal proteins genes: Plakoglobin (JUP), Desmoplakin (DSP), Plakophilin-2 (PKP2), Desmoglein-2 (*DSG2*), and Desmocollin-2 (*DSC2*).[1] Recently, a mutation in a cytoplasmic membrane protein, transmembrane protein 43 (TMEM43), has been described.[340] Mutations in cardiac Ryanodine receptor (RyR-2) and TGF-β (TGF-β3) genes also seems to be associated with an ARVC phenotype.[1]

Plakoglobin, also known as γ-catenin, is the first constituent of cell adhesion junctions to be implicated in the pathogenesis of ARVC. This gene was found by means of molecular studies on a recessive variant of ARVC, known as Naxos disease. This is one of the major syndromic forms of ARVC, characterized by wooly hair and nonepidermolytic palmoplantar keratoderma. The cutaneous manifestations, associated with very high penetrance of cardiac disease by adolescence, facilitated the recognition of affected subjects in this population. Initial mapping of this disorder pointed to the chromosomal locus 17q21.12[341]; subsequently, a two base pair deletion in the Plakoglobin gene was reported as the cause of Naxos disease.[341,342] This mutation results in a frameshift and premature termination of the protein.[342] Homozygous subjects have diffuse palmoplantar keratoderma and wooly hair from infancy. Minor ventricular arrhythmia may occur in children, which are otherwise asymptomatic from a cardiac viewpoint. Symptom onset usually occurs in puberty, often with syncope. The annual mortality from SCD is around 3%, slightly higher than that observed in dominant forms of ARVC.[343]

Another recessive cardiocutaneous syndrome (Carvajal syndrome), consisting of a triad of epidermolytic palmoplantar keratoderma, wooly hair, and apparent DCM was first recognized in India[344] and then further elucidated in several Ecuadorian families.[345] A deletion in Desmoplakin was reported as the causative mutation.[346] This seems to cause truncation of the C-domain in the tail end of the protein. Desmoplakin, a member of the plakin family, is a cytoplasmic protein without a transmembrane domain that serves as an intracellular link between desmosomes and intermediate filaments and is expressed in all desmosomes.[347,348] Another missense mutation in the C-terminal of DSP is described in an Arab family with recessive ARVC, wooly hair, and a pemphigous-like skin disorder.[349] Interestingly, both mutations are located in exon 24 of the desmoplakin gene; however, the cardiomyopathy of Carvajal syndrome shows a predilection for the LV, while the cardiac phenotype in the Arab family appeared to be classic ARVC.

Desmoplakin has also been the first gene abnormality identified in an autosomal-dominant ARVC: a missense mutation in an Italian family with the typical ARVC phenotype.[350] The resulting amino acid substitution modifies a putative phosphorylation site in the N-terminal Plakoglobin binding domain. Interestingly, other missense and nonsense mutations in the Desmoplakin gene have been associated either with isolated dominant ARVC, or with arrhythmogenic LV cardiomyopathy (ALVC), in which affected patients had no hair or skin abnormalities.[350-352] Furthermore, other mutations have been found to cause cutaneous abnormalities without signs of cardiomyopathy.[353,354]

More recently, a variety of mutations in Plakophilin-2, an armadillo-family member gene that is expressed in the heart and interacts directly with plakoglobin and desmoplakin, have been identified in a number of probands with ARVC.[355]

Another ARVC candidate gene is DSG2, encoding Desmoglein-2, which is highly expressed in cardiac tissue. Desmogleins are desmosomal cadherins and together with the desmocollins are essential transmembrane components of the desmosome.[356] There are four related members of the desmoglein family, each with a separate gene localized to chromosome 18p. Sequence analysis led to recognition of DSG2 as the fourth desmosomal gene associated with ARVC.[357,358]

Desmocollin-2 was the fifth major component of the cardiac desmosome to be implicated in ARVC,[359,360] although mutations in the *DSC2* gene seem to be infrequent.[361]

TMEM43 gene mutation has been found in 15 unrelated ARVC families ascertained from a genetically isolated population in Newfoundland. The study suggests that TMEM43 mutation provokes a fully penetrant, sex-influenced morbid, lethal disorder. So far, little is known about the function of the *TMEM43* gene; however, it contains a response element for PPARγ, which may explain the fibrofatty replacement of the myocardium.[340]

2.4.4
Molecular Pathophysiology

Desmosomes are protein complexes that mediate mechanical coupling between cardio-myocytes. Impaired desmosome functioning under conditions of mechanical stress is thought to cause cell detachment and death. The myocardial injury may be accompanied by an inflammatory response. Regeneration of cardiomyocytes is limited; repair by fibro-fatty replacement takes place, with consequent ventricular remodeling. In the normal state, RV has increased distensibility to adapt to wide variations in preload; this appears to confer vulnerability to cell adhesion defects. By Laplace's law, wall tension is inversely pro-portional to wall thickness. Accordingly, early ARVC shows a predilection for the thinnest portions of the RV: inflow, outflow, and apical regions, with typical aneurysm formation in these areas. Similarly, LV involvement is often restricted to the thin posterolateral wall, with sparing of the thicker septum and free wall. Clinical experience suggests that intense and prolonged mechanical stress on the heart during physical training, as occurs in ath-letes, may contribute to disease progression and risk.

Desmosomal dysfunction may also explain the extramyocardial manifestations of syn-dromic ARVC. Cutaneous disease is confined to the palmar and plantar surfaces, which are the areas most exposed to pressure and/or abrasion. It seems that the mutant desmosomal proteins are able to maintain tissue integrity, unless subjected to excessive mechanical stress. A common undercurrent of stress-induced damage to cell surfaces is therefore apparent.

2.4.5
Natural History

ARVC natural history is considered to include four distinct phases, based on clinical and pathological findings.[337]

The early phase is typically described as "concealed," owing to the frequent absence of clinical findings: patients are often asymptomatic, but may nonetheless be at risk of SCD, notably during intense physical exertion. Structural changes, when present, are subtle and may be confined to the thinnest portions of the RV.

The "overt electrical" phase that subsequently develops is characterized by symptom-atic ventricular arrhythmia, accompanied by more obvious morphologic and functional abnormalities of the RV, detectable by imaging. Patients typically present with palpitation, presyncope, or syncope.

The third phase is characterized by further extension of the disease with consequent RV impaired contractility, which results in right-sided HF with LV involvement.

The final, "endstage" phase, is characterized by biventricular pump failure, leading to a phenotype that may be difficult to distinguish from DCM.[337,362,363] When HF is complicated by AF, endocavitary mural thrombosis, especially within aneurysms or in the atrial append-ages may occur, with embolic risk. A multicenter study of patients with evidence of ARVC at transplantation or autopsy found fibrofatty replacement of the LV in 76% of the hearts examined; LV involvement correlated with age, HF, and arrhythmic events.[362]

This clinical picture is representative of the typical severe form of ARVC; however, among the relatives of ARVC probands, disease variants that primarily affect the LV have been identified[364-366] and long-term favorable course of the disease has also been described.[367]

2.4.6
Mechanisms Underlying Arrhythmia

Distinct mechanisms may provoke arrhythmia in ARVC. In the overt stage, myocardial fibrofatty replacement creates reentrant circuits, which lead to sustained monomorphic ventricular tachycardia, with typical LBBB configuration. When the LV is affected, ventricular arrhythmias exhibit morphologies consistent with origins from different cardiac regions.

The phenomenon of "hot phases," during which previously stable patients with mild disease may suffer unheralded arrhythmic events or SCD, is more difficult to explain. ARVC seems to remain quiescent for long periods, until an unknown stimulus triggers inflammation and myocyte loss. This may provide the substrate for arrhythmic exacerbation.

Recent studies have also tested a hypothesis regarding the basis of arrhythmia in "concealed" ARVC.[368-371] Destabilization of cell adhesion complexes at the level of gap junctions, structures very close to desmosomes, may cause inhibition of the preservation of normal numbers of gap junctions. The resultant heterogeneous conduction may be a significant contributor to arrhythmogenesis.[371] According to this hypothesis, clinically significant arrhythmia may occur in the absence of structural heart disease in ARVC. Gap junction remodeling may therefore account for arrhythmogenesis in the "concealed" phase. Whether this mechanism has the potential to produce life-threatening arrhythmia is unresolved.[371]

2.4.7
Clinical Presentation

Clinicians should be alert to the possibility of ARVC in several different circumstances.

Young or middle-aged individuals who die suddenly or who experience palpitation, presyncope, or syncope in the apparent absence of cardiac disease should raise the suspicion of ARVC.[338] Chest pain and dyspnoea may also occur, and symptoms are frequently precipitated by exercise. Arrhythmia of RV origin, which can range from isolated ventricular extrasystoles to ventricular tachycardia, heightens the suspicion. In these cases, the main differential diagnosis is with idiopathic right ventricular outflow tract (RVOT) tachycardia, a focal arrhythmic disorder, not hereditary, that is reported to have an excellent prognosis.[372-374]

Cardiac arrest can be the first manifestation of ARVC and is reported to occur in less than 10% of live index cases.[338,375] However, more than half of the probands in the studies cited had suffered SCD, with the diagnosis established on postmortem.

The under-representation of ventricular fibrillation as a mode of presentation among patients probably reflects the poor rates of survival from out-of-hospital cardiac arrests, coupled with the problems of an accurate diagnosis at post-mortem. The differential diagnosis includes ischemic heart disease, HCM, DCM, Brugada syndrome, long QT syndrome, and anomalous coronary arteries. Inquiry for a family history of premature cardiac symptoms and/or SCD is important.

Presentation with congestive HF, right-sided or biventricular, is uncommon.[362,375] ARVC should be considered in patients with isolated RV failure in the absence of pulmonary hypertension, after excluding RV infarction, valve lesions, left-to-right shunts, and other congenital defects such as Ebstein's anomaly. Cardiac sarcoidosis may mimic ARVC.[376,377] RV fibrofatty replacement induces dilation and chamber remodeling with a resultant drop in EF. As a consequence, the tricuspid valve annulus dilates inducing tricuspid regurgitation with subsequent signs and symptoms of right-sided HF (e.g., elevated jugular venous pressure with clear lung fields, hepathomegaly, ascites, ankle swelling, peripheral edema etc.). At late stages, biventricular HF occurs. Palpitation, dizziness, and syncope can be present: HF itself represents a risk factor for SCD.[378]

ARVC is a recognized cause of SCD during sporting activity. Competitive and endurance athletes seem to be at major risk.[379-382] ARVC is reported to be identified consistently in a substantial proportion of athletes, many of whom are asymptomatic.[383,384] Unfortunately, physiologic adaptations to training may mimic the diagnosis.[385,386] In these unclear cases, serial evaluation and familial evaluation is advised.

2.4.8
Diagnostic Criteria

The gold standard for ARVC diagnosis is the histological demonstration of myocyte loss with transmural fibrofatty replacement of the RV, either by endomyocardial biopsy or surgery, or postmortem examination. This criterion has many limitations in clinical practice and during life relies on invasive procedures. In addition, endomyocardial biopsy is by definition not transmural, and it is usually performed in the interventricular septum, which is often spared by the disease.

To overcome these diagnostic difficulties, standardized criteria for the diagnosis of ARVC were proposed in 1994 by an international task force[335]. These are based on the identification of electrocardiographic repolarization abnormalities, arrhythmias of RV origin, familial disease, RV functional and structural abnormalities and fibro-fatty replacement of the RV myocardium.

Diagnostic criteria are classified as major and minor, according to their specificity for the disease. Based predominantly on tertiary center experience with symptomatic index cases, these guidelines are highly specific but lack sensitivity for early disease. Their main application is therefore in establishing a definitive diagnosis in probands. A modification of these criteria has recently been proposed to improve the diagnosis and management of ARVC[387] (Table 2.2). The presence of two major, or one major plus two minor or four minor criteria from different categories, is considered diagnostic for ARVC. The revised criteria have shown to increase the sensitivity of the classification.

Table 2.2 Proposed Revised Task Force Criteria for the diagnosis of ARVC in probands, modified from[387]

I Global and/or regional dysfunction and structural alterations

MAJOR

By 2D echo:

- Regional RV akinesia, dyskinesia, or aneurysm* *and* 1 of the following at end diastole :
  - PLAX RVOT ≥32 mm (corrected for BSA ≥ 19 mm/m2)
  - PSAX RVOT ≥36 mm (corrected for BSA ≥21 mm/m2)
  - *or* fractional area change ≤33%

By MRI:

- Regional RV akinesia or dyskinesia or dyssynchronous RV contraction* *and* 1 of the following:
  - Ratio of RV end-diastolic volume to BSA ≥110 mL/m2 (♂) or ≥100 mL/m2 (♀)
  - *or* RV ejection fraction ≤40%

By RV angiography:

- Regional RV akinesia, dyskinesia, or aneurysm*

MINOR

By 2D echo:

- Regional RV akinesia or dyskinesia* *and* 1 of the following at end diastole:
  - PLAX RVOT ≥29 to <32 mm (corrected for BSA ≥16 to <19 mm/m2)
  - PSAX RVOT ≥32 to <36 mm (corrected for BSA ≥18 to <21 mm/m2)
  - *or* fractional area change >33% to ≤40%

By MRI:

- Regional RV akinesia or dyskinesia or dyssynchronous RV contraction* *and* 1 of the following:
  - Ratio of RV end-diastolic volume to BSA ≥100 to <110 mL/m2 (♂) or ≥90 to <100 mL/m2 (♀)
  - *or* RV ejection fraction >40% to ≤45%

II Tissue characterisation of walls

MAJOR

- Residual myocytes <60% by morphometric analysis (or <50% if estimated), with fibrous replacement of the RV free wall myocardium in ≥1 sample, with or without fatty replacement of tissue on endomyocardial biopsy

MINOR

- Residual myocytes 60% to 75% by morphometric analysis (or 50% to 65% if estimated), with fibrous replacement of the RV free wall myocardium in ≥1 sample, with or without fatty replacement of tissue on endomyocardial biopsy

(*continued*)

Table 2.2 (continued)

III Repolarisation abnormalities

MAJOR

- Inverted T waves in right precordial leads (V1, V2, and V3) or beyond in individuals >14 years of age (in the absence of complete right bundle-branch block QRS ≥120 ms)

MINOR

- Inverted T waves in leads V1 and V2 in individuals >14 years of age (in the absence of complete right bundle-branch block) or in V4, V5, or V6
- Inverted T waves in leads V1, V2, V3, and V4 in individuals >14 years of age in the presence of complete right bundle-branch block

IV Depolarisation/conduction abnormalities

MAJOR

- Epsilon wave (reproducible low-amplitude signals between end of QRS complex to onset of the T wave) in the right precordial leads (V1 to V3)

MINOR

- Late potentials by SAECG in ≥1 of 3 parameters in the absence of a QRS duration of ≥110 ms on the standard ECG
- Filtered QRS duration (fQRS) ≥114 ms
- Duration of terminal QRS <40 μV (low-amplitude signal duration) ≥38 ms
- Root-mean-square voltage of terminal 40 ms ≤20 μV
- Terminal activation duration of QRS ≥55 ms measured from the nadir of the S wave to the end of the QRS, including R', in V1, V2, or V3, in the absence of complete right bundle-branch block

V Arrhythmias

MAJOR

- Nonsustained or sustained ventricular tachycardia of left bundle-branch morphology with superior axis (negative or indeterminate QRS in leads II, III, and aVF and positive in lead aVL)

MINOR

- Nonsustained or sustained ventricular tachycardia of RV outflow configuration, left bundle-branch block morphology with inferior axis (positive QRS in leads II, III, and aVF and negative in lead aVL) or of unknown axis
- > 500 ventricular extrasystoles per 24 hours (Holter)

VI Family history

MAJOR

- ARVC/D confirmed in a first-degree relative who meets current Task Force criteria
- ARVC/D confirmed pathologically at autopsy or surgery in a first-degree relative
- Identification of a pathogenic mutation categorized as associated or probably associated with ARVC/D in the patient under evaluation

Table 2.2 (continued)

MINOR
• History of ARVC/D in a first-degree relative in whom it is not possible or practical to determine whether the family member meets current Task Force criteria • Premature sudden death (<35 years of age) due to suspected ARVC/D in a first-degree relative • ARVC/D confirmed pathologically or by current Task Force Criteria in second-degree relative

Diagnostic terminology for revised criteria: *Definite diagnosis*: 2 major or 1 major and 2 minor criteria or 4 minor from different categories. *Borderline*: 1 major and 1 minor or 3 minor criteria from different categories. *Possible*: 1 major or 2 minor criteria from different categories.

PLAX parasternal long-axis view; *RVOT* RV outflow tract; *BSA* body surface area; *PSAX* parasternal short-axis view; *aVF* augmented voltage unipolar left foot lead; and *aVL* augmented voltage unipolar left arm lead.
*Hypokinesis is not included in this or subsequent definitions of RV regional wall motion abnormalities for the proposed modified criteria.

2.4.9
Investigations

2.4.9.1
Electrocardiography

Electrocardiography plays a key role in the diagnosis of ARVC.[335,388-390]

T-wave inversion (TWI) in right precordial leads (V1–V3) in males >12 years and in females >14 years, in absence of right bundle bunch block (RBBB), has been described in up to 80% of patients with ARVC.[335,388-390] This pattern is highly specific, being present in less than 3% of healthy adult subjects.

Localized prolongation of QRS complex (>110 ms) in V1–V3 is believed to be related to delayed repolarization of the RV because of myocardial areas of fibro-fatty replacement. It has been described in more than 90% of ARVC patients.[335,388] A prolongation ≥55 ms of the terminal part of the QRS in V1–V3 has been observed in a highly symptomatic population with ARVC and may be a marker in the late stage of the disease.

Epsilon waves, defined as a low-amplitude deflection occurring between the end of the QRS and the beginning of the T wave, are described in up to one third of patients with ARVC.[335] When localized in V1–V3, their presence is highly suggestive of ARVC. Signal-averaged ECG facilitates detection of the equivalent sign of late potentials in 50–80% of established cases.[335,375,391,392] Late potentials are considered strongly suggestive of disease expression in the presence of a confirmed family history of ARVC.[338]

QRS dispersion, defined as a difference ≥40 ms between the QRS duration in V1–V3 and V6, has been reported as a predictor of SCD. Poor R-wave progression in the right precordial leads often associated with TWI and low voltages of the QRS complex in the limbs leads are additional recognized features of ARVC.[335,388]

2.4.9.2
Detection of Arrhythmia

Ambulatory ECG monitoring and maximal exercise testing may help in the identification and quantification of ventricular arrhythmias.

A LBBB configuration tachycardia, indicating probable RV origin, is a minor criterion in probands; many of them are referred on this basis for discrimination of ARVC from idiopathic RVOT arrhythmia. Either >1,000 ventricular extrasystoles in a 24-h period or documented VT are a major diagnostic criterion.[333,335]

Ventricular tachycardia or frequent ventricular extrasystoles can be the sole cardiac abnormality in a small number of relatives. Hence, within the context of a family history of ARVC, the reduced criterion of >200 ventricular extrasystoles in 24 h may imply disease expression.[333,338]

2.4.9.3
Echocardiography

Echocardiography represents the first-line imaging approach for evaluating patients with suspected ARVC or for evaluating family members. Together with pulsed tissue Doppler techniques, it has the benefit of being inexpensive and readily available. However, visualization of the RV by echocardiography is not always satisfactory, leading to high inter-observer and intra-observer variability. Limitations include the complex shape and geometry of the RV, and difficulty applying the standardized reference points for the measurements and their cut-off values. Contrast echocardiography may help to obtain better endocardial definition of the RV and apex of the LV.

Structural abnormalities in ARVC may be localized, in the form of patchy wall thinning and segmental dilation, usually involving the inflow, outflow, and apical regions, or diffuse: ultimately global dilatation of the RV may develop. Functional impairment ranges from mild regional wall motion abnormalities to generalized hypokinesia with reduced EF. Diastolic bulging, due to structural weakness secondary to fibro-fatty infiltration, may be present. When analyzing wall motion, care should be taken for particular areas like moderator band insertion point, which often results in false-positive abnormalities.

Evaluation also includes the LV, which may be affected either in the early or in the late stage of the disease. In a study, hallmark features for ARVC were considered severe in 45% of probands who underwent echocardiography, mild in 26%, and localized aneurysms were found in 10%.[338] Affected relatives had less prominent morphologic abnormalities: in familial ARVC incomplete disease expression may be associated with subtle structural changes that are not detectable by the standard echocardiogram.[338]

2.4.9.4
Cardiac Magnetic Resonance

CMR allows three dimensional imaging of the heart, and its relation with thoracic structures has no need of geometrical assumptions for the quantification of the RV and LV volumes and provides noninvasive tissue characterization, identifying fat and fibrosis. However, postmortem studies demonstrate that fibrofatty replacement is often microscopic rather than overt[393] and hence may not be discernible by imaging. In addition, differentiation between pericardial fat and fatty infiltration may be difficult. Therefore, fatty infiltration and fibrosis detected by CMR are not part of the current diagnostic criteria for ARVC. The lack of knowledge about the normal spectrum of the RV morphology at CMR could potentially lead to over-diagnosis.

2.4.10
Principles of Clinical Management

Endurance training, competitive sports, and extreme physical exertion, as well as ingestion of stimulants are best avoided in subjects in whom a diagnosis of ARVC is confirmed or strongly suspected.

Evidence for the efficacy of antiarrhythmic agents in ARVC is largely anecdotal.[394,395]

Sympathetic stimulation may be a precipitant of arrhythmia, as suggested by the association of arrhythmic events with strenuous activity, together with the observation that VT is often preceded by an increased HR.[396] Therefore, the use of β-blockers is standard when there are no contraindications. Amiodarone or sotalol can also be effective is suppressing VT.[395]

Optimal protection against SCD is conferred by ICD. In current practice, it is recommended for cardiac arrest survivors and is offered as primary prevention to selected ARVC patients with arrhythmic syncope, SVT resistant to drug treatment, severe RV dilation, LV involvement and congestive HF.[343,397-399] In ARVC patients, appropriate interventions occur frequently, confirming the likely survival benefit.[400,401] Antitachycardia pacing is frequently able to terminate SVT.[400] Restrictions to more widespread use of ICD include risks of inappropriate intervention, infection, potential complications of lead insertion into the diseased RV and psychological repercussions associated with the device.[400] ICD therapy may allow cutback or discontinuation of drugs; however, in some cases, medication is continued after device placement to reduce the likelihood of discharge.

Catheter ablation has been used in VT refractory to drug treatment.[402] However, this procedure is palliative: the treatment may be effective in the short term, but is associated with high rate of recurrence.[402]

2.4.11
Heart Failure in ARVC

The earlier identification of affected probands unmasks the problem of HF in patients with a longer disease history.

HF in ARVC patients is usually described as a rare event,[403] but recent studies suggest its increased prevalence.[404,405] In large clinical series reported up to 2005, patients who died due to HF or underwent heart transplantation represented 47–66% of all cases of cardiac terminal events.[378,405-407] The mean age of such patients was significantly higher than those who died suddenly.[408] In this series, the high prevalence of death due to HF may be explained by a change in the cause of death because of aggressive therapeutic management of tachyarrhythmias.

Isolated RV failure in ARVC represents a unique clinical situation where RV failure is not associated with high pulmonary pressures. This implies that damage of the RV muscle has no apparent effect on hemodynamics, as a low pressure difference is sufficient to provide adequate pulmonary flow. Right atrial contraction and paradoxical ventricular septum motion provide functional compensation enabling normal physical activity for a long time.[409] At this stage, the mechanisms which may trigger symptoms of RV failure are LV damage, AF, SVT, superimposed myocarditis, and RV thrombosis.[409]

LV damage is increasingly observed and in some patients (e.g., Desmoplakin mutations), it may appear early and lead to a clinical picture of congestive HF.[351] A history of congestive HF and the presence of LV involvement are independent risk factors for an adverse outcome.[378] Biventricular HF occurs at late stages of the disease.

ARVC patients with long disease duration may develop supraventricular tachycardia.[378,411] Frequently AF, provoking lack of atrial contraction, may precipitate symptoms. Advanced HF may be complicated by thrombosis, usually in patients with concomitant AF.[412] The annual incidence of thromboembolic complications in ARVC seems to be less frequent than in patients with HF for other causes.[412] Anticoagulation should be recommended in ARVC patients with AF, marked ventricular dilation, or ventricular aneurysms, as both pulmonary and cerebral embolism are recognized complications.[362,413]

Management of HF in ARVC patients includes diuretics, ACE-Is, ARBs, β-blockers, and aldosterone antagonists. Sinus rhythm control is essential: the therapeutic goal is to postpone permanent AF as long as possible. Amiodarone is usually effective in prophylaxis. In patients with refractory HF symptoms and long-lasting AF, rhythm conversion should be attempted. In recurrent AF, refractory to pharmacological prevention, pulmonary vein ablation can be considered.

In the rare patient with predominantly RV failure refractory to pharmacological therapy, a surgical approach has been proposed: the conventional LV cardiomyoplasty procedure using the *latissimus dorsi* muscle was modified to perform RV cardiomyoplasty, with satisfactory results in a 10-year follow-up.[414]

Recently, RV exclusion surgery (Fontan-type repair) has been used. This can be an alternative treatment for refractory right-sided HF before heart transplantation is considered, or a "bridge to transplant" in critically ill patients.[415,416] In refractory congestive biventricular HF, cardiac transplantation becomes the only therapeutic option.[362]

2.4.12
Family Screening

Relatives of patients with a confirmed diagnosis on clinical assessment or postmortem examination should be evaluated. Serial periodic evaluation from early adolescence is recommended as presentation in childhood is rare.[417] Evolution of characteristic ECG features over years has been documented.[390] Age and family history are useful to determine the interval between assessments; adolescents may be seen every 6–12 months as the disease often becomes manifest in this age group. Older relatives may require less frequent follow-up. A clinical diagnosis of ARVC was confirmed in 10–40% of the family members investigated in two major studies.[338,375]

In terms of risk stratification in relatives, clinical experience suggests that the onset of symptoms such as sustained palpitation, dizziness, or syncope may herald an active phase of a previously "concealed" disease. In such situation, prompt reevaluation of the patient is imperative.

References

1. Elliott P, Andersson B, Arbustini E, et al. Classification of the cardiomyopathies: a position statement from the European society of cardiology working group on myocardial and pericardial diseases. *Eur Heart J.* 2008;29(2):270-276.
2. Dickstein K, Cohen-Solal A, Filippatos G, et al. ESC guidelines for the diagnosis and treatment of acute and chronic heart failure 2008: the Task Force for the diagnosis and treatment of acute and chronic heart failure 2008 of the European Society of Cardiology. Developed in collaboration with the Heart Failure Association of the ESC (HFA) and endorsed by the European Society of Intensive Care Medicine (ESICM). *Eur J Heart Fail.* 2008;10(10):933-989.
3. Harris KM, Spirito P, Maron MS, et al. Prevalence, clinical profile, and significance of left ventricular remodeling in the end-stage phase of hypertrophic cardiomyopathy. *Circulation.* 2006;114(3):216-225.
4. Richardson P, McKenna W, Bristow M, et al. Report of the 1995 World Health Organization/International Society and Federation of Cardiology task force on the definition and classification of cardiomyopathies. *Circulation.* 1996;93:841-842.
5. Maron BJ, McKenna WJ, Danielson GK, et al.; Task Force on Clinical Expert Consensus Documents. American College of Cardiology; Committee for Practice Guidelines. European Society of Cardiology. American College of Cardiology/European Society of Cardiology clinical expert consensus document on hypertrophic cardiomyopathy. A report of the American College of Cardiology Foundation Task Force on Clinical Expert Consensus Documents and the European Society of Cardiology Committee for Practice Guidelines. *J Am Coll Cardiol.* 2003;42(9):1687-1713.
6. Maron BJ, Towbin JA, Thiene G, et al. Contemporary definitions and classification of the cardiomyopathies: an American Heart Association Scientific Statement from the Council on Clinical Cardiology, Heart Failure and Transplantation Committee; Quality of Care and Outcomes Research and Functional Genomics and Translational Biology Interdisciplinary Working Groups; and Council on Epidemiology and Prevention. *Circulation.* 2006;113(14): 1807-1816.
7. Elliott P, McKenna WJ. Hypertrophic cardiomyopathy. *Lancet.* 2004;363:1881-1891.
8. Morita H, Rehm HL, Menesses A, et al. Shared genetic causes of cardiac hypertrophy in children and adults. *N Engl J Med.* 2008;358(18):1899-1908.
9. Seidman JG, Seidman C. The genetic basis for cardiomyopathy: from mutation identification to mechanistic paradigms. *Cell.* 2001;104:557-567.
10. Richard P, Charron P, Carrier L, et al. Hypertrophic cardiomyopathy: distribution of disease genes, spectrum of mutations, and implications for a molecular diagnosis strategy. *Circulation.* 2003;107:2227-2232.

11. Sanbe A, Nelson D, Gulick J, et al. In vivo analysis of an essential myosin light chain mutation linked to familial hypertrofic cardiomyopathy. *Circ Res*. 2000;87:296-302.

12. Sachdev B, Takenaka T, Teraguchi H, et al. Prevalence of Anderson-Fabry disease in male patients with late onset hypertrophic cardiomyopathy. *Circulation*. 2002;105(12): 1407-1411.

13. DiMauro S, Schon EA. Mitochondrial respiratory-chain diseases. *N Engl J Med*. 2003; 348(26):2656-2668.

14. Blair E, Redwood C, Ashrafian H, et al. Mutations in the gamma(2) subunit of AMP-activated protein kinase cause familial hypertrophic cardiomyopathy: evidence for the central role of energy compromise in disease pathogenesis. *Hum Mol Genet*. 2001;10(11):1215-1220.

15. Arad M, Maron BJ, Gorham JM, et al. Glycogen storage diseases presenting as hypertrophic cardiomyopathy. *N Engl J Med*. 2005;352:362-372.

16. Geier C, Perrot A, Özcerlik C, et al. Mutations in the human muscle LIM protein gene in families with hypertrophic cardiomyopathy. *Circulation*. 2003;107:1390-1395.

17. Charron P, Villard E, Sébillon P, et al. Danon's disease as a cause of hypertrophic cardiomyopathy: a systematic survey. *Heart*. 2004;90(8):842-846.

18. Minamisawa S, Sato Y, Tatsuguchi Y, et al. Mutation of the phospholamban promoter associated with hypertrophic cardiomyopathy. *Biochem Biophys Res Commun*. 2003;304:1-4.

19. Raymen I, Holden HM, Sellers JR, et al. Structural interpretation of the mutations in the beta-cardiac myosin that have been implicated in familial hypertrophic cardiomyopathy. *Proc Natl Acad Sci USA*. 1995;92:3864-3868.

20. Raymen I, Holden HM, Whittaker M, et al. Structure of the actin-myosin complex and its implications for muscle contraction. *Science*. 1993;261:58-65.

21. Schiaffino S, Reggiani C. Molecular diversity of myofibrillar proteins: gene regulation and functional significance. *Physiol Rev*. 1996;76:371-396.

22. Marian AJ, Wu Y, Lim DS, et al. A transgenic rabbit model for human hypertrophic cardiomyopathy. *J Clin Invest*. 1999;104:1683-1692.

23. Geisterfer-Lowrance AA, Christe M, Conner DA, et al. A mouse model of familial hypertrophic cardiomyopathy. *Science*. 1996;272:731-734.

24. Yang Q, Sanbe A, Osinska H, Hewett TE, Klevitsky R, Robbins J. A mouse model of myosin binding protein C human familial hypertrophic cardiomyopathy. *J Clin Invest*. 1998; 102(7):1292-1300.

25. Oberst L, Zhao G, Park JT, Brugada R, et al. Dominant-negative effect of a mutant cardiac troponin T on cardiac structure and function in transgenic mice. *J Clin Invest*. 1998;102(8):1498-1505.

26. Tardiff JC, Factor SM, Tompkins BD, et al. A truncated cardiac troponin T molecule in transgenic mice suggests multiple cellular mechanisms for familial hypertrophic cardiomyopathy. *J Clin invest*. 1998;101:2800-2811.

27. Redwood CS, Moolman-Smook JC, Watkins H. Properties of mutant contractile proteins that cause hypertrophic cardiomyopathy. *Cardiovasc Res*. 1999;44(1):20-36.

28. Watkins H. Genetic clues to disease pathways in hypertrophic and dilated cardiomyopathies. *Circulation*. 2003;107(10):1344.

29. Gomes AV, Potter JD. Molecular and cellular aspects of troponin cardiomyopathies. *Ann N Y Acad Sci*. 2004;1015:214-224.

30. Knollmann BC, Kirchhof P, Sirenko SG, et al. Familial hypertrophic cardiomyopathy-linked mutant troponin T causes stress-induced ventricular tachycardia and Ca2+-dependent action potential remodeling. *Circ Res*. 2003;92(4):428-436.

31. Olsson MC, Palmer BM, Stauffer BL, et al. Morphological and functional alterations in ventricular myocytes from male transgenic mice with hypertrophic cardiomyopathy. *Circ Res*. 2004;94:201-207.

32. Harris SP, Bartley CR, Hacker TA, et al. Hypertrophic cardiomyopathy in çardiac myosin binding protein-C knockout mice. *Circ Res*. 2002;90:594-601.

33. Alpert NR, Mohiddin SA, Tripodi D, et al. Molecular and phenotypic effects of heterozygous, homozygous, and compound heterozygote myosin heavy-chain mutations. *Am J Physiol Heart Circ Physiol.* 2005;288(3):H1097-H1102.
34. Nagueh SF, Chen S, Patel R, et al. Evolution of expression of cardiac phenotypes over a 4-year period in the beta-myosin heavy chain-Q403 transgenic rabbit model of human hypertrophic cardiomyopathy. *J Mol Cell Cardiol.* 2004;36(5):663-673.
35. Doolan A, Tebo M, Ingles J, et al. Cardiac troponin I mutations in Australian families with hypertrophic cardiomyopathy: clinical, genetic and functional consequences. *J Mol Cell Cardiol.* 2005;38(2):387-393.
36. Schwartz K, Carrier L, Guicheney P, Komajda M. Molecular basis of familial cardiomyopathies. *Circulation.* 1995;91:532-540.
37. Gomes AV, Liang J, Potter JD. Mutations in human cardiac troponin I that are associated with restrictive cardiomyopathy affect basal ATPase activity and the calcium sensitivity of force development. *J Biol Chem.* 2005;280(35):30909-30915.
38. Gomes AV, Harada K. PotterJD. A mutation in the N-terminus of troponin I that is associated with hypertrophic cardiomyopathy affects tha Ca(2+)-sensitivity, phosphorilastion kinetics and proteolytic susceptibility of troponin. *J Mol Cell Cardiol.* 2005;39:754-765.
39. Gomes AV, Barnes JA, Harada K, Potter JD. Role of troponin T in disease. *Mol Cell Biochem.* 2004;263(1–2):115-129.
40. Gomes AV, Potter JD. Cellular and molecular aspects of familial hypertrophic cardiomyopathy caused by mutations in the cardiac troponin I gene. *Mol Cell Biochem.* 2004;263(1–2):99-114.
41. Redwood C, Lohmann K, Bing W, et al. Investigation of a truncated cardiac troponin T that causes familial hypertrophic cardiomyopathy: Ca(2+) regulatory properties of reconstituted thin filaments depend on the ratio of mutant to wild-type protein. *Circ Res.* 2000; 86(11):1146-1152.
42. Crilley JG, Boehm EA, Blair E, et al. Hypertrophic cardiomyopathy due to sarcomeric gene mutations is characterized by impaired energy metabolism irrespective of the degree of hypertrophy. *J Am Coll Cardiol.* 2003;41(10):1776-1782.
43. Marian AJ, Roberts R. The molecular genetic basis for hypetrophic cardiomyopathy. *J Mol Cell Cardiol.* 2001;33:655-670.
44. Murphy RT, Mogensen J, McGarry K, et al. Adenosine monophosphate-activated protein kinase disease mimicks hypertrophic cardiomyopathy and Wolff-Parkinson-White syndrome: natural history. *J Am Coll Cardiol.* 2005;45(6):922-930.
45. Ashrafian H, Redwood C, Blair E, et al. Hypertrophic cardiomyopathy: a paradigm for myocardial energy depletion. *Trends Genet.* 2003;19(5):263-268.
46. Kirschner SE, Becker E, Antognozzi M, et al. Hypertrophic cardiomyopathy-related β-myosin mutations cause highly varable calcium sensitivity with functional imbalances among individual muscle cells. *Am J Physiol Heart Circ Physiol.* 2005;288:H1242-H1251.
47. Pfeufer A, Osterziel KJ, Urata H, et al. Angiotensin-converting enzyme and heart chymase gene polymorphisms in hypertrophic cardiomyopathy. *Am J Cardiol.* 1996;78(3):362-364.
48. Yoneya K, Okamoto H, Machida M, et al. Angiotensin-converting enzyme gene polymorphism in Japanese patients with hypertrophic cardiomyopathy. *Am Heart J.* 1995; 130(5):1089-1093.
49. Lechin M, Quiñones MA, Omran A, et al. Angiotensin-I converting enzyme genotypes and left ventricular hypertrophy in patients with hypertrophic cardiomyopathy. *Circulation.* 1995; 92(7):1808-1812.
50. Tesson F, Dufour C, Moolman JC. The influence of the angiotensin I converting enzyme genotype in familial hypertrophic cardiomyopathy varies with the disease gene mutation. *J Mol Cell Cardiol.* 1997;29(2):831-838.
51. Richard P, Charron P, Leclercq C, et al. Homozygotes for a R869G mutation in the beta -myosin heavy chain gene have a severe form of familial hypertrophic cardiomyopathy. *J Mol Cell Cardiol.* 2000;32(8):1575-1583.

52. Maron BJ, Spirito P, Green KJ, Wesley YE, Bonow RO, Arce J. Noninvasive assessment of left ventricular diastolic function by pulsed Doppler echocardiography in patients with hypertrophic cardiomyopathy. *J Am Coll Cardiol.* 1987;10:733-742.

53. Chikamori T, Dickie S, Poloniecki JD, Myers MJ, Lavender JP, McKenna WJ. Prognostic significance of radionuclide-assessed diastolic dysfunction in hypertrophic cardiomyopathy. *Am J Cardiol.* 1990;65:478-482.

54. Bonow RO, Dilsizian V, Rosing DR, et al. Verapamil induced improvement in left ventricular filling and increased exercise tolerance in patients with hypertrophic cardiomyopathy. Short and long-term effects. *Circulation.* 1985;72:853-864.

55. Pak PH, Maughan L, Baughman KL, Kass DA. Marked discordance between dynamic and passive diastolic pressure volume relations in idiopathic hypertrophic cardiomyopathy. *Circulation.* 1996;94(1):52-60.

56. Glancy DL, O'Brien KP, Gold HK, Epstein SE. Atrial fibrillation in patients with idiopathic hypertrophic subaortic stenosis. *Br Heart J.* 1970;32(5):652-659.

57. Fassbach M, Schwartzkopff B. Elevated serum markers for collagen synthesis in patients with hypertrophic cardiomyopathy and diastolic dysfunction. *Z Kardiol.* 2005;94(5): 328-335.

58. Lombardi R, Betocchi S, Losi MA, et al. Myocardial collagen turnover in hypertrophic cardiomyopathy. *Circulation.* 2003;108(12):1455-1460.

59. Mundhenke M, Schwartzkopff B, Stark P, et al. Myocardial collagen type I and impaired left ventricular function under exercise in hypertrophic cardiomyopathy. *Thorac Cardiovasc Surg.* 2002;50(4):216-222.

60. Henry WL, Clarke CE, Epstein SE. Asymmetrical septal hypertrophy (ASH): Echocardiographic identification of the pathognomonic anatomic abnormality of IHSS. *Circulation.* 1973;42: 225-233.

61. Shah PM, Gramiak R, Kramer DH. Ultrasound localization of left ventricular outflow obstruction in hypertrophic obstructive cardiomyopathy. *Circulation.* 1969;40(1):3-11.

62. Popp RL, Harrison DC. Ultrasound in the diagnosis and evaluation of therapy of idiopathic hypertrophic subaortic stenosis. *Circulation.* 1969;40(6):905-914.

63. Maron BJ, Gottdiener JS, Epstein SE. Patterns and significance of distribution of left ventricular hypertrophy in hypertrophic cardiomyopathy. A wide angle, two dimensional echocardiographic study of 125 patients. *Am J Cardiol.* 1981;48(3):418-428.

64. Mogensen J, Kubo T, Duque M, et al. Idiopathic restrictive cardiomyopathy is part of the clinical expression of cardiac troponin I mutations. *J Clin Invest.* 2003;111(2):209-216.

65. Betocchi S, Bonow RO, Bacharach SL, et al. Isovolumic relaxation period in hypertrophic cardiomyopathy: assessment by radionuclide angiography. *J Am Coll Cardiol.* 1986;7(1): 74-81.

66. Bonow RO, Frederick TM, Bacharach SL, et al. Atrial systole and left ventricular filling in hypertrophic cardiomyopathy: effect of verapamil. *Am J Cardiol.* 1983;51(8):1386-1391.

67. Betocchi S, Hess OM. LV hypertrophy and diastolic heart failure. *Heart Fail Rev.* 2000; 5(4):333-336.

68. Ito T, Suwa M, Imai M, Nakamura T, Kitaura Y. Assessment of regional left ventricular filling dynamics using color kinesis in patients with hypertrophic cardiomyopathy. *J Am Soc Echocardiogr.* 2004;17(2):146-151.

69. McKenna WJ, Stewart JT, Nihoyannopoulos P, et al. Hypertrophic cardiomyopathy without hypertrophy: two families with myocardial disarray in the absence of increased myocardial mass. *Br Heart J.* 1990;63(5):287-290.

70. Waller BF, Maron BJ, Morrow AG, et al. Hypertrophic cardiomyopathy mimicking pericardial constriction or myocardial restriction. *Am Heart J.* 1981;102(4):790-792.

71. Thaman R, Gimeno JR, Murphy RT, et al. Prevalence and clinical significance of systolic impairment in hypertrophic cardiomyopathy. *Heart.* 2005;91:920-925.

72. Thaman R, Gimeno JR, Reith S, et al. Progressive left ventricular remodeling in patients with hypertrophic cardiomyopathy and severe left ventricular hypertrophy. *J Am Coll Cardiol.* 2004;44:398-405.

73. Sengupta PP, Mehta V, Arora R, et al. Quantification of regional nonuniformity and paradoxical intramural mechanics in hypertrophic cardiomyopathy by high frame rate ultrasound myocardial strain mapping. *J Am Soc Echocardiogr.* 2005;18(7):737-742.

74. Tabata T, Oki T, Yamada H, et al. Subendocardial motion in hypertrophic cardiomyopathy: assessment from long- and short-axis views by pulsed tissue Doppler imaging. *J Am Soc Echocardiogr.* 2000;13(2):108-115.

75. Yamada H, Oki T, Tabata T, et al. Assessment of left ventricular systolic wall motion velocity with pulsed tissue Doppler imaging: comparison with peak dP/dt of the left ventricular pressure curve. *J Am Soc Echocardiogr.* 1998;11(5):442-449.

76. Matsumura Y, Elliott PM, Virdee MS, et al. Left ventricular diastolic function assessed using Doppler tissue imaging in patients with hypertrophic cardiomyopathy: relation to symptoms and exercise capacity. *Heart.* 2002;87(3):247-251.

77. Nagueh SF, Bachinski LL, Meyer D, et al. Tissue Doppler imaging consistently detects myocardial abnormalities in patients with hypertrophic cardiomyopathy and provides a novel means for an early diagnosis before and independently of hypertrophy. *Circulation.* 2001; 104(2):128-130.

78. Losi MA, Betocchi S, Aversa M, et al. Dobutamine stress echocardiography in hypertrophic cardiomyopathy. *Cardiology.* 2003;100(2):93-100.

79. Okeie K, Shimizu M, Yoshio H, et al. Left ventricular systolic dysfunction during exercise and dobutamine stress in patients with hypertrophic cardiomyopathy. *J Am Coll Cardiol.* 2000; 36(3):856-863.

80. Kawano S, Iida K, Fujieda K, et al. Response to isoproterenol as a prognostic indicator of evolution from hypertrophic cardiomyopathy to a phase resembling dilated cardiomyopathy. *J Am Coll Cardiol.* 1995;25(3):687-692.

81. Briguori C, Betocchi S, Manganelli F, et al. Determinants and clinical significance of natriuretic peptides and hypertrophic cardiomyopathy. *Eur Heart J.* 2001;22(15):1328-1336.

82. Maron BJ, Tholakanahalli VN, Zenovich AG, et al. Usefulness of B-type natriuretic peptide assay in the assessment of symptomatic state in hypertrophic cardiomyopathy. *Circulation.* 2004;109(8):984-989.

83. Noji Y, Shimizu M, Ino H, Higashikata T, et al. Increased circulating matrix metalloproteinase-2 in patients with hypertrophic cardiomyopathy with systolic dysfunction. *Circ J.* 2004;68(4):355-360.

84. Zen K, Irie H, Doue T, Takamiya M, et al. Analysis of circulating apoptosis mediators and proinflammatory cytokines in patients with idiopathic hypertrophic cardiomyopathy: comparison between nonobstructive and dilated-phase hypertrophic cardiomyopathy. *Int Heart J.* 2005;46(2):231-244.

85. Högye M, Mándi Y, Csanády M, Sepp R, Buzás K. Comparison of circulating levels of interleukin-6 and tumor necrosis factor-alpha in hypertrophic cardiomyopathy and in idiopathic dilated cardiomyopathy. *Am J Cardiol.* 2004;94(2):249-251.

86. Maron BJ, Olivotto I, Spirito P, et al. Epidemiology of hypertrophic cardiomyopathy-related death: revisited in a large non-referral-based patient population. *Circulation.* 2000;102(8): 858-864.

87. Ikeda H, Maki S, Yoshida N, et al. Predictors of death from congestive heart failure in hypertrophic cardiomyopathy. *Am J Cardiol.* 1999;83(8):1280-1283, A9.

88. Frank S, Braunwald E. Idiopathic hypertrophic subaortic stenosis. Clinical analysis of 126 patients with emphasis on the natural history. *Circulation.* 1968;37(5):759-788.

89. Goodwin JF, Hollman A, Cleland WP, Teare D. Obstructive cardiomyopathy simulating aortic stenosis. *Br Heart J.* 1960;22:403-414.

90. Wigle ED, Heimbecker RO, Gunton RW. Idiopathic ventricular septal hypertrophy causing muscular subaortic stenosis. *Circulation*. 1962;26:325-340.
91. Wigle ED, Sasson Z, Henderson MA, et al. Hypertrophic cardiomyopathy. The importance of the site and the extent of hypertrophy. A review. *Prog Cardiovasc Dis*. 1985;28:1-83.
92. Maron BJ, Nishimura RA, Danielson GK. Pitfalls in clinical recognition and a novel operative approach for hypertrophic cardiomyopathy with severe outflow obstruction due to anomalous papillary muscle. *Circulation*. 1998;98:2505-2508.
93. Klues HG, Roberts WC, Maron BJ. Anomalous insertion of papillary muscle directly into anterior mitral leaflet in hypertrophic cardiomyopathy. Significance in producing left ventricular outflow obstruction. *Circulation*. 1991;84:1188-1197.
94. Davies MJ, McKenna WJ. Hypertrophic cardiomyopathy: pathology and pathogenesis. *Histopathology*. 1995;26:493-500.
95. Shapiro LM, McKenna WJ. Distribution of left ventricular hypertrophy in hypertrophic cardiomyopathy: a two-dimensional echocardiographic study. *J Am Coll Cardiol*. 1983; 2:437-444.
96. Delling FN, Sanborn DY, Levine RA, et al. Frequency and mechanism of persistent systolic anterior motion and mitral regurgitation after septal ablation in obstructive hypertrophic cardiomyopathy. *Am J Cardiol*. 2007;100(11):1691-1695.
97. He S, Hopmeyer J, Lefebvre XP, Schwammenthal E, Yoganathan AP, Levine RA. Importance of leaflet elongation in causing systolic anterior motion of the mitral valve. *J Heart Valve Dis*. 1997;6(2):149-159.
98. Levine RA, Vlahakes GJ, Lefebvre X, et al. Papillary muscle displacement causes systolic anterior motion of the mitral valve. Experimental validation and insights into the mechanism of subaortic obstruction. *Circulation*. 1995;91(4):1189-1195.
99. Maron BJ, Harding AM, Spirito P, et al. Systolic anterior motion of the posterior mitral leaflet: a previously unrecognized cause of dynamic subaortic obstruction in patients with hypertrophic cardiomyopathy. *Circulation*. 1983;68(2):282-293.
100. Spirito P, Maron BJ. Patterns of systolic anterior motion of the mitral valve in hypertrophic cardiomyopathy: assessment by two-dimensional echocardiography. *Am J Cardiol*. 1984; 54(8):1039-1046.
101. Spirito P, Maron BJ. Significance of left ventricular outflow tract cross-sectional area in hypertrophic cardiomyopathy: a two-dimensional echocardiographic assessment. *Circulation*. 1983;67(5):1100-1108.
102. Reis RL, Bolton MR, King JF, et al. Anterion-superior displacement of papillary muscles producing obstruction and mitral regurgitation in idiopathic hypertrophic subaortic stenosis. Operative relief by posterior-superior realignment of papillary muscles following ventricular septal myectomy. *Circulation*. 1974;50(2 suppl):II181-II188.
103. Klues HG, Roberts WC, Maron BJ. Morphological determinants of echocardiographic patterns of mitral valve systolic anterior motion in obstructive hypertrophic cardiomyopathy. *Circulation*. 1993;87(5):1570-1579.
104. Klues HG, Proschan MA, Dollar AL, et al. Echocardiographic assessment of mitral valve size in obstructive hypertrophic cardiomyopathy. Anatomic validation from mitral valve specimen. *Circulation*. 1993;88(2):548-555.
105. Cannon RO, Dilsizian V, O'Gara PT, et al. Myocardial metabolic, hemodynamic, and electrocardiographic significance of reversible thallium-201 abnormalities in hypertrophic cardiomyopathy. *Circulation*. 1991;83(5):1660-1667.
106. Pasternac A, Noble J, Streulens Y, et al. Pathophysiology of chest pain in patients with cardiomyopathies and normal coronary arteries. *Circulation*. 1982;65(4):778-789.
107. Camici P, Chiriatti G, Lorenzoni R, et al. Coronary vasodilation is impaired in both hypertrophied and nonhypertrophied myocardium of patients with hypertrophic cardiomyopathy: a study with nitrogen-13 ammonia and positron emission tomography. *J Am Coll Cardiol*. 1991; 17(4):879-886.

108. Elliott PM, Rosano GM, Gill JS, et al. Changes in coronary sinus pH during dipyridamole stress in patients with hypertrophic cardiomyopathy. *Heart*. 1996;75(2):179-183.

109. Cannon RO III, Rosing DR, Maron BJ, et al. Myocardial ischemia in patients with hypertrophic cardiomyopathy: contribution of inadequate vasodilator reserve and elevated left ventricular filling pressures. *Circulation*. 1985;71(2):234-243.

110. Morioka N, Shigematsu Y, Hamada M, Higaki J. Circulating levels of heart-type fatty acid-binding protein and its relation to thallium-201 perfusion defects in patients with hypertrophic cardiomyopathy. *Am J Cardiol*. 2005;95(11):1334-1337.

111. Elliott PM, Kaski JC, Prasad K, et al. Chest pain during daily life in patients with hypertrophic cardiomyopathy: an ambulatory electrocardiographic study. *Eur Heart J*. 1996;17(7): 1056-1064.

112. Cecchi F, Olivotto I, Gistri R, et al. Coronary microvascular dysfunction and prognosis in hypertrophic cardiomyopathy. *N Engl J Med*. 2003;349(11):1027-1035.

113. Shimizu M, Ino H, Okeie K, et al. Exercise-induced ST-segment depression and systolic dysfunction in patients with nonobstructive hypertrophic cardiomyopathy. *Am Heart J*. 2000;140(1):52-60.

114. Dilsizian V, Bonow RO, Epstein SE, Fananapazir L. Myocardial ischemia detected by thallium scintigraphy is frequently related to cardiac arrest and syncope in young patients with hypertrophic cardiomyopathy. *J Am Coll Cardiol*. 1993;22(3):796-804.

115. Lipshultz SE, Sleeper LA, Towbin JA, et al. The incidence of pediatric cardiomyopathy in two regions of the United States. *N Engl J Med*. 2003;348(17):1647-1655.

116. Nugent AW, Daubeney PE, Chondros P, et al; National Australian Childhood Cardiomyopathy Study. The epidemiology of childhood cardiomyopathy in Australia. *N Engl J Med*. 2003; 348(17):1639-1646.

117. Maron BJ. Hypertrophic cardiomyopathy in childhood. *Pediatr Clin North Am*. 2004;51(5): 1305-1346.

118. Maron BJ, Spirito P, Wesley Y, Arce J. Development and progression of left ventricular hypertrophy in children with hypertrophic cardiomyopathy. *N Engl J Med*. 1986;315(10): 610-614.

119. Topol EJ, Traill TA, Fortuin NJ. Hypertensive hypertrophic cardiomyopathy of the elderly. *N Engl J Med*. 1985;312(5):277-283.

120. Chikamori T, Doi YL, Yonezawa Y, Dickie S, Ozawa T, McKenna WJ. Comparison of clinical features in patients greater than or equal to 60 years of age to those less than or equal to 40 years of age with hypertrophic cardiomyopathy. *Am J Cardiol*. 1990;66(10):875-878.

121. Maron BJ, Schiffers A, Klues HG. Comparison of phenotypic expression of hypertrophic cardiomyopathy in patients from the United States and Germany. *Am J Cardiol*. 1999;83(4):626-627, A10.

122. Fay WP, Taliercio CP, Ilstrup DM, et al. Natural history of hypertrophic cardiomyopathy in the elderly. *J Am Coll Cardiol*. 1990;16(4):821-826.

123. Gilligan DM, Chan WL, Ang EL, Oakley CM. Effects of a meal on hemodynamic function at rest and during exercise in patients with hypertrophic cardiomyopathy. *J Am Coll Cardiol*. 1991;18:429-436.

124. Lewis JF, Maron BJ. Clinical and morphologic expression of hypertrophic cardiomyopathy in patients > or = 65 years of age. *Am J Cardiol*. 1994;73(15):1105-1111.

125. McKenna WJ, Franklin RCG, Nihoyannopoulos P, et al. Arrhythmia and prognosis in infants, children and adolescents with hypertrophic cardiomyopathy. *J Am Coll Cardiol*. 1988;11: 147-153.

126. Maron BJ, Casey SA, Poliac LC, Gohman TE, Almquist AK, Aeppli DM. Clinical course of hypertrophic cardiomyopathy in a regional United States cohort. *JAMA*. 1999;281(7): 650-655.

127. Spirito P, Chiarella F, Carratino L, et al. Clinical course and prognosis of hypertrophic cardiomyopathy in an outpatient population. *N Engl J Med*. 1989;320(12):749-755.

128. Prasad K, Williams L, Campbell R, Elliott PM, McKenna WJ, Frenneaux M. Episodic syncope in hypertrophic cardiomyopathy: evidence for inappropriate vasodilation. *Heart.* 2008; 94(10):1312-1317.

129. Paz R, Jortner R, Tunick PA, et al. The effect of the ingestion of ethanol on obstruction of the left ventricular outflow tract in hypertrophic cardiomyopathy. *N Engl J Med.* 1996;335: 938-941.

130. Savage DD, Seides SF, Clark CE, et al. Electrocardiographic findings in patients with obstructive and non-obstructive hypertrophic cardiomyopathy. *Circulation.* 1978;58: 402-409.

131. Maron BJ, Wolfson JK, Ciro E, Spirito P. Relation of electrocardiographic abnormalities and patterns of left ventricular hypertrophy identified by 2-dimensional echocardiography in patients with hypertrophic cardiomyopathy. *Am J Cardiol.* 1983;51:189-194.

132. Lemery R, Kleinebenne A, Nihoyannopoulos P, Alfonso F, McKenna WJ. Q-waves in hypertrophic cardiomyopathy in relation to the distribution and severity of right and left ventricular hypertrophy. *J Am Coll Cardiol.* 1990;16:368-374.

133. Fananapazir L, Tracey CM, Leon MB, et al. Electrophysiological abnormalities in patients with hypertrophic cardiomyopathy: a consecutive analysis in 155 patients. *Circulation.* 1989; 80:1259.

134. Yamaguchi H, Ishimura T, Nishiyama S, et al. Hypertrophic nonobstructive cardiomyopathy with giant negative T-waves (apical hypertrophy): ventriculographic and echocardiographic features in 30 patients. *Am J Cardiol.* 1979;44:401-412.

135. Krikler DM, Davies MJ, Rowland E, Goodwin JF, Evans RC, Shaw DB. Sudden death in hypertrophic cardiomyopathy: associated accessory atrioventricular pathways. *Br Heart J.* 1980;43:245-251.

136. Adabag AS, Casey SA, Kuskowski MA, et al. Spectrum and prognostic significance of arrhythmias on ambulatory Holter electrocardiogram in hypertrophic cardiomyopathy. *J Am Coll Cardiol.* 2005;45(5):697-704.

137. McKenna WJ, England D, Doi Y, Deanfield JE, Oakley CM, Goodwin JF. Arrhythmia in hypertrophic cardiomyopathy. 1. Influence on prognosis. *Br Heart J.* 1981;46:168-172.

138. Maron BJ, Savage DD, Wolfson JK, Epstein SE. Prognostic significance of 24 hour ambulatory electrocardiographic monitoring in patients with hypertrophic cardiomyopathy: a prospective study. *Am J Cardiol.* 1981;48:252-257.

139. Robinson K, Frenneaux MP, Stockins B, Karatasakis G, Poloniecki J, McKenna WJ. Atrial fibrillation in hypertrophic cardiomyopathy: a longitudinal study. *J Am Coll Cardiol.* 1990; 15:1279-1285.

140. Alfonso F, Frenneaux MP, McKenna WJ. Clinical sustained uniform ventricular tachycardia in hypertrophic cardiomyopathy: association with left ventricular apical aneurysm. *Br Heart J.* 1989;61:178-181.

141. Losi MA, Betocchi S, Aversa M, et al. Determinants of atrial fibrillation development in patients with hypertrophic cardiomyopathy. *Am J Cardiol.* 2004;94(7):895-900.

142. Topol EJ, Califf RM, Prystowsky EN, et al. *Textbook of Cardiovascular Medicine.* 3rd ed. Philadelphia: Lippincott Williams & Wilkins; 2007 [chapter 29].

143. Klues HG, Schiffers A, Maron BJ. Phenotypic spectrum and patterns of left ventricular hypertrophy in hypertrophic cardiomyopathy: morphologic observations and significance as assessed by two-dimensional echocardiography in 600 patients. *J Am Coll Cardiol.* 1995;26: 1699-1708.

144. Doi YL, McKenna WJ, Gehrke J, et al. M mode echocardiography in hypertrophic cardiomyopathy: diagnostic criteria and prediction of obstruction. *Am J Cardiol.* 1980;45(1):6-14.

145. Spirito P, Bellone P, Harris KM, Bernabo P, Bruzzi P, Maron BJ. Magnitude of left ventricular hypertrophy and risk of sudden death in hypertrophic cardiomyopathy. *N Engl J Med.* 2000;342(24):1778-1785.

146. Spirito P, Maron BJ. Relation between extent of left ventricular hypertrophy and age in hypertrophic cardiomyopathy. *J Am Coll Cardiol.* 1989;13(4):820-823.

147. Panza JA, Petrone RK, Fananapazir L, Maron BJ. Utility of continuous wave Doppler echocardiography in the non-invasive assessment of left ventricular outflow tract pressure gradient in patients with hypertrophic cardiomyopathy. *J Am Coll Cardiol.* 1991; 19:91-99.

148. Nishimura RS, Appleton CP, Redfield MM, et al. Nonivasive Doppler echocardiographic evaluation of left ventricular filling pressures in patients with cardiomyopathies: a simultaneous Doppler echocardiographic and cardiac catheterization study. *J Am Coll Cardiol.* 1996;28:1226-1233.

149. Spirito P, Maron BJ, Bonow RO, Epstein SE. Occurrence and significance of progressive left ventricular wall thinning and relative cavity dilatation in hypertrophic cardiomyopathy. *Am J Cardiol.* 1987;60:123-139.

150. Sharma S, Elliott P, Whyte G, et al. Utility of cardiopulmonary exercise in the assessment of clinical determinants of functional capacity in hypertrophic cardiomyopathy. *Am J Cardiol.* 2000;86:162-168.

151. Jones S, Elliott PM, Sharma S, McKenna WJ, Whipp BJ. Cardiopulmonary responses to exercise in patients with hypertrophic cardiomyopathy. *Heart.* 1998;80:60-67.

152. Sadoul N, Prasad K, Elliott PM, Banerjee S, Frenneaux MP, McKenna WJ. Prospective prognostic assessment of blood pressure response during exercise in patients with hypertrophic cardiomyopathy. *Circulation.* 1997;96:2987-2991.

153. Maki S, Ikeda H, Muro A, et al. Predictors of sudden cardiac death in hypertrophic cardiomyopathy. *Am J Cardiol.* 1998;82:774-778.

154. Olivotto I, Maron BJ, Montereggi A, et al. Prognostic value of systemic blood pressure response during exercise in a community based population with hypertrophic cardiomyopathy. *J Am Coll Cardiol.* 1999;33:2044-2051.

155. Counihan PJ, Frenneaux MP, Webb DJ, McKenna WJ. Abnormal vascular responses to supine exercise in hypertrophic cardiomyopathy. *Circulation.* 1991;84:686-696.

156. Ciampi Q, Betocchi S, Lombardi R, et al. Hemodynamicv determinants of exercise-induced abnormal blood pressure response in hypertrophic cardiomyopathy. *J Am Coll Cardiol.* 2002;40:278-284.

157. Moon JCC, McKenna WJ, McCrohon JA, et al. Towards clinical risk assessment in hypertrophic cardiomyopathy with gadolinium cardiovascular magnetic resonance. *J Am Coll Cardiol.* 2003;41:1561-1567.

158. Choudhury L, Mahrholdt H, Wagner A, et al. Myocardial scarring in asymptomatic or mildly symptomatic patients with hypertrophic cardiomyopathy. *J Am Coll Cardiol.* 2002;53: 121-123.

159. Moon JC, Reed E, Sheppard MN, et al. The histologic basis of late gadolinium enhancement cardiovascular magnetic resonance in hypertrophic cardiomyopathy. *J Am Coll Cardiol.* 2004;43(12):2260-2264.

160. Amano Y, Takayama M, Takahama K, et al. Delayed hyper-enhancement of myocardium in hypertrophic cardiomyopathy with asymmetrical septal hypertrophy: comparison with global and regional cardiac MR imaging appearances. *J Magn Reson Imaging.* 2004;20(4):595-600.

161. Moon JC, Mogensen J, Elliott PM, et al. Myocardial late gadolinium enhancement cardiovascular magnetic resonance in hypertrophic cardiomyopathy caused by mutations in troponin I. *Heart.* 2005;91(8):1036-1040.

162. Teraoka K, Hirano M, Ookubo H, et al. Delayed contrast enhancement of MRI in hypertrophic cardiomyopathy. *Magn Reson Imaging.* 2004;22(2):155-161.

163. Sipola P, Lauerma K, Jääskeläinen P, et al. Cine MR imaging of myocardial contractile impairment in patients with hypertrophic cardiomyopathy attributable to Asp175Asn mutation in the alpha-tropomyosin gene. *Radiology.* 2005;236(3):815-824.

164. Spirito P, Seidman CE, McKenna WJ, Maron BJ. The management of hypertrophic cardio-myopathy. *N Engl J Med*. 1997;336:775-785.
165. Maron BJ. Hypertrophic cardiomyopathy. A systematic review. *JAMA*. 2002;287:1308-1320.
166. Cohen LS, Braunwald E. Amelioration of angina pectoris in idiopathic hypertrophic subaortic stenosis with beta-adrenergic blockade. *Circulation*. 1967;35(5):847-851.
167. Wigle ED, Rakowski H, Kimball BP, Williams WG. Hypertrophic cardiomyopathy. Clinical spectrum and treatment. *Circulation*. 1995;92(7):1680-1692.
168. Gilligan DM, Chan WL, Joshi J, et al. A double-blind, placebo-controlled crossover trial of nadolol and verapamil in mild and moderately symptomatic hypertrophic cardiomyopathy. *J Am Coll Cardiol*. 1993;21(7):1672-1679.
169. Sherrid MV, Pearle G, Gunsburg DZ. Mechanism of benefit of negative inotropes in obstructive hypertrophic cardiomyopathy. *Circulation*. 1998;97(1):41-47.
170. Ostman-Smith I, Wettrell G, Riesenfeld T. A cohort study of childhood hypertrophic cardio-myopathy: improved survival following high-dose beta-adrenoceptor antagonist treatment. *J Am Coll Cardiol*. 1999;34(6):1813-1822.
171. Kaltenbach M, Hopf R, Kober G, Bussmann WD, Keller M, Petersen Y. Treatment of hyper-trophic obstructive cardiomyopathy with verapamil. *Br Heart J*. 1979;42(1):35-42.
172. Rosing DR, Kent KM, Maron BJ, et al. Verapamil therapy: a new approach to the pharmaco-logic treatment of hypertrophic cardiomyopathy. II. Effects on exercise capacity and symp-tomatic status. *Circulation*. 1979;60(6):1208-1213.
173. Bonow RO, Rosing DR, Bacharach SL, et al. Effects of verapamil on left ventricular systolic function and diastolic filling in patients with hypertrophic cardiomyopathy. *Circulation*. 1981;64(4):787-796.
174. Spicer RL, Rocchini AP, Crowley DC, Rosenthal A. Chronic verapamil therapy in pediatric and young adult patients with hypertrophic cardiomyopathy. *Am J Cardiol*. 1984;53(11): 1614-1619.
175. Udelson JE, Bonow RO, O'Gara PT, et al. Verapamil prevents silent myocardial perfusion abnormalities during exercise in asymptomatic patients with hypertrophic cardiomyopathy. *Circulation*. 1989;79(5):1052-1060.
176. Gistri R, Cecchi F, Choudhury L, et al. Effect of verapamil on absolute myocardial blood flow in hypertrophic cardiomyopathy. *Am J Cardiol*. 1994;74(4):363-368.
177. Iwase M, Sotobata I, Takagi S, et al. Effects of diltiazem on left ventricular diastolic behavior in patients with hypertrophic cardiomyopathy: evaluation with exercise pulsed Doppler echocardiography. *J Am Coll Cardiol*. 1987;9(5):1099-1105.
178. Pollick C. Muscular subaortic stenosis: hemodynamic and clinical improvement after disopy-ramide. *N Engl J Med*. 1982;307:997-999.
179. Pollick C, Kimball B, Henderson M, Wigle ED. Disopyramide in hypertrophic cardiomyopa-thy. I. Hemodynamic assessment after intravenous administration. *Am J Cardiol*. 1988;62: 1248-1251.
180. Matsubara H, Nakatani S, Nagata S, et al. Salutary effect of disopyramide on left ventricular diastolic function in hypertrophic obstructive cardiomyopathy. *J Am Coll Cardiol*. 1995;26: 768-775.
181. Sherrid MV, Barac I, McKenna WJ, et al. Multicenter study of the efficacy and safety of disopyramide in obstructive hypertrophic cardiomyopathy. *J Am Coll Cardiol*. 2005;45(8): 1251-1258.
182. Schulte HD, Bircks WH, Loesse B, Godehardt EA, Schwartzkopff B. Prognosis of patients with hypetrophic cardiomyopathy after transaortic myectomy. Late results up to twenty five years. *J Thorac Cardiovasc Surg*. 1993;106:709-717.
183. Morrow AG, Reitz BA, Epstein SE, et al. Operative treatment in hypertrophic subaortic steno-sis: techniques and the results of pre and post-operative assessments in 83 patients. *Circulation*. 1975;52:88-102.

184. Maron BJ, Epstein SE, Morrow AG. Symptomatic status and prognosis of patients after operation for hypertrophic cardiomyopathy: efficacy of ventricular septal myotomy/myectomy. *Eur Heart J.* 1983;4(suppl F):175-180.
185. Williams WG, Wigle ED, Rakowski H, Smallhorn J, LeBlanc J, Trusler GA. Results of surgery for hypertrophic obstructive cardiomyopathy. *Circulation.* 1987;76:V104-V108.
186. Schoendube FA, Klues HG, Reith S, Flachskampf FA, Hanrath P, Messmer BJ. Long-term clinical and echocardiographic follow-up after surgical correction of hypertrophic obstructive cardiomyopathy with extended myectomy and reconstruction of the subvalvular mitral apparatus. *Circulation.* 1995;92:II122-II127.
187. Lakkis NM, Nagueh SF, Dunn JK, Killip D, Spencer WH III. Nonsurgical septal reduction therapy for hypertrophic obstructive cardiomyopathy: one-year follow-up. *J Am Coll Cardiol.* 2000;36:852-855.
188. Faber L, Meissner A, Ziemssen P, Seggewiss H. Percutaneous transluminal septal myocardial ablation for hypertrophic obstructive cardiomyopathy: long term follow up of the first series of 25 patients. *Heart.* 2000;83:326-331.
189. Faber L, Seggewiss H, Gleichmann U. Percutaneous transluminal septal myocardial ablation in hypertrophic obstructive cardiomyopathy: results with respect to intraprocedural myocardial contrast echocardiography. *Circulation.* 1998;98:2415-2421.
190. Gietzen FH, Leuner CJ, Raute-Kreinsen U, et al. Acute and long-term results after transcoronary ablation of septal hypertrophy (TASH). Catheter interventional treatment for hypertrophic obstructive cardiomyopathy. *Eur Heart J.* 1999;20:1342-1354.
191. Knight C, Kurbaan AS, Seggewiss H, et al. Nonsurgical septal reduction for hypertrophic obstructive cardiomyopathy: outcome in the first series of patients. *Circulation.* 1997;95:2075-2081.
192. Seggewiss H, Gleichmann U, Faber L, Fassbender D, Schmidt HK, Strick S. Percutaneous transluminal septal myocardial ablation in hypertrophic obstructive cardiomyopathy: acute results and 3-month follow-up in 25 patients. *J Am Coll Cardiol.* 1998;31:252-258.
193. Mazur W, Nagueh SF, Lakkis NM, et al. Regression of left ventricular hypertrophy after nonsurgical septal reduction therapy for hypertrophic cardiomyopathy. *Circulation.* 2001;103:1492-1496.
194. Nagueh SF, Ommen SR, Lakkis NM, et al. Comparison of ethanol septal reduction therapy with surgical myectomy for the treatment of hypertrophic obstructive cardiomyopathy. *J Am Coll Cardiol.* 2001;38:1701-1706.
195. Qin JX, Shiota T, Lever HM, et al. Outcome of patients with hypertrophic obstructive cardiomyopathy after percutaneous transluminal septal myocardial ablation and septal myectomy surgery. *J Am Coll Cardiol.* 2001;38:1994-2000.
196. Firoozi S, Elliott P, Sharma S, et al. Septal myotomy-myectomy and transcoronary septal alcohol ablation in hypertrophic obstructive cardiomyopathy. A comparison of clinical, haemodynamic and exercise outcomes. *Eur Heart J.* 2002;23:1617.
197. Gietzen FH, Leuner CJ, Obergassel L, et al. Transcoronary ablation of septal hypertrophy for hypertrophic obstructive cardiomyopathy: feasibility, clinical benefit, and short term results in elderly patients. *Heart.* 2004;90(6):638-644.
198. Fernandes VL, Nagueh SF, Wang W, et al. A prospective follow-up of alcohol septal ablation for symptomatic hypertrophic obstructive cardiomyopathy–the Baylor experience (1996–2002). *Clin Cardiol.* 2005;28(3):124-130.
199. Chang SM, Lakkis NM, Franklin J, et al. Predictors of outcome after alcohol septal ablation therapy in patients with hypertrophic obstructive cardiomyopathy. *Circulation.* 2004;109(7):824-827.
200. Ralph-Edwards A, Woo A, McCrindle BW, et al. Hypertrophic obstructive cardiomyopathy: comparison of outcomes after myectomy or alcohol ablation adjusted by propensity score. *J Thorac Cardiovasc Surg.* 2005;129(2):351-358.

201. Talreja DR, Nishimura RA, Edwards WD, et al. Alcohol septal ablation versus surgical septal myectomy: comparison of effects on atrioventricular conduction tissue. *J Am Coll Cardiol.* 2004;44(12):2329-2332.

202. Jeanrenaud X, Goy JJ, Kappenberger L. Effects of dual-chamber pacing in hypertrophic obstructive cardiomyopathy. *Lancet.* 1992;339:1318-1323.

203. Nishimura RA, Trusty JM, Hayes DL, et al. Dual chamber pacing for hypertrophic cardiomyopathy: a randomised double-blind crossover trial. *J Am Coll Cardiol.* 1997; 29:435-441.

204. Kappenberger L, Linde C, Daubert C, et al. Pacing in hypertrophic obstructive cardiomyopathy. A randomized crossover study. PIC Study Group. *Eur Heart J.* 1997;18:1249-1256.

205. Gadler F, Linde C, Daubert C, et al. Significant improvement of quality of life following atrioventricular synchronous pacing in patients with hypertrophic obstructive cardiomyopathy. Data from 1 year of follow-up. PIC study group. Pacing in cardiomyopathy. *Eur Heart J.* 1999;20:1044-1050.

206. Maron BJ, Nishimura RA, McKenna WJ, Rakowski H, Josephson ME, Kieval RS. Assessment of permanent dual-chamber pacing as a treatment for drug-refractory symptomatic patients with obstructive hypertrophic cardiomyopathy. A randomized, double-blind, crossover study (M-PATHY). *Circulation.* 1999;99:2927-2933.

207. Betocchi S, Elliott PM, Briguori C, et al. Dual chamber pacing in hypertrophic cardiomyopathy: long-term effects on diastolic function. *Pacing Clin Electrophysiol.* 2002;25:1433-1440.

208. Fananapazir L, Epstein ND, Curiel RV, et al. Long-term results of dual-chamber (DDD) pacing in obstructive hypertrophic cardiomyopathy. Evidence for progressive symptomatic and hemodynamic improvement and reduction of left ventricular hypertrophy. *Circulation.* 1994;90(6):2731-2742.

209. Megevand A, Ingles J, Richmond DR, et al. Long-term follow-up of patients with obstructive hypertrophic cardiomyopathy treated with dual-chamber pacing. *Am J Cardiol.* 2005; 95(8):991-993.

210. Ruzyłło W, Chojnowska L, Demkow M, et al. Left ventricular outflow tract gradient decrease with non-surgical myocardial reduction improves exercise capacity in patients with hypertrophic obstructive cardiomyopathy. *Eur Heart J.* 2000;21(9):770-777.

211. Biagini E et al. Dilated-hypokinetic evolution of hypertrophic cardiomyopathy: prevalence, incidence, risk factors, and prognostic implications in pediatric and adult patients. *J Am Coll Cardiol.* 2005;46:1543-1550.

212. Shirani J, Pick R, Roberts WC, Maron BJ. Morphology and significance of the left ventricular collagen network in young patients with hypertrophic cardiomyopathy and sudden cardiac death. *J Am Coll Cardiol.* 2000;35:36-44.

213. Chien KR. Genotype, phenotype: upstairs, downstairs in the family of cardiomyopathies. *J Clin Invest.* 2003;111:175-178.

214. Maron BJ, Shen W-K, Link MS, et al. Efficacy of implantable cardioverter defibrillators for the prevention of sudden death in patients with hypertrophic cardiomyopathy. *N Engl J Med.* 2000;342:365-373.

215. Maron BJ, Estes NAM III, Maron MS, Almquist AK, Link MS, Udelson JE. Primary prevention of sudden death as a novel treatment strategy in hypertrophic cardiomyopathy. *Circulation.* 2003;107:2872-2875.

216. Elliott PM, Poloniecki J, Dickie S, et al. Sudden death in hypertrophic cardiomyopathy: identification of high risk patients. *J Am Coll Cardiol.* 2000;36:2212-2218.

217. Rogers DP, Marazia S, Chow AW, Lambiase PD, et al. Effect of biventricular pacing on symptoms and cardiac remodelling in patients with end stage hypertrophic cardiomyopathy. *Eur J Heart Fail.* 2008;10(5):507-513.

218. Ashrafian H, Mason MJ, Mitchell AG. Regression of dilated-hypokinetic hypertrophic cardiomyopathy by biventricular cardiac pacing. *Europace.* 2007;9:50-54.

219. Shirani J, Maron BJ, Cannon RO III, Shahin S, Roberts WC. Clinicopathologic features of hypertrophic cardiomyopathy managed by cardiac transplantation. *Am J Cardiol.* 1993;72:434-440.
220. Olivotto I, Cecchi F, Casey SA, Dolara A, Traverse JH, Maron BJ. Impact of atrial fibrillation on the clinical course of hypertrophic cardiomyopathy. *Circulation.* 2001;104:2517-2524.
221. Maron BJ, Olivotto I, Bellone P, et al. Clinical profile of stroke in 900 patients with hypertrophic cardiomyopathy. *J Am Coll Cardiol.* 2002;39:301-307.
222. Cecchi F, Olivotto I, Montereggi A, Santoro G, Dolara A, Maron BJ. Hypertrophic cardiomyopathy in Tuscany: clinical course and outcome in an unselected regional population. *J Am Coll Cardiol.* 1995;26:1529-1536.
223. McKenna WJ, Deanfield JE. Hypertrophic cardiomyopathy: an important cause of sudden death. *Arch Dis Child.* 1984;59:971-975.
224. Elliott PM, Gimeno Blanes JR, Mahon NG, McKenna WJ. Relation between the severity of left ventricular hypertrophy and prognosis in patients with hypertrophic cardiomyopathy. *Lancet.* 2001;357:420-424.
225. Kofflard MJ, Ten Cate FJ, van der Lee C, et al. Hypertrophic cardiomyopathy in a large community-based population: clinical outcome and identification of risk factors for sudden cardiac death and clinical deterioration. *J Am Coll Cardiol.* 2003;41:987-993.
226. Stafford WJ, Trohman RG, Bilsker M, Zaman L, Catellanos A, Myerburg RJ. Cardiac arrest in an adolescent with atrial fibrillation and hypertrophic cardiomyopathy. *J Am Coll Cardiol.* 1986;7:701-704.
227. Maron BJ, Robert WC, Epstein SE. Sudden death in hypertrophic cardiomyopathy: a profile of 78 patients. *Circulation.* 1982;65:1388-1394.
228. Elliott PM, Sharma S, Varnava A, Poloniecki J, Rowland E, McKenna WJ. Survival after cardiac arrest or sustained ventricular tachycardia in patients with hypertrophic cardiomyopathy. *J Am Coll Cardiol.* 1999;33:1596-1601.
229. Cecchi F, Maron BJ, Epstein SE. Long-term outcome of patients with hypertrophic cardiomyopathy successfully resuscitated after cardiac arrest. *J Am Coll Cardiol.* 1989;13:1283-1288.
230. Olivotto I, Gistri R, Petrone P, Pedemonte E, Vargiu D, Cecchi F. Maximum left ventricular thickness and risk of sudden death in patients with hypertrophic cardiomyopathy. *J Am Coll Cardiol.* 2003;41:315-321.
231. Saumarez RC, Chojnowska L, Derksen R, et al. Sudden death in noncoronary heart disease is associated with delayed paced ventricular activation. *Circulation.* 2003;107:2595-2600.
232. Silka MJ, Kron J, Dunnigan A, et al. Sudden cardiac death and the use of implantable cardioverter-defibrillators in pediatric patients. The Pediatric Electrophysiology Society. *Circulation.* 1993;87(3):800-807.
233. Kron J, Oliver RP, Norsted S, Silka MJ. The automatic implantable cardioverter-defibrillator in young patients. *J Am Coll Cardiol.* 1990;16(4):896-902.
234. Maron BJ, Spirito P, Shen WK, et al. Implantable cardioverter-defibrillators and prevention of sudden cardiac death in hypertrophic cardiomyopathy. *JAMA.* 2007;298(4):405-412.
235. Taylor MR, Carniel E, Mestroni L. Cardiomyopathy, familial dilated. *Orphanet J Rare Dis.* 2006;1:27.
236. Bowles NE, Bowles KR, Towbin JA. Viral genomic detection and outcome in myocarditis. *Heart Fail Clin.* 2005;1(3):407-417.
237. Cooper LT, Baughman KL, Feldman AM, et al. The role of endomyocardial biopsy in the management of cardiovascular disease: a scientific statement from the American Heart Association, the American College of Cardiology, and the European Society of Cardiology. Endorsed by the Heart Failure Society of America and the Heart Failure Association of the European Society of Cardiology. *J Am Coll Cardiol.* 2007;50(19):1914-1931.
238. Weber MA, Ashworth MT, Risdon RA, et al. Clinicopathological features of paediatric deaths due to myocarditis: an autopsy series. *Arch Dis Child.* 2008;93(7):594-598.

239. Burkett EL, Hershberger RE. Clinical and genetic issues in familial dilated cardiomyopathy. *J Am Coll Cardiol.* 2005;45:969-981.
240. Dec GM, Fuster V. Idiopathic dilated cardiomyopathy. *N Engl J Med.* 1994;331:1564-1575.
241. Mestroni L, Rocco C, Gregori D, et al. Familial dilated cardiomyopathy: evidence for genetic and phenotypic heterogeneity. *J Am Coll Cardiol.* 1999;34:181-190.
242. Politano L, Nigro V, Nigro G, et al. Development of cardiomyopathy in female carriers of Duchenne and Becker muscular dystrophies. *JAMA.* 1996;275:1335-1338.
243. Bione S, D'Adamo P, Maestrini E, et al. A novel X-linked gene, G4.5. is responsible for Barth syndrome. *Nat Genet.* 1996;12(4):385-389.
244. Fatkin D, MacRae C, Sasaki T, et al. Missense mutations in the rod domain of the lamin A/C gene as causes of dilated cardiomyopathy and conduction-system disease. *N Engl J Med.* 1999;341:1715-1724.
245. Hershberger RE, Hanson E, Jakobs PM, et al. A novel lamin A/C mutation in a family with dilated cardiomyopathy, prominent conduction system disease, and need for permanent pacemaker implantation. *Am Heart J.* 2002;144:1081-1086.
246. Towbin JA, Bowles NE. The failing heart. *Nature.* 2002;415(6868):227-233.
247. Towbin JA. The role of cytoskeletal proteins in cardiomyopathies. *Curr Opin Cell Biol.* 1998;10:131-139.
248. Bowles NE, Bowles KR, Towbin JA. The "Final Common Pathway" hypothesis and inherited cardiovascular disease: the role of cytoskeletal proteins in dilated cardiomyopathy. *Herz.* 2000;25:168-175.
249. Towbin JA, Bowles NE. Dilated cardiomyopathy: a tale of cytoskeletal proteins and beyond. *J Cardiovasc Electrophysiol.* 2006;17(8):919-926.
250. Cox GF, Kunkel LM. Dystrophies and heart disease. *Curr Opin Cardiol.* 1997;12:329-343.
251. Feng J, Yan J, Buzin CH, et al. Mutations in the dystrophin gene are associated with sporadic dilated cardiomyopathy. *Mol Genet Metab.* 2002;77(1–2):119-126.
252. Feng J, Yan JY, Buzin CH, et al. Comprehensive mutation scanning of the dystrophin gene in patients with nonsyndromic X-linked dilated cardiomyopathy. *J Am Coll Cardiol.* 2002;40(6):1120-1124.
253. Taylor MR, Slavov D, Ku L, et al. Prevalence of desmin mutations in dilated cardiomyopathy. *Circulation.* 2007;115(10):1244-1251.
254. Van Tintelen JP, Hofstra RM, Katerberg H, et al. High yield of LMNA mutations in patients with dilated cardiomyopathy and/or conduction disease referred to cardiogenetics outpatient clinics. *Am Heart J.* 2007;154(6):1130-1139.
255. Parks SB, Kushner JD, Nauman D, et al. Lamin A/C mutation analysis in a cohort of 324 unrelated patients with idiopathic or familial dilated cardiomyopathy. *Am Heart J.* 2008;156(1):161-169.
256. Tsubata S. et al.Mutations in the human d-sarcoglycan gene in familial and sporadic dilated cardiomyopathy. *J Clin Invest.* 2000;106:655-662.
257. Barresi R, Di Blasi C, Negri T, et al. Disruption of heart sarcoglycan complex and severe cardiomyopathy caused by beta sarcoglycan mutations. *J Med Genet.* 2000;37(2):102-107.
258. Olson TM, Illenberger S, Kishimoto NY, et al. Metavinculin mutations alter actin interaction in dilated cardiomyopathy. *Circulation.* 2002;105(4):431-437.
259. Kärkkäinen S, Peuhkurinen K. Genetics of dilated cardiomyopathy. *Ann Med.* 2007;39(2):91-107.
260. Kamisago M et al. Mutations in sarcomeric protein genes as a cause of dilated cardiomyopathy. *N Engl J Med.* 2000;343:1688-1696.
261. Chang AN, Potter JD. Sarcomeric protein mutations in dilated cardiomyopathy. *Heart Fail Rev.* 2005;10(3):225-235.
262. Chang AN, Parvatiyar MS, Potter JD. Troponin and cardiomyopathy. *Biochem Biophys Res Commun.* 2008;369(1):74-81.
263. Murphy RT, Mogensen J, Shaw A, et al. Novel mutation in cardiac troponin I in recessive idiopathic dilated cardiomyopathy. *Lancet.* 2004;363(9406):371-372.

264. Olson TM, Kishimoto NY, Whitby FG, Michels VV. Mutations that alter the surface change of a-tropomyosin are associated with dilated cardiomyopathy. *J Mol Cell Cardiol.* 2001;33: 723-732.

265. Pyle WG, Solaro RJ. At the crossroads of myocardial signaling: the role of Z-discs in intracellular signaling and cardiac function. *Circ Res.* 2004;94(3):296-305.

266. Vatta M, Mohapatra B, Jimenez S, et al. Mutations in Cypher/ZASP in patients with dilated cardiomyopathy and left ventricular non- compaction. *J Am Coll Cardiol.* 2003;42(11): 2014-2027.

267. Mohapatra B, Jimenez S, Lin JH, et al. Mutations in the muscle LIM protein and alpha-actinin-2 genes in dilated cardiomyopathy and endocardial fibroelastosis. *Mol Genet Metab.* 2003;80(1–2):207-215.

268. Knöll R, Hoshijima M, Hoffman HM, et al. The cardiac mechanical stretch sensor machinery involves a Z disc complex that is defective in a subset of human dilated cardiomyopathy. *Cell.* 2002;111(7):943-955.

269. Duboscq-Bidot L, Xu P, Charron P, et al. Mutations in the Z-band protein myopalladin gene and idiopathic dilated cardiomyopathy. *Cardiovasc Res.* 2008;77(1):118-125.

270. Hayashi T, Arimura T, Itoh-Satoh M, et al. Tcap gene mutations in hypertrophic cardiomyopathy and dilated cardiomyopathy. *J Am Coll Cardiol.* 2004;44(11):2192-2201.

271. Schmitt JP, Kamisago M, Asahi M, et al. Dilated cardiomyopathy and heart failure caused by a mutation in phospholamban. *Science.* 2003;299(5611):1410-1413.

272. Haghighi K, Kolokathis F, Pater L, et al. Human phospholamban null results in lethal dilated cardiomyopathy revealing a critical difference between mouse and human. *J Clin Invest.* 2003;111(6):869-876.

273. McNair WP, Ku L, Taylor MR, et al. SCN5A mutation associated with dilated cardiomyopathy, conduction disorder and arrhythmia. *Circulation.* 2004;100:2163-2167.

274. Nguyen TP, Wang DW, Rhodes TH, et al. Divergent biophysical defects caused by mutant sodium channels in dilated cardiomyopathy with arrhythmia. *Circ Res.* 2008;102: 364-371.

275. Olson TM, Michels VV, Ballew JD, et al. Sodium channel mutations and susceptibility to heart failure and atrial fibrillation. *JAMA.* 2005;293(4):447-454.

276. Arimura T, Hayashi T, Kimura A. Molecular etiology of idiopathic cardiomyopathy. *Acta Myol.* 2007;26(3):153-158.

277. LeWinter MM. Functional consequences of sarcomeric protein abnormalities in failing myocardium. *Heart Fail Rev.* 2005;10(3):249-257.

278. Towbin JA. Inflammatory cardiomyopathy: there is a specific matrix destruction in the course of the disease. *Ernst Schering Res Found Workshop.* 2006;(55):219-250.

279. Ahmad F, Seidman JG, Seidman CE. The genetic basis for cardiac remodeling. *Annu Rev Genomics Hum Genet.* 2005;6:185-216.

280. Robinson P, Griffiths PJ, Watkins H, et al. Dilated and hypertrophic cardiomyopathy mutations in troponin and alpha-tropomyosin have opposing effects on the calcium affinity of cardiac thin filaments. *Circ Res.* 2007;101(12):1266-1273.

281. Arber S, Hunter JJ, Ross J Jr, et al. MLP-deficient mice exhibit a disruption of cardiac cytoarchitectural organization, dilated cardiomyopathy, and heart failure. *Cell.* 1997;88(3): 393-403.

282. Zolk O, Caroni P, Böhm M, et al. Decreased expression of the cardiac LIM domain protein MLP in chronic human heart failure. *Circulation.* 2000;101(23):2674-2677.

283. Zhou Q, Chu PH, Huang C, et al. Ablation of Cypher, a PDZ-LIM domain Z-line protein, causes a severe form of congenital myopathy. *J Cell Biol.* 2001;155(4):605-612.

284. Granzier HL, Labeit S. The giant protein titin: a major player in myocardial mechanics, signaling, and disease. *Circ Res.* 2004;94(3):284-295.

285. Knowlton KU. CVB infection and mechanisms of viral cardiomyopathy. *Curr Top Microbiol Immunol.* 2008;323:315-335.

286. Badorff C, Knowlton KU. Dystrophin disruption in enterovirus-induced myocarditis and dilated cardiomyopathy: from bench to bedside. *Med Microbiol Immunol.* 2004;193(2–3): 121-126.

287. Vatta M, Stetson SJ, Perez-Verdia A, et al. Molecular remodeling of dystrophin in patients with end-stage cardiomyopathies and reversal in patients on assistance-device therapy. *Lancet.* 2002;359(9310):936-941.

288. Vatta M, Stetson SJ, Jimenez S, et al. Molecular normalization of dystrophin in the failing left and right ventricle of patients treated with either pulsatile or continuous flow-type ventricular assistdevices. *J Am Coll Cardiol.* 2004;43(5):811-817.

289. Parnaik VK. Role of nuclear lamins in nuclear organization, cellular signaling, and inherited diseases. *Int Rev Cell Mol Biol.* 2008;266:157-206.

290. Brodsky G, Muntoni F, Miocic S, Sinagra G, Sewry C, Mestroni L. Lamin A/C gene mutation associated with dilated cardiomyopathy with variable skeletal muscle involvement. *Circulation.* 2000;101:473-476.

291. Becane HM, Bonne G, Varnous S, et al. High incidence of sudden death with conduction system and myocardial disease due to lamins A and C gene mutation. *Pacing Clin Electrophysiol.* 2000;23:1661-1666.

292. Jakobs PM, Hanson E, Crispell KA, et al. Novel lamin A/C mutations in two families with dilated cardiomyopathy and conduction system disease. *J Card Fail.* 2001;7:249-256.

293. Arbustini E, Pilotto A, Repetto A, et al. Autosomal dominant dilated cardiomyopathy with atrioventricular block: a lamin A/C defectrelated disease. *J Am Coll Cardiol.* 2002;39:981-990.

294. Taylor MR, Fain PR, Sinagra G, et al. Natural history of dilated cardiomyopathy due to lamin A/C gene mutations. *J Am Coll Cardiol.* 2003;41:771-780.

295. Sebillon P, Bouchier C, Bidot LD, et al. Expanding the phenotype of LMNA mutations in dilated cardiomyopathy and functional consequences of these mutations. *J Med Genet.* 2003;40:560-567.

296. Berko BA, Swift M. X-linked dilated cardiomyopathy. *N Engl J Med.* 1987;316(19):1186-1191.

297. Hoffman EP, Brown RH, Kunkel LM. Dystrophin: the protein product of the Duchenne muscular dystrophy locus. *Cell.* 1987;51:919-928.

298. Towbin JA, Hejtmancik JF, Brink P, et al. X-linked dilated cardiomyopathy. Molecular genetic evidence of linkage to the Duchenne muscular dystrophy (dystrophin) gene at the Xp21 locus. *Circulation.* 1993;87(6):1854-1865.

299. Ervasti JM, Sonnemann KJ. Biology of the striated muscle dystrophin-glycoprotein complex. *Int Rev Cytol.* 2008;265:191-225.

300. Kaprielian RR, Stevenson S, Rothery SM, et al. Distinct patterns of dystrophin organization in myocyte sarcolemma and transverse tubules of normal and diseased human myocardium. *Circulation.* 2000;101(22):2586-2594.

301. Ségalat L, Grisoni K, Archer J, et al. CAPON expression in skeletal muscle is regulated by position, repair, NOS activity, and dystrophy. *Exp Cell Res.* 2005;302(2):170-179.

302. Petrof BJ, Shrager JB, Stedman HH, et al. Dystrophin protects the sarcolemma from stresses developed during muscle contraction. *Proc Natl Acad Sci USA.* 1993;90(8):3710-3714.

303. Deconinck N, Dan B. Pathophysiology of duchenne muscular dystrophy: current hypotheses. *Pediatr Neurol.* 2007;36(1):1-7.

304. Davies KE, Nowak KJ. Molecular mechanisms of muscular dystrophies: old and new players. *Nat Rev Mol Cell Biol.* 2006;7(10):762-773.

305. Barth PG, Valianpour F, Bowen VM, et al. X-linked cardioskeletal myopathy and neutropenia (Barth syndrome): an update. *Am J Med Genet A.* 2004;126A(4):349-354.

306. Houtkooper RH, Vaz FM. Cardiolipin, the heart of mitochondrial metabolism. *Cell Mol Life Sci.* 2008;65(16):2493-2506.

307. Izawa H, Murohara T, Nagata K, et al. Mineralocorticoid receptor antagonism ameliorates left ventricular diastolic dysfunction and myocardial fibrosis in mildly symptomatic

patients with idiopathic dilated cardiomyopathy: a pilot study. *Circulation.* 2005;112: 2940-2945.

308. Goldman L, Ausiello D, eds. *Cecil Medicine.* 23 ed. Philadelphia: Saunders Elsevier; 2007 [chapters 59-68].

309. Kathy A, Crispell MD, Wray A, et al. Clinical profiles of four large pedigrees with familial dilated cardiomyopathy: preliminary recommendations for clinical practice. *J Am Coll Cardiol.* 1999;34(3):837-847.

310. Kilic T, Vural A, Ural D, et al. Cardiac resynchronization therapy in a case of myotonic dystrophy (Steinert's disease) and dilated cardiomyopathy. *Pacing Clin Electrophysiol.* 2007;30(7):916-920.

311. Groh WJ, Groh MR, Saha C, et al. Electrocardiographic abnormalities and sudden death in myotonic dystrophy type 1. *N Engl J Med.* 2008;358(25):2688-2697.

312. Lainscak M, von Haehling S, Springer J, Anker SD. Biomarkers for chronic heart failure. *Heart Fail Monit.* 2007;5(3):77-82.

313. Price JF, Thomas AK, Grenier M, et al. B-type natriuretic peptide predicts adverse cardiovascular events in pediatric outpatients with chronic left ventricular systolic dysfunction. *Circulation.* 2006;114(10):1063-1069.

314. Heidecker B, Kasper EK, Wittstein IS, et al. Transcriptomic biomarkers for individual risk assessment in new-onset heart failure. *Circulation.* 2008;118(3):238-246.

315. Hamdan A, Shapira Y, Bengal T, et al. Tissue Doppler imaging in patients with advanced heart failure: relation to functional class and prognosis. *J Heart Lung Transplant.* 2006;25(2):214-218.

316. McMahon CJ, Nagueh SF, Eapen RS, et al. Echocardiographic predictors of adverse clinical events in children with dilated cardiomyopathy: a prospective clinical study. *Heart.* 2004; 90(8):908-915.

317. Assomull RG, Prasad SK, Lyne J, et al. Cardiovascular magnetic resonance, fibrosis, and prognosis in dilated cardiomyopathy. *J Am Coll Cardiol.* 2006;48(10):1977-1985.

318. Yokokawa M, Tada H, Koyama K, et al. The characteristics and distribution of the scar tissue predict ventricular tachycardia in patients with advanced heart failure. *Pacing Clin Electrophysiol.* 2009;32(3):314-322.

319. Shimizu I, Iguchi N, Watanabe H, et al. Delayed enhancement cardiovascular magnetic resonance as a novel technique to predict cardiac events in dilated cardiomyopathy patients. *Int J Cardiol.* 2009;[Epub ahead of print]

320. Yokokawa M, Tada H, Toyama T, et al. Magnetic resonance imaging is superior to cardiac scintigraphy to identify nonresponders to cardiac resynchronization therapy. *Pacing Clin Electrophysiol.* 2009;32(suppl 1):S57-S62.

321. Cohn JN, Johnson G, Ziesche S, et al. A comparison of enalapril with hydralazine-isosorbide dinitrate in the treatment of chronic congestive heart failure. *N Engl J Med.* 1991; 325(5):303-310.

322. Taylor AL, Ziesche S, Yancy C, et al.; African-American Heart Failure Trial Investigators. Combination of isosorbide dinitrate and hydralazine in blacks with heart failure. *N Engl J Med.* 2004;351(20):2049-2057.

323. Loeb HS, Johnson G, Henrick A, et al. Effect of enalapril, hydralazine plus isosorbide dinitrate, and prazosin on hospitalization in patients with chronic congestive heart failure. The V-HeFT VA Cooperative Studies Group. *Circulation.* 1993;87(6 suppl):VI78-VI87.

324. Vinge LE, Raake PW, Koch WJ. Gene therapy in heart failure. *Circ Res.* 2008;102(12): 1458-1470.

325. Yamada S, Nelson TJ, Crespo-Diaz RJ, et al. Stem Embryonic stem cell therapy of heart failure in genetic cardiomyopathy. *Cells.* 2008;26(10):2644-2653.

326. Townsend D, Yasuda S, Li S, et al. Emergent dilated cardiomyopathy caused by targeted repair of dystrophic skeletal muscle. *Mol Ther.* 2008;16(5):832-835.

327. Crispell K, Wray A, Ni H, Nauman D, Hershberger R. Clinical profiles of four large pedigrees with familial dilated cardiomyopathy: preliminary recommendations for clinical practice. *J Am Coll Cardiol*. 1999;34:837-847.
328. Hanson E, Hershberger RE. Genetic counseling and screening issues in familial dilated cardiomyopathy. *J Genet Counseling*. 2001;10:397-415.
329. Baig MK, Goldman JH, Caforio AP, Coonar AS, Keeling PJ, McKenna WJ. Familial dilated cardiomyopathy: cardiac abnormalities are common in asymptomatic relatives and may represent early disease. *J Am Coll Cardiol*. 1998;31:195-201.
330. Hershberger RE, Ni H, Crispell KA. Familial dilated cardiomyopathy: echocardiographic diagnostic criteria for classification of family members as affected. *J Cardiac Fail*. 1999; 51:203-212.
331. The SOLVD Investigators. Effect of enalapril on mortality and the development of heart failure in asymptomatic patients with reduced left ventricular ejection fractions. *N Engl J Med*. 1992;327:685-691.
332. Crispell KA, Hanson E, Coates K, Toy W, Hershberger R. Periodic rescreening is indicated for family members at risk of developing familial dilated cardiomyopathy. *J Am Coll Cardiol*. 2002;39:1503-1507.
333. Sen-Chowdhry S, Lowe MD, Sporton SC, McKenna WJ. Arrhythmogenic right ventricular cardiomyopathy: clinical presentation, diagnosis, and management. *Am J Med*. 2004;117:685-695.
334. Sen-Chowdhry S, Syrris P, McKenna WJ. Genetics of right ventricular cardiomyopathy. *J Cardiovasc Electrophysiol*. 2005;16(8):927-935.
335. McKenna WJ, Thiene G, Nava A, et al. Diagnosis of arrhythmogenic right ventricular dysplasia/cardiomyopathy. *Br Heart J*. 1994;71:215-218.
336. Thiene G, Nava A, Corrado D, et al. Right ventricular cardiomyopathy and sudden death in young people. *N Engl J Med*. 1988;318:129-133.
337. Corrado D, Fontaine G, Marcus FI, et al. Arrhythmogenic right ventricular dysplasia/cardiomyopathy: need for an international registry. Study Group on Arrhythmogenic Right Ventricular Dysplasia/Cardiomyopathy of the Working Groups on Myocardial and Pericardial Disease and Arrhythmias of the European Society of Cardiology and of the Scientific Council on Cardiomyopathies of the World Heart Federation. *Circulation*. 2000; 101(11):E101-E106.
338. Hamid MS, Norman M, Quraishi A, et al. Prospective evaluation of relatives for familial arrhythmogenic right ventricular cardiomyopathy reveals a need to broaden diagnostic criteria. *J Am Coll Cardiol*. 2002;40:1445-1450.
339. Nava A, Thiene G, Canciani B, et al. Familial occurrence of right ventricular dysplasia: a study involving nine families. *J Am Coll Cardiol*. 1988;12:1222-1228.
340. Merner ND, Hodgkinson KA, Haywood AF, et al. Arrhythmogenic right ventricular cardiomyopathy type 5 is a fully penetrant, lethal arrhythmic disorder caused by a missense mutation in the TMEM43 gene. *Am J Hum Genet*. 2008;82:809-821.
341. Coonar AS, Protonotarios N, Tsatsopoulou A, et al. Gene for arrhythmogenic right ventricular cardiomyopathy with diffuse nonepidermolytic palmoplantar keratoderma and woolly hair (Naxos disease) maps to 17q21. *Circulation*. 1998;97:2049-2058.
342. McKoy G, Protonotarios N, Crosby A, et al. Identification of a deletion in plakoglobin in arrhythmogenic right ventricular cardiomyopathy with palmoplantar keratoderma and woolly hair (Naxos disease). *Lancet*. 2000;355:2119-2124.
343. Protonotarios N, Tsatsopoulou A, Anastasakis A, et al. Genotype-phenotype assessment in autosomal recessive arrhythmogenic right ventricular cardiomyopathy (Naxos disease) caused by a deletion in plakoglobin. *J Am Coll Cardiol*. 2001;38:1477-1484.
344. Rao BH, Reddy IS, Chandra KS. Familial occurrence of a rare combination of dilated cardiomyopathy with palmoplantar keratoderma and curly hair. *Indian Heart J*. 1996;48: 161-162.

345. Carvajal-Huerta L. Epidermolytic palmoplantar keratoderma with woolly hair and dilated cardiomyopathy. *J Am Acad Dermatol*. 1998;39:418-421.

346. Norgett EE, Hatsell SJ, Carvajal-Huerta L, et al. Recessive mutation in desmoplakin disrupts desmoplakin-intermediate filament interactions and causes dilated cardiomyopathy, woolly hair and keratoderma. *Hum Mol Genet*. 2000;9:2761-2766.

347. Getsios S, Huen AC, Green KJ. Working out the strength and flexibility of desmosomes. *Nat Rev Mol Cell Biol*. 2004;5:271-281.

348. Smith EA, Fuchs E. Defining the interactions between intermediate filaments and desmosomes. *J Cell Biol*. 1998;141:1229-1241.

349. Alcalai R, Metzger S, Rosenheck S, Meiner V, Chajek-Shaul T. A recessive mutation in desmoplakin causes arrhythmogenic right ventricular dysplasia, skin disorder, and woolly hair. *J Am Coll Cardiol*. 2003;42:319-327.

350. Rampazzo A, Nava A, Malacrida S, et al. Mutation in human desmoplakin domain binding to plakoglobin causes a dominant form of arrhythmogenic right ventricular cardiomyopathy. *Am J Hum Genet*. 2002;71:1200-1206.

351. Bauce B, Basso C, Rampazzo A, et al. Clinical profile of four families with arrhythmogenic right ventricular cardiomyopathy caused by dominant desmoplakin mutations. *Eur Heart J*. 2005;26:1666-1675.

352. Norman M, Simpson M, Mogensen J, et al. Novel mutation in desmoplakin causes arrhythmogenic left ventricular cardiomyopathy. *Circulation*. 2005;112:636-642.

353. Jonkman MF, Pasmooij AM, Pasmas SG, et al. Loss of desmoplakin tail causes lethal acantholytic epidermolysis bullosa. *Am J Hum Genet*. 2005;77:653-660.

354. Whittock NV, Wan H, Morley SM, et al. Compound heterozygosity for non-sense and missense mutations in desmoplakin underlies skin fragility/woolly hair syndrome. *J Invest Dermatol*. 2002;118:232-238.

355. Gerull B, Heuser A, Wichter T, et al. Mutations in the desmosomal protein plakophilin-2 are common in arrhythmogenic right ventricular cardiomyopathy. *Nat Genet*. 2004;36: 1162-1164.

356. Schwarz MA, Owaribe K, Kartenbeck J, Franke WW. Desmosomes and hemidesmosomes: constitutive molecular components. *Annu Rev Cell Biol*. 1990;6:461-491.

357. Awad MM, Dalal D, Cho E, et al. DSG2 mutations contribute to arrhythmogenic right ventricular dysplasia/cardiomyopathy. *Am J Hum Genet*. 2006;79:136-142.

358. Pilichou K, Nava A, Basso C, et al. Mutations in desmoglein-2 gene are associated with arrhythmogenic right ventricular cardiomyopathy. *Circulation*. 2006;113:1171-1179.

359. Heuser A, Plovie ER, Ellinor PT, et al. Mutant desmocollin-2 causes arrhythmogenic right ventricular cardiomyopathy. *Am J Hum Genet*. 2006;79:1081-1088.

360. Syrris P, Ward A, Evans A, et al. Arrhythmogenic right ventricular dysplasia/cardiomyopathy associated with mutations in the desmosomal gene desmocollin-2. *Am J Hum Genet*. 2006; 79:978-984.

361. Beffagna G, De Bortoli M, Nava A, et al. Missense mutations in desmocollin-2 N-terminus, associated with arrhythmogenic right ventricular cardiomyopathy, affect intracellular localization of desmocollin-2 in vitro. *BMC Med Genet*. 2007;8:65.

362. Corrado D, Basso C, Thiene G, et al. Spectrum of clinicopathologic manifestations of arrhythmogenic right ventricular cardiomyopathy/dysplasia: a multicenter study. *J Am Coll Cardiol*. 1997;30:1512-1520.

363. Nemec J, Edwards BS, Osborn MJ, Edwards WD. Arrhythmogenic right ventricular dysplasia masquerading as dilated cardiomyopathy. *Am J Cardiol*. 1999;84:237-239, A9.

364. De Pasquale CG, Heddle WF. Left sided arrhythmogenic ventricular dysplasia in siblings. *Heart*. 2001;86:128-130.

365. Michalodimitrakis M, Papadomanolakis A, Stiakakis J, Kanaki K. Left side right ventricular cardiomyopathy. *Med Sci Law*. 2002;42:313-317.

366. Suzuki H, Sumiyoshi M, Kawai S, et al. Arrhythmogenic right ventricular cardiomyopathy with an initial manifestation of severe left ventricular impairment and normal contraction of the right ventricle. *Jpn Circ J*. 2000;64:209-213.
367. Buja G, Estes N III, Wichter T, Corrado D, Marcus F, Thiene G. Arrhythmogenic Right Ventricular Cardiomyopathy/Dysplasia: Risk Stratification and Therapy. *Prog Cardiovasc Dis*. 2008;50(4):282-293.
368. Protonotarios N, Tsatsopoulou A. Naxos disease and Carvajal syndrome: Cardiocutaneous disorders that highlight the pathogenesis and broaden the spectrum of arrhythmogenic right ventricular cardiomyopathy. *Cardiovasc Pathol*. 2004;13:185-194.
369. Kaplan SR, Gard JJ, Carvajal-Huerta L, Ruiz-Cabezas JC, Thiene G, Saffitz JE. Structural and molecular pathology of the heart in Carvajal syndrome. *Cardiovasc Pathol*. 2004;13:26-32.
370. Duran M, Avellan F, Carvajal L. Dilated cardiomyopathy in the ectodermal dysplasia. Electro-echocardiographic observations in palmoplantar keratoderma with woolly hair. *Rev Esp Cardiol*. 2000;53:1296-1300.
371. Kaplan SR, Gard JJ, Protonotarios N, et al. Remodeling of myocyte gap junctions in arrhythmogenic right ventricular cardiomyopathy due to a deletion in plakoglobin (Naxos disease). *Heart Rhythm*. 2004;1:3-11.
372. Lemery R, Brugada P, Bella PD, et al. Nonischemic ventricular tachycardia. Clinical course and long-term follow-up in patients without clinically overt heart disease. *Circulation*. 1989; 79:990-999.
373. Buxton AE, Waxman HL, Marchlinski FE, et al. Right ventricular tachycardia: clinical and electrophysiologic characteristics. *Circulation*. 1983;68:917-927.
374. Wilber DJ, Baerman J, Olshansky B, et al. Adenosine-sensitive ventricular tachycardia: clinical characteristics and response to catheter ablation. *Circulation*. 1993;87:126-134.
375. Nava A, Bauce B, Basso C, et al. Clinical profile and long-term follow-up of 37 families with arrhythmogenic right ventricular cardiomyopathy. *J Am Coll Cardiol*. 2000;36:2226-2233.
376. Ott P, Marcus FI, Sobonya RE, et al. Cardiac sarcoidosis masquerading as right ventricular dysplasia. *Pacing Clin Electrophysiol*. 2003;26:1498-1503.
377. Shiraishi J, Tatsumi T, Shimoo K, et al. Cardiac sarcoidosis mimicking right ventricular dysplasia. *Circ J*. 2003;67:169-171.
378. Lemola K, Brunckhorst C, Helfenstein U, et al. Predictors of adverse outcome in patients with arrhythmogenic right ventricular dysplasia/cardiomyopathy: long-term experience of a tertiary care center. *Heart*. 2005;91:1167-1172.
379. Fontaine G, Fontaliran F, Frank R, et al. Causes of sudden death in athletes. *Arch Mal Coeur Vaiss*. 1989;82:107-111.
380. Tabib A, Miras A, Taniere P, Loire R. Undetected cardiac lesions cause unexpected sudden cardiac death during occasional sport activity. A report of 80 cases. *Eur Heart J*. 1999;20: 900-903.
381. Corrado D, Thiene G, Nava A, et al. Sudden death in young competitive athletes: clinico-pathologic correlations in 22 cases. *Am J Med*. 1990;89:588-596.
382. Furlanello F, Bertoldi A, Dallago M, et al. Cardiac arrest and sudden death in competitive athletes with arrhythmogenic right ventricular dysplasia. *Pacing Clin Electrophysiol*. 1998; 21(1 pt 2):331-335.
383. Heidbuchel H, Hoogsteen J, Fagard R, et al. High prevalence of right ventricular involvement in endurance athletes with ventricular arrhythmias. Role of an electrophysiologic study in risk stratification. *Eur Heart J*. 2003;24:1473-1480.
384. Biffi A, Pelliccia A, Verdile L, et al. Long-term clinical significance of frequent and complex ventricular tachyarrhythmias in trained athletes. *J Am Coll Cardiol*. 2002;40:446-452.
385. Henriksen E, Kangro T, Jonason T, et al. An echocardiographic study of right ventricular adaptation to physical exercise in elite male orienteers. *Clin Physiol*. 1998;18:498-503.
386. Sciomer S, Vitarelli A, Penco M, et al. Anatomico-functional changes in the right ventricle of the athlete. *Cardiologia*. 1998;43:1215-1220.

387. F.I. Marcus; W.J. McKenna; D. Sherrill; et al. Diagnosis of Arrhythmogenic Right Ventricular Cardiomyopathy/Dysplasia. Proposed Modification of the Task Force Criteria. *Circulation*. 2010;121(13):1533-1541.

388. Peters S, Trummel M. Diagnosis of arrhythmogenic right ventricular dysplasia-cardiomyopathy: value of standard ECG revisited. *Ann Noninvasive Electrocardiol*. 2003;8:238-245.

389. Fontaine G, Fontaliran F, Hebert JL, et al. Arrhythmogenic right ventricular dysplasia. *Annu Rev Med*. 1999;50:17-35.

390. Jaoude SA, Leclercq JF, Coumel P. Progressive ECG changes in arrhythmogenic right ventricular disease. Evidence for an evolving disease. *Eur Heart J*. 1996;17:1717-1722.

391. Turrini P, Angelini A, Thiene G, et al. Late potentials and ventricular arrhythmias in arrhythmogenic right ventricular cardiomyopathy. *Am J Cardiol*. 1999;83:1214-1219.

392. Kinoshita O, Fontaine G, Rosas F, et al. Time and frequency-domain analyses of the signal-averaged ECG in patients with arrhythmogenic right ventricular dysplasia. *Circulation*. 1995;91:715-721.

393. Burke AP, Robinson S, Radentz S, et al. Sudden death in right ventricular dysplasia with minimal gross abnormalities. *J Forensic Sci*. 1999;44:438-443.

394. Marcus FI, Fontaine GH, Frank R, et al. Long-term follow-up in patients with arrhythmogenic right ventricular disease. *Eur Heart J*. 1989;10(suppl D):68-73.

395. Wichter T, Borggrefe M, Haverkamp W, et al. Efficacy of antiarrhythmic drugs in patients with arrhythmogenic right ventricular disease. Results in patients with inducible and noninducible ventricular tachycardia. *Circulation*. 1992;86:29-37.

396. Leclercq JF, Potenza S, Maison-Blanche P, et al. Determinants of spontaneous occurrence of sustained monomorphic ventricular tachycardia in right ventricular dysplasia. *J Am Coll Cardiol*. 1996;28:720-724.

397. Peters S, Peters H, Thierfelder L. Risk stratification of sudden cardiac death and malignant ventricular arrhythmias in right ventricular dysplasia-cardiomyopathy. *Int J Cardiol*. 1999; 71:243-250.

398. Turrini P, Corrado D, Basso C, et al. Dispersion of ventricular depolarisation-repolarisation: a non-invasive marker for risk stratification in arrhythmogenic right ventricular cardiomyopathy. *Circulation*. 2001;103:3075-3080.

399. Turrini P, Corrado D, Basso C, et al. Noninvasive risk stratification in arrhythmogenic right ventricular cardiomyopathy. *Ann Noninvasive Electrocardiol*. 2003;8:161-169.

400. Tavernier R, Gevaert S, De Sutter J, et al. Long term results of cardioverter-defibrillator implantation in patients with right ventricular dysplasia and malignant ventricular tachyarrhythmias. *Heart*. 2001;85:53-56.

401. Link MS, Wang PJ, Haugh CJ, et al. Arrhythmogenic right ventricular dysplasia: clinical results with implantable cardioverter defibrillators. *J Interv Card Electrophysiol*. 1997;1:41-48.

402. Wichter T, Paul M, Eckardt L, et al. Arrhythmogenic right ventricular cardiomyopathy. Antiarrhythmic drugs, catheter ablation, or ICD? *Herz*. 2005;30:91-101.

403. Blomström-Lundqvist C, Sabel KG, Olsson SB. A long term follow up of 15 patients with arrhythmogenic right ventricular dysplasia. *Br Heart J*. 1987;58(5):477-488.

404. Pinamonti B, Sinagra G, Salvi A, et al. Left ventricular involvement in right ventricular dysplasia. *Am Heart J*. 1992;123(3):711-724.

405. Peters S, Peters H, Thierfelder L. Heart failure in arrhythmogenic right ventricular dysplasia-cardiomyopathy. *Int J Cardiol*. 1999;71(3):251-256.

406. Corrado D, Leoni L, Link MS, et al. Implantable cardioverter-defibrillator therapy for prevention of sudden death in patients with arrhythmogenic right ventricular cardiomyopathy/dysplasia. *Circulation*. 2003;108(25):3084-3091.

407. Hulot JS, Jouven X, Empana JP, et al. Natural history and risk stratification of arrhythmogenic right ventricular dysplasia/cardiomyopathy. *Circulation*. 2004;110:1879-1884.

408. Peters S. Age related dilatation of the right ventricle in arrhythmogenic right ventricular dysplasia-cardiomyopathy. *Int J Cardiol*. 1996;56(2):163-167.

409. Marcus F, Nava A, Thiene G, et al. *Arrhythmogenic RV Cardiomyopathy/Dysplasia, Recent Advances*. Italia: Springer; 2007.
410. Pinamonti B, Miani D, Sinagra G, et al. Familial right ventricular dysplasia with biventricular involvement and inflammatory infiltration. Heart Muscle Disease Study Group. *Heart*. 1996;76(1):66-69.
411. Tonet JL, Castro-Miranda R, Iwa T, et al. Frequency of supraventricular tachyarrhythmias in arrhythmogenic right ventricular dysplasia. *Am J Cardiol*. 1991;67(13):1153.
412. Wlodarska EK, Wozniak O, Konka M, et al. Thromboembolic complications in patients with arrhythmogenic right ventricular dysplasia/cardiomyopathy. *Europace*. 2006;8(8):596-600.
413. Antonini-Canterin F, Sandrini R, Pavan D, et al. Right ventricular thrombosis in arrhythmogenic cardiomyopathy. A case report. *Ital Heart J*. 2000;1:415-418.
414. Chachques JC, Argyriadis PG, Fontaine G, et al. Right ventricular cardiomyoplasty: 10-year follow-up. *Ann Thorac Surg*. 2003;75:1464-1468.
415. Takagaki M, Ishino K, Kawada M, et al. Total right ventricular exclusion improves left ventricular function in patients with end-stage congestive right ventricular failure. *Circulation*. 2003;9:108.
416. Motta P, Mossad E, Savage R. Right ventricular exclusion surgery for arrhythmogenic right ventricular dysplasia with cardiomyopathy. *Anesth Analg*. 2003;96(6):1598-1602.
417. Pawel BR, de Chadarevian JP, Wolk JH, et al. Sudden death in childhood due to right ventricular dysplasia: report of two cases. *Pediatr Pathol*. 1994;14:987-995.

Valvular Heart Disease in Heart Failure

3

Farouk Mookadam, Sherif E. Moustafa, and Joseph F. Malouf

Congestive heart failure (CHF) is a significant health burden whose impact is increasing globally. An aging population, coupled with advances in medical technology, has extended the average life expectancy. The result is greater numbers of people living with chronic cardiac disease than ever before. As a result, surgical techniques for valvular repair or replacement have evolved.[1,2]

3.1
Aortic Valve Disease

3.1.1
Aortic Stenosis

Aortic stenosis (AS) is the most common valvular lesion in Europe and North America. It primarily presents as calcific AS in 2–7% of the population aged >65 years. About 1–2% of the population are born with a congenital bicuspid aortic valve, and as populations are aging AS is becoming more common.[3,4] Approximately 25% of patients over age 65 years have evidence of aortic sclerosis, and 4% of the North American population above 75 years has AS. Approximately 16% of persons with aortic sclerosis progresses to hemodynamically severe AS, and in individuals with mild-to-moderate AS, 50% progress to hemodynamically severe AS.[5–9]

3.1.1.1
Diagnosis of AS and Grading of Severity

On the basis of two-dimensional echocardiography and Doppler measurements, AS can be graded as mild, moderate, and severe (Table 3.1).[10] Because noninvasive transvalvular gradients show excellent correlation with invasive transvalvular gradients, cardiac

F. Mookadam (✉)
Mayo Clinic, Scottsdale, AZ, USA
e-mail: mookadam.farouk@mayo.edu

M.Y. Henein (ed.), *Heart Failure in Clinical Practice*,
DOI: 10.1007/978-1-84996-153-0_3, © Springer-Verlag London Limited 2010

Table 3.1 AS Severity Grading (adapted from 10)

	Mild As	Moderate As	Severe As
AVA (cm^2)	>1.5	1.5–1.0	<1.0
AVA index (cm^2/m^2)			<0.6
Mean gradient (mmHg)	<25	25–40	>40
Aortic jet velocity (m/s)	<3.0	3.0–4.0	>4.0

catheterization is rarely used to diagnose AS. More recently, three-dimensional echocardiography, cardiac computerized tomography, and cardiac magnetic resonance imaging are ancillary techniques that may be used to quantify aortic valve area (AVA) and AS severity in selected cases.

3.1.1.2
Pathophysiology of Heart Failure in AS

The development of CHF in patients with AS is associated with a high mortality, and aortic valve replacement can help ameliorate this high morbidity and mortality. The pathophysiology of CHF in patients with AS occurs as a result of several compensatory changes. Hypertrophic remodeling is a mechanism by which the left ventricle can generate increased systolic pressures while maintaining normal systolic wall stress (afterload) and a normal ejection fraction (EF). If the hypertrophic remodeling is inadequate, systolic wall stress will be increased. There is an inverse relation between wall stress and the EF: the presence of afterload excess results in a decline in the EF. Aortic valve replacement (AVR) can increase the EF by correcting the afterload excess created by a truly stenotic valve. A second mechanism causing a depressed EF in AS patients is a decrease in the intrinsic contractility of the myocardium; in this instance, AVR may have little or no effect on the EF if decreased contractility coexists with "relative" AS (or "pseudo" aortic stenosis) or if there is a primary cardiomyopathy.[12,13]

3.1.1.3
Predictors of Clinical Outcome

Cardiac Biomarkers

In asymptomatic severe AS, patients with brain natriuretic peptide (BNP) or N-terminal BNP concentrations of <130 pg/mL and 80 pmol/L, respectively, subjects had a 9-month symptom-free survival of almost 90%. Patients with higher natriuretic peptide concentrations frequently required surgery (symptom-free survival <50%). Kaplan–Meier analysis in patients with BNP levels <130 pg/mL ($n=25$) vs. ≥130 pg/mL ($n=18$) showed symptom-free survival of 100 vs. $94\pm5\%$ at 3 months, 90 ± 7 vs. $64\pm12\%$ at 6 months, 90 ± 7 vs. $45\pm14\%$ at 9 months, and $66\pm16\%$ vs. $34\pm14\%$ at 12 months ($p<0.05$).[14] Only N-terminal BNP independently predicted symptom-free survival. Serial measurements of these markers might therefore add incremental information in defining optimal timing for AVR.[15]

Echocardiography

Patients with asymptomatic severe AS and a reduced LVEF (<50%) have a higher relative risk (RR) of sustaining cardiac events (AVR; cardiac death second to AS; RR: 5.6; 95% CI: 1.46–21.3; $p<0.01$).[16] With regard to AVA, the RR of a cardiac event (AVR; cardiac death) has been found to increase per 0.2 cm^2 decrease in AVA (RR: 1.20; 95% CI: 1.06–1.36; $p<0.006$).[17]

In true severe aortic stenosis, the AVA is constant (or nearly constant) and is proportional to the stroke volume divided by the square root of the pressure gradient. Therefore, if the stroke volume declines, as it does in some patients with AS in whom heart failure has developed, there is a proportional decline in the pressure gradient. Under these low-flow conditions, the calculated effective AVA may indicate the presence of severe aortic stenosis, despite a low transvalvular pressure gradient. A mean pressure gradient that is less than 30 mmHg in a patient with clinically suspected severe AS (an AVA of <1 cm^2) indicates what is referred to as "low-gradient AS."[13]

Low-Flow, Low-Gradient AS

Patients with LV systolic dysfunction and low-flow, low-gradient AS (LFLG-AS) represent a challenging subset of AS patients in terms of surgical recommendations for AVR. The specific criteria for LFLG-AS vary widely in the literature, but generally include at least two of the following hemodynamic measurements: AVA ≤0.7–1.2 cm^2, mean transvalvular pressure gradient ≤30–40 mmHg, and LVEF ≤30–45%.[18–20] The most challenging management decision occurs in those patients with an LVEF <40%, AVA <1.0 cm^2 and a mean pressure gradient <30 mmHg. In this group, the "true" hemodynamic severity of valve stenosis may be difficult to determine; AVR is associated with a high operative risk, and benefits of AVR to improve symptoms and improve prognosis may be limited.[19]

The challenge in low-flow, low-gradient severe AS is to distinguish whether the patient has "true" severe AS' (TSAS), where the aortic valve is severely stenotic and afterload mismatch exists, or "pseudo-severe" AS (PSAS), where the aortic valve is not severely stenotic but the valve area calculation appears severely stenotic because of inherent limitations in the valve area equation under low-flow conditions, or because of an inability of the poorly functioning ventricle to provide sufficient force to open the valve cusps completely. Afterload reduction with AVR would be expected to result in an improvement in symptoms, LV function and survival in TSAS patients, but may not be beneficial in PSAS patients where the valve stenosis is not the primary problem. The prevalence of PSAS in studies of LFLG-AS has varied with the specific diagnostic criteria employed and ranges from 5 to 35% of patients.[18,19,21,22]

Dobutamine Stress Echocardiography to Distinguish TSAS and PSAS

Augmenting cardiac output in the patient with low-flow, low-gradient severe AS and reevaluating the valve hemodynamics at a normal transvalvular flow rate should assist in distinguishing the patient with TSAS and PSAS.[19]

The utility of dobutamine echocardiography to differentiate TSAS and PSAS was first reported by deFilippi et al In 18 patients with symptomatic severe low-gradient AS (effective orifice area (EOA) ≤0.5 cm^2/m^2, ΔP_{mean} ≤30 mmHg, LVEF <45%), dobutamine infusion up to 20 μg/kg/min identified three distinct hemodynamic responses. In 12 patients, dobutamine infusion resulted in an improvement in LV function. Seven of these 12 patients had an increase in transvalvular pressure gradient, little change in EOA (increase <0.3 cm^2) and a peak EOA <1.0 cm^2 and were thus labeled as having "fixed" severe AS. Severe AS was confirmed in the four patients undergoing surgery. In contrast, 5 of the 12 patients had little change in transvalvular pressure gradient, an increase in EOA ≥0.3 cm^2 and peak EOA>1.0 cm^2, and were labeled as having relative (pseudo-severe) AS. None of these five patients underwent surgery. Four were alive at 1 year with an outcome better than expected for severe symptomatic severe AS. In the remaining six patients, dobutamine infusion resulted in no improvement in LV function and no change in the hemodynamic indices. These patients were labeled as having indeterminate AS because of the lack of contractile reserve and the 1-year outcome was poor.[21]

Nishimura et al demonstrated the utility of dobutamine challenge during cardiac catheterization to distinguish TSAS and PSAS in 32 patients with LFLG-AS (EOA <1.0 cm^2, ΔP_{mean} <40 mmHg, LVEF <40%). Surgery was performed on 21 patients based on the results of graded dobutamine infusion up to 40 μg/kg/min. All patients with a mean transvalvular pressure gradient >30 mmHg and a Gorlin AVA ≤1.2 cm^2 at peak dobutamine infusion were found to have severe AS at surgery. Of the subset of 11 patients who underwent surgery with a mean transvalvular pressure gradient <30 mmHg at rest, ten patients had severe AS and they all had a mean pressure gradient >30 mmHg during dobutamine challenge. The one patient with only mild–moderate AS at surgery had a mean pressure gradient of 22 mmHg during dobutamine challenge. These data suggests the presence of TSAS if the mean pressure gradient is >30 mmHg at rest or during dobutamine challenge, in conjunction with a Gorlin AVA ≤1.2 cm^2.[22]

A potential limitation of dobutamine challenge to distinguish patients with TSAS and PSAS relates to the individual variability in hemodynamic response or flow augmentation. since increases in transvalvular pressure gradient and valve area are largely dependent on the magnitude of the transvalvular flow augmentation, any interpretation of the underlying AS severity using the response of these indices to dobutamine challenge will be complicated by differences in flow augmentation.[18,23]

To address this limitation, a new index, the projected valve area at 250 mL/s (EOAproj), has been proposed to better distinguish patients with TSAS and PSAS.[18] This index attempts to predict EOA at a standardized transvalvular flow rate of 250 mL/s, the typical flow rate observed in AS patients with normal LV systolic function.[24] Studies have largely demonstrated a linear relationship between transvalvular flow rate and Gorlin AVA or continuity equation EOA.[23,25] The slope of the valve area and transvalvular flow rate relationship, however, frequently referred to as valve compliance, varies between AS patients depending on whether the degree of valve obstruction is relatively "fixed" (shallow slope) or "flexible" (steep slope). Using dobutamine echocardiography, multiple EOA and trans-valvular flow rate measurements can be obtained in an individual patient at different infusion rates to derive the valve compliance.[18,23,25] Valve compliance can then be used to predict EOA at the standardized transvalvular flow rate of 250 mL/s, using the equation[18]:

$$EOAproj = EOArest + VC \times (250 - Qrest),$$

where EOAproj=projected EOA at 250 mL/s, EOArest=resting EOA, Qrest=resting transvalvular flow rate and VC=valve compliance or slope of the valve area and transval-vular flow relationship. Thus, EOAproj corrects for the individual variation in the magni-tude of flow augmentation during dobutamine challenge and provides an index that can be compared between individuals within the framework of the ACC/AHA guidelines.[10]

The potential utility of EOAproj to discriminate TSAS and PSAS was investigated in 23 patients with LFLG-AS undergoing AVR (27%).[18] Based on surgical inspection, 15 patients (65%) had TSAS, and eight patients (35%) had PSAS. An EOAproj ≤ 1.0 cm^2 correctly classified 83% of patients. Indexing EOAproj to body surface area improved the discriminatory value with an EOAproj ≤ 0.55 cm^2/m^2 correctly classifying 91% of patients. All patients with TSAS were identified using an EOAproj ≤ 0.55 cm^2/m^2. The discriminatory ability of EOAproj was superior to that achieved using previously pro-posed indices during dobutamine challenge (Fig. 3.1). The discriminatory ability of EOAproj may, however, be worse if there is minimal increase in transvalvular flow (<15%) during dobutamine challenge due to the difficulty in accurately measuring valve compliance over a narrow range of transvalvular flow rates.[18]

The utility of the EOAproj to identify the determinants of survival, functional status, and change in LVEF during follow-up of patients with LFLG-AS was investigated by the same group using the Duke Activity Status Index. Significant predictors of mortality

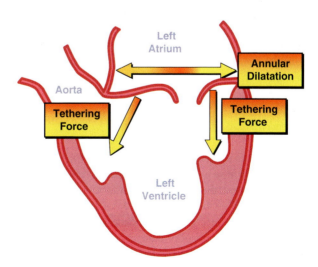

Fig. 3.1 The abnormal mitral valve apparatus in a dilated heart (*CT* chordae tendinae; *MV* mitral valve; *PM* papillary muscle

during follow-up were a Duke Activity Status Index ≤20 ($p=0.0005$) or 6-min walk test distance ≤320 m ($p<0.0001$, EOAproj at a normal transvalvular flow rate ≤1.2 cm^2 ($p=0.03$), and peak dobutamine stress echocardiography LVEF ≤35% ($p=0.03$). The Duke Activity Status Index, 6-min walk test, and LVEF improved significantly during follow-up in the AVR group, but remained unchanged or decreased in the no-AVR group.[26]

Implications of Contractile Reserve Using Dobutamine on Prognosis

Dobutamine challenge can provide additional information on the presence or absence of LV contractile reserve, a strong predictor of both perioperative mortality rate and long-term survival of patients with LFLG-AS.[19,20,22,27] Several measures have been used to define contractile reserve, including an improvement in wall motion score,[21] EF,[28] transvalvular flow rate,[29] or stroke volume[22,27] during dobutamine challenge. The impact of contractile reserve on clinical outcome has been most extensively studied using the change in stroke volume during dobutamine challenge. An absence of contractile reserve, defined as a <20% increase in stroke volume during dobutamine challenge, has been associated with a perioperative mortality rate of 33% after AVR.[19,20,22,27] In contrast, perioperative mortality rate was only 5–8% in patients with contractile reserve, defined as a ≥20% increase in stroke volume during dobutamine challenge.[19,20,22,27] The lack of contractile reserve was the strongest predictor of operative mortality with an odds ratio of 10.9 in the largest series of LFLG-AS patients.[27,30]

The presence of contractile reserve is also a strong predictor of long-term survival. In 136 patients with LFLG-AS (median AVA=0.7 cm^2, $\Delta P_{mean}=29$ mmHg and cardiac index=0.11 L/min/m^2), 3-year survival after AVR was 79% in patients with contractile reserve compared with only 35% in patients with no contractile reserve.[27] Furthermore, patients with contractile reserve did significantly better with AVR than medical management, which had a poor 3-year survival of <25%.[27] The presence of contractile reserve and AVR were the only two independent predictors of long-term survival with hazard ratios of 0.4 and 0.3, respectively.[20,27]

Thus, the absence of contractile reserve should not be used to preclude surgery, but rather to identify the patient with a higher operative mortality rate and reduced long-term survival who may still benefit from AVR.

Paradoxical LFLG-AS with Preserved EF

Recent studies suggest that subset of patients with severe AS on the basis of AVA area may paradoxically have a relatively low gradient despite the presence of a preserved LVEF. In the same context, the clinical observation that an important proportion of elderly patients with severe AS on the basis of AVA calculations (e.g., indexed AVA <0.6 cm^2/m^2) tend to have low gradients (e.g., mean gradient <30 mmHg) despite a preserved LVEF (>50%).[31] The clinical management of these patients can be confusing and raises the specter of the reliability of the Doppler measurements although the same patients are often symptomatic.

The problem may be further compounded when these patients may be sent to cardiac catheterization, where the signs of AS severity may be masked by the presence of concomitant hypertension.[32] This may lead to a situation in which symptomatic patients without a clear indication for surgery are left with no treatment strategy.

Hachicha et al[31] retrospectively studied the clinical and Doppler echocardiographic data of 512 consecutive patients with severe AS (indexed AVA ≤ 0.6 cm^2/m^2) and preserved LVEF ($\geq 50\%$). Of these patients, 65% had normal LV flow output defined as a stroke volume index >35 mL/m^2, and 35% had paradoxically low-flow output defined as stroke volume index ≤ 35 mL/m^2. When compared with normal flow patients, low-flow patients were females with a lower transvalvular gradient (32 ± 17 vs. 40 ± 15 mmHg; $p<0.001$), a lower LV diastolic volume index, a lower LVEF (62 ± 8 vs. $68 \pm 7\%$; $p<0.001$), a higher level of LV global afterload reflected by a higher valvulo-arterial impedance (represents the valvular and arterial factors that oppose ventricular ejection by absorption of the mechanical energy developed by the LV), and a lower overall 3-year survival (76 vs. 86%; $p=0.006$). Only age, valvulo-arterial impedance and medical treatment were independently associated with increased mortality.[31]

3.1.1.4
Management and Predictors of Outcome

When symptoms develop, mortality rises sharply; so standard therapeutic guidelines recommend surgery.[10,33] No effective drug treatment exists for severe AS, and only a few drugs are available to alleviate symptoms. Patients with evidence of pulmonary congestion can benefit from cautious treatment with digitalis,diuretics, or both. In addition, the afterload reduction caused by angiotensin-converting enzyme inhibitors is partially blunted by a parallel increase in the transvalvular pressure gradient. However, angiotensin-converting enzyme inhibitors favorably affect stress hemodynamic variables in most hypertensive patients with AS.[4] A prospective, single-blinded study showed that in patients with acute pulmonary edema, LV systolic dysfunction, and severe AS, nitroprusside infusion may help to reduce congestion and improve symptoms.[34] Atrial fibrillation has an adverse effect on atrial pump function and ventricular rate; hence, prompt cardioversion is beneficial. The association of AS with clinical features similar to atherosclerosis has led to the hypothesis that aggressive modification of risk factors, as for coronary heart disease, may slow or prevent disease progression in the valve leaflets. Despite this hope, recent reports using statins have shown mixed results: one study failed to show a beneficial effect, whereas another study showed that rosuvastatin can slow the hemodynamic progression of AS.[35,36]

Aortic Valve Replacement: Predictors of Outcome

AS is a mechanical obstruction, hence requires mechanical correction. Studies have shown that once symptoms develop, a patient's life span is severely shortened unless the valve is replaced.[4,6,10] Therefore, in the absence of any serious comorbid conditions, AVR is indicated in virtually all symptomatic patients with severe AS, even in the very elderly. Once heart failure supervenes, AVR should be performed as soon as the patient is medically stable.[10] Balloon valvuloplasty is not recommended in adults but can be used as a bridge to surgery in hemodynamically unstable patients who are at high risk when contemplating noncardiac surgery.[33] Preliminary reports show that percutaneous AVR is feasible, but this procedure is restricted to in-protocol management in select centers only; its role is evolving as data accrues.[37]

In patients with LV dysfunction and severe AS, the outcome after valve replacement is excellent despite a low preoperative EF. Excessive afterload may contribute to the LV dysfunction, which often returns to normal once obstruction is relieved.[4,38] In a systematic review of the outcome of AVR in patients with AS, increase in EF after surgery is more pronounced in patients with a low preoperative EF ($28\pm4.3\%$ preop vs. $40\pm9.4\%$ 6–41 months follow-up). Patients with normal or high preoperative EF have variable outcomes. However, regression of LV mass is uniformly achieved regardless of age, gender, or type of valve prosthesis used.[38]

AVR should be considered in LFLG-AS patients with TSAS, but avoided in patients with PSAS as the valve stenosis is not the primary problem. Perioperative mortality rates for patients with LFLG-AS have ranged from 8 to 33% in various studies.[19,39–41] Advanced age,[39] prior myocardial infarction,[41] mean pressure gradient <20 mmHg[27] and the absence of LV contractile reserve[22,27,40] are preoperative patient characteristics predictive of a higher operative mortality rate. Survival 3–5 years after AVR has ranged from 39 to 78%[39,40] with coronary artery disease[39] and the lack of contractile reserve[27,40] predictive of a worse longer-term outcome. However, the lack of contractile reserve should not be interpreted as an absolute contraindication to AVR as the majority of survivors will have an improvement in symptoms and LV function. This was enforced by a recent European multicenter trial by Levy et al[30] In a total of 217 consecutive patients with LFLG-AS severe AS who underwent AVR between 1990 and 2005, perioperative mortality was 16% and decreased dramatically from 20% in the 1990–1999 period compared to 10% in the 2000–2005 period. Higher European System for Cardiac Operative Risk Evaluation score (EuroSCORE), very low mean gradient and EF, New York Heart Association functional class III or IV, history of CHF, and multivessel coronary artery disease were associated with perioperative mortality. On multivariate analysis, very low preoperative mean gradient and multivessel coronary artery disease were predictors of excess perioperative mortality. In the subgroup of patients with dobutamine stress echocardiography, the absence of contractile reserve was a strong predictor of perioperative mortality.[30]

Potentially modifiable factors related to the operative procedure have also been associated with worse perioperative and long-term outcomes. Connolly et al[39] identified smaller aortic prosthesis size as an independent risk factor for perioperative mortality. This increased risk may have been a result of prosthesis–patient mismatch, which has been identified as an independent predictor of perioperative mortality in patients undergoing AVR, especially in those patients with LV dysfunction.[42] Furthermore, prosthesis–patient mismatch, defined as an indexed EOA ≤0.85 cm^2/m^2, had a negative impact on the long-term outcome of LFLG-AS patients with an observed increased incidence of CHF or CHF-related death, less LV mass regression, and a trend toward increased late mortality.[43] Thus, it appears that patients with LFLG-AS are sensitive to increased

LV afterload, and a failure to adequately reduce afterload with AVR will result in a worse outcome. Further investigation is needed to determine whether more extensive surgical procedures such as enlargement of the aortic root or implantation of a stentless prosthesis with the associated improved hemodynamics can lead to improved outcomes.[44]

Postoperative Heart Failure

Despite early symptomatic improvement following AVR for AS, there is a significant incidence of late CHF despite early improvement.[2,45] The cause of this is likely multifactorial related to intrinsic and extrinsic patient factors. In patients who had obtained complete freedom from functional disability 1 year after AVR, the recurrence of CHF noted at 10-year follow up is exclusively related to the starting point (i.e., to advanced symptomatic disease before the operation). Almost two-thirds of deaths occurring more than 12 years after AVR, when the late excess mortality becomes prevalent, are caused by CHF.[2,46,47] This was enforced recently by Vanky et al[48] In addition to the previously mentioned preoperative factors, four preoperative (hypertension, history of CHF, pulmonary hypertension, preoperative hemodynamic instability) and two intraoperative (aortic cross-clamp time, intraoperative myocardial infarction) variables were identified as independent risk factors for postoperative heart failure. Interestingly, patient–prosthesis mismatch did not influence the risk of postoperative heart failure.[48]

3.1.2
Aortic Regurgitation

The most common cause of aortic regurgitation (AR) in developing countries is rheumatic disease, with clinical presentation in the second or third decade of life. Commonly, an acute presentation of AR occurs and is attributable to endocarditis or aortic dissection.[49,50] Other common disorders of the aortic root leading to AR include idiopathic dilatation, Marfan syndrome, or aortopathy associated with a bicuspid aortic valve.[49,51] The overall prevalence of AR was 4.9% in the Framingham Heart Study[52] and 10% in the Strong Heart Study[53]; the prevalence of AR of moderate or greater severity was 0.5 and 2.7%, respectively.[54]

3.1.2.1
Pathophysiology and Compensation for Volume Overload

In AR, both volume overload and pressure overload occurs.[51] The volume overload results in compensatory eccentric hypertrophy, whereas the pressure overload results in superimposed concentric hypertrophy. The compensatory hypertrophy normalizes the mass-to-volume ratio in the compensated stages of the disease. Through chamber dilatation, the LV accommodates the increased end-diastolic volume without an increase in end-diastolic pressure. If preload reserve or compensatory hypertrophy is inadequate, however, further increases in afterload result in afterload mismatch, with a reduction in systolic performance and subsequent reduction in EF.[51,55] Depressed LV EF is initially a reversible process due to the afterload mismatch.[47] If the onset of severe AR is rapid with acute pulmonary edema supervening, detection of the clinical findings can be challenging because the bedside findings of severe AR may be absent. There is a sudden and severe increase in LV diastolic pressure but relatively little change in aortic pressure or pulse contour. Forward stroke volume is reduced, so heart rate rises to preserve cardiac output. The LV becomes hyperdynamic but cannot respond in the short term with dilataion in an effort to lower the LVEDP.[56] LVEDP and LA pressure and pulmonary venous pressures all rise acutely resulting in pulmonary edema.

3.1.2.2
Evaluation of AR

Classifying the severity of regurgitation is the first step in evaluating patients with AR.[11] Clinical findings of a hyperdynamic state with bounding pulses are easily recognized.[49,50] Doppler echocardiography has become the mainstay of the assessment of the severity of AR. Uncommonly transesophageal echocardiography or angiography of the aortic root is necessary to determine the severity of AR. LV size and function (particularly, the end-systolic diameter and EF) should be routinely assessed, as should dilatation of the ascending aorta. Exercise testing may be warranted in asymptomatic patients with limited physical activity to evaluate functional limitations and may also provide information about changes of LV function with stress.[50,57]

3.1.2.3
Management and Predictors of Outcome

Symptomatic patients with chronic severe AR managed nonsurgically have a mortality rate greater than 10% per year.[56,57] In contrast, asymptomatic patients with severe AR fair better over the long term with an observed rate of sudden death of less than 0.2% per year. Once symptoms of dyspnea, anginal, presyncope, or syncope develop, the average survival is only 3–5 years. The rate of progression to depressed LV EF (without symptoms) is less than 3.5% per year, and the rate of progression to symptoms (usually, heart failure) without LV dysfunction is less than 6% per year. Once systolic dysfunction supervenes, the rate of progression to cardiac symptoms is greater than 25% per year.[2,49]

Aortic Valve Replacement: Predictors of Outcome

Surgery relieves the AR but is not appropriate for all patients because of the defined risks of the procedure and complications that can result from the aortic prostheses or anticoagulation.[49,50] There are no data from randomized trials comparing surgical management of AR with nonsurgical therapy, and data on the benefits and risks of surgery are derived only from observational studies. These studies have demonstrated lower morbidity and mortality among high-risk patients who undergo surgery than among those who do not.[49,50,54] The severity of regurgitation, the symptoms and degree of functional impairment, the degree of LV dysfunction, and the degree of aortic enlargement are central to clinical decision making.[50] Recommendations for operative thresholds in patients with AR pivot on symptoms, exercise testing, LVEF, LV systolic dimensions, changes in LV dimensions, and serial evaluations. Any symptoms of CHF represent a class I indication for surgery.[10,33]

In cases of acute AR, the decision for urgent AVR is clear. The decision to proceed with aortic valve surgery for chronic AR remains controversial and difficult because (1) a large number of patients do well in the long term without surgery, (2) patients undergoing aortic valve surgery after the onset of severe LV decompensation are less likely to improve symptomatically and are at increased risk of developing advanced heart failure within 5 years after surgery, and (3) asymptomatic patients who have AR may progress to irreversible LV dysfunction without perceptible symptomatic deterioration.[2] Thus, asymptomatic or minimally symptomatic patients who have AR should be prospectively identified and offered aortic valve surgery prior to the occurrence of irreversible LV dysfunction. Several studies show that the overwhelming majority of symptomatic patients at risk of death from heart failure after operation have preoperative LV systolic dysfunction. In symptomatic patients undergoing aortic valve surgery for AR, the postoperative survival, incidence of postoperative CHF, and likelihood of postoperative reversal of LV dilation can be predicted on the basis of preoperative LV systolic function, systolic size, and systolic wall stress.[2] These same variables also identify asymptomatic patients who have severe chronic AR and normal LV systolic function and who are likely to require AR over the course of the next 4 years because of the development of symptoms or the onset of LV dysfunction.[2,58] In spite of these surveillance recommendations and close follow up, there remains a poorly studied subset of patients who receive no survival benefit from the surgery and their long-term results are not as good.[2] LV systolic dysfunction at rest is a sensitive means of detecting patients at risk, it is not specific, and improvement and even normalization LV systolic function can occur in patients after operation despite severe depression of systolic function before operation. LV function during exercise and exercise capacity has been used as additional indices to determine timing of operation for AR and provide prognostic information following surgery. Preserved exercise capacity before operation predicts improved survival after surgery and predicts postoperative reversibility of LV dysfunction. Further, abnormal EF during exercise may precede the onset of symptoms or the onset of resting LV dysfunction in many patients. However, LV dysfunction present only with exercise should not be an indication for aortic valve surgery, but may identify a group of patients who need closer surveillance for other indices of LV dysfunction.[2,57,59]

Medical Therapy

Nitroprusside and inotropic agents (dopamine or dobutamine) may be used before surgery in patients with poorly tolerated acute AR to stabilize their clinical condition. In patients with chronic severe AR and heart failure, ACE-inhibitors are the treatment of choice when surgery is contraindicated or in cases with persistent postoperative LV dysfunction. In asymptomatic patients with high blood pressure, the indication for antihypertensive treatment with vasodilators such as ACE-inhibitors or dihydropyridine calcium channel blockers is warranted. The role of vasodilators in the asymptomatic patients without high blood pressure in order to delay surgery remains unproven. In patients with severe AR, the use of beta-blockers should be used with caution because the lengthening of diastole increases the regurgitant volume. However, they can be used in patients with severe LV dysfunction.[33,58]

3.2
Mitral Valve Disease

3.2.1
Mitral Regurgitation

In addressing the current therapy for mitral regurgitation (MR), it is important to discriminate between primary and secondary (functional) MR. If this overload is severe enough and prolonged enough, it results in LV remodeling, dysfunction, pulmonary hypertension, heart failure, and eventually death.[60] An LV, previously damaged by coronary artery disease and myocardial infarction or by dilated cardiomyopathy, develops papillary muscle displacement and annular dilatation, causing the mitral valve to leak. Thus, although the treatment for primary MR is relatively straightforward, the therapy for secondary MR is considerably more controversial.[60]

3.2.1.1
Primary MR

Pathophysiology and Mechanisms of LV Decompensation

When a patient survives the acute episode of MR or has slowly progressive mitral valve disease, chronic compensation occurs, often resulting in few symptoms till LV decompensation occurs. There is also a modest increase in LV mass that contributes to the compensatory process. Eccentric hypertrophy, enhanced preload, normal wall stress, and normal contractile function allow normal LV performance.[51,60,61] Patients who have compensated MR may remain in this phase for varying periods, often for decades. If the regurgitation is severe enough, however, decompensation may eventually result. EF can be misleading as a measure of compensation in this disorder, and advanced myocardial dysfunction may occur while LVEF fraction is still well in the normal range. The causes of LV decompensation at the cellular level in this disorder are multifactorial and highly complex. The loss of contractile elements results in reduced mechanical function of the sarcomeres, with reduced sarcomere shortening and velocity of shortening at any given workload. Insufficient hypertrophy of the myocytes has also been proposed as a mechanism of eventual LV failure. Unlike patients who have pressure overload in whom mass greatly exceeds volume, in patients who have MR the ratio of mass to volume is less than 1.[51,60,61] Thus, the increase in LV wall stress that accompanies the increase in LV volume is not associated with an appropriate hypertrophic response to normalize wall stress. The increased systolic wall stress further taxes the left ventricle's contractile elements.[51,60,61] β-Adrenergic stimulation is a compensatory mechanism in all forms of heart failure that results in increased LV contractility and stroke volume. Over time, however, excessive β-adrenergic stimulation contributes to the decline in LV function. There is evidence of increased sympathetic nervous system activity in chronic MR.[51,60–62]

3.2.1.2
Evaluation of MR

Echocardiography with Doppler is the principal examination and must include an assessment of severity, mechanisms and repairability, and consequences. Several methods can be used to determine the severity of MR.[10,11] It should be emphasized that the assessment of severity should not rely entirely on one single parameter, but requires an approach integrating blood flow data from Doppler with morphologic information and careful cross-checking of the validity of such data against the consequences on LV and pulmonary pressures.[11]

3.2.1.3
Management and Predictors of Outcome

Acute MR is poorly tolerated and carries a poor prognosis in the absence of intervention. The natural history of chronic MR has greatly improved. In addition to symptoms, age, atrial fibrillation, degree of MR (particularly ERO), left atrial dilatation, LV dilatation, and low LVEF are all predictors of poor outcome.[10,33]

Medical Therapy

Vasodilators are effective in reducing regurgitant flow in acute MR. This occurs as vasodilators preferentially increase the forward flow while reducing the regurgitant flow, by reducing the aortic impedance and also by reducing the regurgitant orifice area.[60,63] However, medical therapies in the form of ACE-inhibitors or angiotensin receptor blockers for chronic MR have produced conflicting results and are not recommended for the prevention of LV dysfunction in MR.[64,65] However, they should be used to manage heart failure, whether or not MR is present. Beta-blockers are effective in reversing the LV dysfunction caused by experimental MR where the mechanism is one of restoration of sarcomere structure and function.[66] Whether these results apply to humans awaits confirmation.[60]

Surgical Therapy: Indications and Timing

MR is a mechanical problem that can only be corrected with a mechanical solution by restoration of valve competence, thereby removing the volume overload and its deleterious consequences. There is near unanimity that mitral valve repair (MVP), instead of mitral valve replacement (MVR), is the preferred method of MR correction in nonrheumatic valves.[10,67,68] Most reports show a lower operative mortality with MVP compared with MVR and better long-term survival.[60,68] It is important to recognize that the mitral valve is an important component of the LV, serving a major role in LV function by helping to maintain LV shape and chamber contractility. Destruction of the mitral valve apparatus at the time of MVR causes an immediate decrease in chamber contractility and an increase in afterload as the radial measure in the Laplace equation increases.[60,69] In fact, MVP also removes the low-impedance left atrium ejection pathway but causes only minor changes in EF, indicating that the large decrease in EF after MVR is caused by destruction in the mitral valve apparatus instead of its effect on ejection into the left atrium.[60,69]

In symptomatic patients with normal LV function, ventricular function is a key determinant of outcome (as in all valvular heart disease), symptoms have a major impact on prognosis even when LV function is normal. Thus, surgery, preferably MVP, should be performed once even mild symptoms develop [10,60,70]

In asymptomatic patients with LV dysfunction, although LV function may improve after MVP it is not a guarantee, and while sophisticated measures of LV function are available, they are impractical for daily use. However, when EF normalizes towards 60% or when end-systolic dimension approaches 40 mm, postoperative outcome worsens, suggesting that these are fairly reliable markers for clinically important LV dysfunction.[18,28,29] Thus, irrespective of symptomatic status, surgery, preferably MVP, should be performed once these objective benchmarks for LV dysfunction are reached.[10,60,71]

Patients with asymptomatic severe MR with normal LV function have excellent short-term prognosis. Many clinicians would support regular observation for subjective and objective changes in LV function However, patients with severe MR are likely to develop symptoms, LV dysfunction, or atrial fibrillation within a relatively short period of time (2–3 years), especially in the face of a flail leaflet.[60,72] Evidence suggest repairing such valves shortly after discovery in centers with excellent surgical skills toward repair offers low mortality (<1% in experienced centers)[67] and reduces the risk of unwanted sequelae and the need for close longitudinal follow-up for the onset of symptoms or LV dysfunction. Indeed, the recent American Heart Association/American College of Cardiology guidelines on valvular heart disease recommend surgery for such patients at a IIa level (most would favor surgery); where there is a >90% likelihood the valve can be repaired.[10]

3.2.1.4
Secondary (Functional) MR

The pathophysiology of secondary MR is more complex in comparison to the pathophysiology of primary MR. Here, myocardial damage, either through ischemic events or from dilated cardiomyopathy, results in an anatomically normal valve to leak. Even if the MR is corrected, the underlying muscle disease persists and is likely responsible for the poor prognosis in patients with secondary MR. Thus, the advantages of correction of secondary MR are less clear.[60,73]

Pathophysiology and Mechanisms of LV Decompensation

Understanding the functional anatomy of the mitral valve is fundamental to the management of MR in heart failure. The mitral valve apparatus consists of the annulus, leaflets, chordae tendineae, and papillary muscles, as well as the entire LV. Thus, the maintenance of chordal, annular, and subvalvular continuity is essential for the preservation of mitral geometric relationships and overall ventricular function. As the ventricle fails, the progressive dilatation of the LV gives rise to MR, which begets more MR and further ventricular dilatation. With postinfarction remodeling and lateral wall dysfunction, similar processes combine to result in ischemic MR. If untreated, the end result of progressive MR and global ventricular remodeling is similar regardless of the etiology of cardiomyopathy. Incomplete leaflet coaptation, loss of the zone of coaptation, and regurgitation develop secondary to alterations in the annular–ventricular apparatus and ventricular geometry.[2,74] As more mitral leaflet tissue is used for the closure of the mitral valve orifice, a critical reduction in leaflet tissue available for coaptation is reached so that there is no longer an established zone of coaptation, and a central regurgitant jet of insufficiency begins to develop. This pathologic process has been referred to as "functional" MR. Thus, reconstruction of this geometric abnormality serves to not only restore valvular competency but also improve ventricular function (Fig. 3.1).[2,75,76] It is clear that the presence of MR in ischemic and dilated cardiomyopathies worsens prognosis.[60,73]

3.2.1.5
Evaluation

Echocardiographic examination is useful for establishing the diagnosis and differentiating true functional MR, where valves are normal; from primary MR. The use of quantitative methods adds important information (Table 3.2). In ischemic MR, lower thresholds of severity, using quantitative methods, have been proposed (20 mm^2 for ERO and 30 mL for regurgitant volume).[33,77]

3.2.1.6
Management and Predictors of Outcome

Because the MR is not the primary problem, the indications for mitral valve intervention are less certain. Although the treatment for primary MR is relatively straightforward, the therapy for secondary MR is considerably more controversial.[60]

Medical Therapy

It must be recognized that almost all patients with secondary MR have heart failure and should be treated with standard heart failure therapy, which typically includes ACE-inhibitors (or angiotensin receptor blockers), beta-blockers, diuretics, and aldosterone

Table 3.2 Classification of the MR severity (adapted from[10,11])

	Mild	Moderate	Severe
Qualitative			
Angiographic grade	1+	2+	3–4+
Color Doppler jet area	Small, central jet (less than 4 cm² or less than 20% LA area)	Signs of MR greater than mild present, but no criteria for severe MR	Vena contracta width greater than 0.7 cm with large central MR jet (area greater than 40% of LA area) or with a wall-impinging jet of any size, swirling in LA
Doppler vena contracta width (cm)	Less than 0.3	0.3–0.69	Greater than or equal to 0.70
Quantitative (cath or echo)			
Regurgitant volume (mL/beat)	Less than 30	30–59	Greater than or equal to 60
Regurgitant fraction (%)	Less than 30	30–49	Greater than or equal to 50
Regurgitant orifice area (cm²)	Less than 0.20	0.2–0.39	Greater than or equal to 0.40
Additional essential criteria			
Left atrial size			Enlarged
Left ventricular size			Enlarged

antagonists. Although these agents may alter regurgitant volume, their major thrust is at the antecedent heart failure.[33,60]

Cardiac Resynchronization Therapy

LV dilatation, distortion, and dyssynchrony are linked to functional MR in patients with heart failure and LV dysfunction. Thus, in patients with increased QRS duration and intra-ventricular asynchrony, cardiac resynchronization therapy may reduce MR severity and improve LV function.[33,78,79]

Surgical Therapy

In treating patients with heart failure, the most significant determinant of leaflet coaptation and MR is the diameter of the mitral valve annulus. The LV dimension is of less importance in functional MR, because the lengths of the chordae and papillary muscles are similar in myopathic hearts regardless of the presence of MR. The complex relationship between mitral annular area and leaflet coaptation may thus explain why an undersized "valvular" repair may help a "ventricular" problem. This restoration of the mitral apparatus and ventricle is the basis for geometric mitral reconstruction for the treatment of heart failure.[2]

Partial correction of secondary MR using a restrictive annuloplasty ring has been successful.[80] By reducing annular diameter, this simple procedure significantly reduced the amount of MR present and was well tolerated with an operative mortality of <5%. A 75% 1-year survival was noted,[80] In the Acorn trial, patients with secondary MR were randomized to receive either MVP alone or MVP plus an external restraint device. Importantly, substantial reverse remodeling occurred in the MVP only group, as it has in other reports.[60,81,82]

Question is whether surgery in ischemic MR improves survival and/or long-term quality of life.[60,83] It is clear from the conflicting published literature that a large randomized trial is needed to identify the role of MVR and MVP in the treatment of patients with secondary MR.[60] Indications of surgery in ischemic MR are incorporated in current European guidelines,[33] including severe MR with LVEF >30% undergoing CABG, moderate MR undergoing CABG if repair is feasible, severe symptomatic MR with LVEF <30% and an option for CABG and finally with severe MR, LVEF >30% with no option for CABG, refractory to medial therapy and low comorbidities.[33]

In coronary revascularization alone vs. combined revascularization and mitral surgery, general consensus suggests correction of severe MR during coronary revascularization surgery, but no convincing data supports this practice.[60,84,85] The first human percutaneous MVPs have been performed using either implants introduced via the coronary sinus or stitches mimicking the Alfieri operation (edge-to-edge method) introduced transseptally. Further evaluation is needed before defining the potential role of these approaches.[33,86,87]

3.2.2
Mitral Stenosis

Rheumatic fever as a leading cause of valvular heart disease has declined over the last 50 years. Mitral stenosis (MS) is the major valvular sequelae of rheumatic fever observed in adults. Although there are numerous other causes of MS, including severe mitral annular calcification, carcinoid tumor, methylsergide therapy, Fabry's disease, Whipple's disease, systemic lupus erythematous, and mucopolysaccharidosis, more than 99% of MS is still due to prior rheumatic disease.[88,89]

3.2.2.1
Evaluation

Echocardiography remains the most common method to assess the severity and consequences of MS, valve morphology, as well as the extent of anatomic lesions. Severity of

MS should be quantified using two-dimensional planimetry and the pressure half-time method, which are complementary approaches for measuring valve area. In patients with no or doubtful symptoms, stress testing aids decision making by unmasking symptoms. Exercise echocardiography provides other information by assessing the evolution of mitral gradient and pulmonary pressures.[10,33,90]

3.2.2.2
CHF with MS

The overwhelming majority of patients presenting with hemodynamically significant MS have preserved LV wall thickness, LV volume, and systolic and diastolic function in the absence of associated coronary artery disease.[2,91] Symptoms of CHF are due to elevated pulmonary venous pressures as a result of obstruction to blood flow at the level of the mitral valve. Patients with long-standing hemodynamically significant MS may develop fixed and elevated pulmonary vascular resistance. As pulmonary vascular resistance rises, the pulmonary arteriolar bed becomes protected from sudden elevations in pressure associated with exertion, with the result that pulmonary edema does not occur, and patients subsequently experience less symptoms of dyspnea. These patients, however, develop symptoms of right-heart failure including peripheral coldness, cyanosis, hepatic enlargement and pulsation, elevated jugular venous pressure, ascites, and peripheral edema. The risk of valve surgery in these patients is a consequence of pulmonary hypertension and right-heart dysfunction and not the failure of the LV.

The prevalence of LV dysfunction with MS is controversial. Much of the research performed on this topic is several decades old secondary because of the declining prevalence of rheumatic heart disease. Although it is generally believed that LV contractility is normal in most cases of MS,[92] some studies have suggested otherwise. Several studies have reported that the prevalence of a reduced LVEF in patients with pure MS may be as high as 33%.[89]

In some patients with long-standing MS, mild to modest degrees of posterobasal regional wall contraction abnormalities may develop and may be attributed to a rigid mitral valve annulus and subvalvular apparatus.[2,93] However, significant impairment of LV function in association with hemodynamically significant MS requiring operative treatment is an unusual finding but is present in a small proportion of elderly patients. These patients have severe posterobasal segmental wall contraction abnormalities, anterolateral segmental contraction abnormalities, or diffuse hypokinesis.[2,93–96] The basis for the regional wall motion abnormalities may be related to diffuse scarring and retraction of the papillary muscles, and/or markedly decreased compliance of the LV. Chronic low cardiac output with significantly decreased coronary flow reserves may contribute to diffuse hypokinesis and decreased LV compliance.[89]

3.2.2.3
Management and Predictors of Outcome

In patients with mitral stenosis, symptoms of right-sided heart failure usually resolve with the appropriate management. The treatment of MS with LV dysfunction, the only invasive treatment that works well, involves chordal excision.[89,97] No studies have provided clear evidence of improved ejection performance after surgical therapy. Little data exists regarding the outcomes in patients who have reduced EF with MVR.[89] Medical therapy of these conditions is currently limited. Although standard of care involves β-blockade for prolongation of diastolic filling time, which also provides benefit in LV dysfunction, there is data regarding ACE inhibition. Regardless, a reduced EF does not appear to alter long-term outcomes, either surgical or percutaneous.[89]

3.3
Tricuspid Valve Disease

3.3.1
Tricuspid Regurgitation

Trivial tricuspid regurgitation (TR) is frequently detected by echocardiography in normal subjects. Pathological TR is more often functional rather than due to a primary valve lesion. Functional TR is due to annular dilatation and secondary to right ventricular pressure and/or volume overload. Predominant symptoms are those of associated diseases and even severe TR may be well tolerated for many years. Although load-dependent, clinical signs of right heart failure are of value in evaluating the severity of TR.[33,98] Echocardiography is the ideal technique to evaluate TR.[11] Evaluation of the right ventricle and measurement of peak right ventricular systolic pressure as an estimate of pulmonary pressure are crucial for complete echocardiographic assessment of TR.[11,33]

The limited data that are available on the natural history of primary TR suggest that severe TR has a poor prognosis even if it is well tolerated for years.[33] Functional TR may diminish or disappear as right ventricular failure improves following the treatment of its cause. However, TR may persist even after successful correction of left-sided lesions. Predicting the evolution of functional TR after surgical treatment of mitral valve disease remains a challenge.[99] Pulmonary hypertension, increased right ventricular pressure and dimension, reduced right ventricular function, and the diameter of the tricuspid annulus are important risk factors for persistence or late worsening of TR.[100,101] However, TR may persist even after successful correction of left-sided lesions.[33]

3.3.1.1
Management and Predictors of Outcome

The timing of surgical intervention and the appropriate technique remain controversial mostly because of the limited data available and their heterogeneous nature (Table 3.1).[33] As general principles, if technically possible, conservative surgery is preferable to valve replacement, and surgery should be carried out early enough to avoid irreversible right ventricular dysfunction. The possible need for correction of TR is usually considered at the time of surgical correction of left-sided valvular lesions. In these circumstances, the relative simplicity of tricuspid valve repair and the high risk of secondary surgical correction are incentives to earlier indications for tricuspid repair. Surgery limited to the tricuspid valve can be required in patients with severe primary TR resulting from endocarditis or trauma who remain symptomatic or in those with mild symptoms who have objective signs of significant impairment of right ventricular function. Medical therapy in the form of diuretics improve signs of congestion; however, specific treatment directed to the underlying disease is warranted.[33]

3.3.2
Tricuspid Stenosis

Tricuspid stenosis (TS), which is almost exclusively of rheumatic origin, is rarely observed in developed countries, although it is still seen in developing countries.[33,102] Detection requires careful evaluation, as it is almost always associated with left-sided valve lesions that dominate the presentation. Clinical signs are often masked by those of the associated valvular lesions, especially MS.[98] Echocardiography provides the most useful information. TS is often overlooked and requires careful evaluation.[33]

3.3.2.1
Management and Predictors of Outcome

In the presence of heart failure, diuretics are useful but of limited efficacy. Intervention on the tricuspid valve is usually carried out at the time of intervention on the other valves in patients who are symptomatic despite medical therapy. Conservative surgery or valve replacement, according to anatomy and surgical expertise in valve repair, is preferred to balloon commissurotomy.[33,103]

3.3.3
Ebstein Anomaly

Ebstein anomaly is a spectrum of tricuspid valve and right ventricular dysplasia. The TV usually is insufficient but occasionally can be stenotic. Atrial septal defect or patent foramen ovale occurs in 30–70% of cases, and ventricular preexcitation is associated with approximately 15% of cases.[104] Less commonly, LV dysfunction and ventricular septal defects can be part of the anomaly. Morbidity and mortality are thought to be related to the degree of TR or TS; the size, thickness, and function of the right ventricle; and the presence or absence of an ASD.[104] In two recently published retrospective studies by the Mayo Clinic, the medical records of 539 patients with Ebstein anomaly were reviewed from 1972 to 2006. Ebstein anomaly can be surgically treated with low perioperative mortality.[105,106] Patients have good long-term survival and functional outcomes after surgery. Both tricuspid valve repair and tricuspid valve replacement are associated with good long-term survival. Risk factors for poorer outcome include right or left ventricular systolic dysfunction, increased hematocrit values, male gender, right ventricular outflow tract obstruction, or hypoplastic pulmonary arteries.[105,106]

3.4
Pulmonary Valve Disease

3.4.1
Pulmonary Regurgitation

The deleterious effect of chronic pulmonary regurgitation (PR) is most clearly seen in the syndrome of exercise intolerance or arrhythmias associated with low pressure dilated right ventricles after repair of tetralogy of Fallot. During surgical repair, these patients may have received a transannular patch, compounded by damage to the right ventricular outflow tract caused by a ventriculotomy, right ventricular patching, extensive muscle resection, or damage to coronary branches. Although PR is a major mechanism, the right ventricular dilatation is often multifactorial in origin. The management strategy in this group of patients has generally been directed to first relieve obstructive lesions and subsequently turning attention to dealing with volume loading when dilatation is progressive. Homografts, valved conduits and xenograft valves all have limited durability and these patients require multiple procedures during their lifetime. Percutaneous pulmonary valve insertion is an important technological advancement, but the long-term fate of the first generation valves remains unclear. In addition to finding improved materials for valve replacement, the major challenge lies in timing an intervention on a dilating ventricle and the management of these patients during the periods of recurrent progressive volume overload in the intervals between procedures. Markers of the reversibility of ventricular dilatation remain elusive.[107]

3.4.2
Congenital Pulmonary Stenosis

Obstruction may occur at the valvular, subvalvular, or supravalvular levels. Regardless of the level of obstruction, the right ventricle undergoes significant hypertrophy, the degree of which varies with the magnitude of obstruction, which ultimately may lead to right ventricular dysfunction and failure. Relief of the obstruction leads to improvement of symptoms and right ventricular function. Percutaneous balloon valvulopasty is increasingly becoming an option in appropriate patient subsets.[108]

References

1. Sarris GE, Cahill PD, Hansen DE, Derby GC, Miller DC. Restoration of left ventricular systolic performance after reattachment of the mitral chordae tendineae. The importance of valvular-ventricular interaction. *J Thorac Cardiovasc Surg*. 1988;95(6):969-979.
2. Spoor MT, Bolling SF. Valve pathology in heart failure: which valves can be fixed? *Heart Fail Clin*. 2007;3(3):289-298.

3. Lung B, Baron G, Butchart EG, et al. A prospective survey of patients with valvular heart disease in Europe: The Euro Heart Survey on Valvular Heart Disease. *Eur Heart J.* 2003; 24(13):1231-1243.

4. Ramaraj R, Sorrell VL. Degenerative aortic stenosis. *BMJ.* 2008;336(7643):550-555.

5. Cosmi JE, Kort S, Tunick PA, et al. The risk of the development of aortic stenosis in patients with "benign" aortic valve thickening. *Arch Intern Med.* 2002;162(20):2345-2347.

6. Dal-Bianco JP, Khandheria BK, Mookadam F, Gentile F, Sengupta PP. Management of asymptomatic severe aortic stenosis. *J Am Coll Cardiol.* 2008;52(16):1279-1292.

7. Nkomo VT, Gardin JM, Skelton TN, Gottdiener JS, Scott CG, Enriquez-Sarano M. Burden of valvular heart diseases: a population-based study. *Lancet.* 2006;368(9540):1005-1011.

8. Rosenhek R, Klaar U, Schemper M, et al. Mild and moderate aortic stenosis. Natural history and risk stratification by echocardiography. *Eur Heart J.* 2004;25(3):199-205.

9. Stewart BF, Siscovick D, Lind BK, et al. Clinical factors associated with calcific aortic valve disease. Cardiovascular Health Study. *J Am Coll Cardiol.* 1997;29(3):630-634.

10. Bonow RO, Carabello BA, Chatterjee K, et al. ACC/AHA 2006 guidelines for the management of patients with valvular heart disease: a report of the American College of Cardiology/ American Heart Association Task Force on Practice Guidelines (writing Committee to Revise the 1998 guidelines for the management of patients with valvular heart disease) developed in collaboration with the Society of Cardiovascular Anesthesiologists endorsed by the Society for Cardiovascular Angiography and Interventions and the Society of Thoracic Surgeons. *J Am Coll Cardiol.* 2006;48(3):e1-e148.

11. Zoghbi WA, Enriquez-Sarano M, Foster E, et al. Recommendations for evaluation of the severity of native valvular regurgitation with two-dimensional and Doppler echocardiography. *J Am Soc Echocardiogr.* 2003;16(7):777-802.

12. Carabello BA. Aortic stenosis: from pressure overload to heart failure. *Heart Fail Clin.* 2006;2(4):435-442.

13. Zile MR, Gaasch WH. Heart failure in aortic stenosis - improving diagnosis and treatment. *N Engl J Med.* 2003;348(18):1735-1736.

14. Bergler-Klein J, Klaar U, Heger M, et al. Natriuretic peptides predict symptom-free survival and postoperative outcome in severe aortic stenosis. *Circulation.* 2004;109(19):2302-2308.

15. Baumgartner H. Aortic stenosis: medical and surgical management. *Heart.* 2005;91(11):1483-1488.

16. Pellikka PA, Nishimura RA, Bailey KR, Tajik AJ. The natural history of adults with asymptomatic, hemodynamically significant aortic stenosis. *J Am Coll Cardiol.* 1990;15(5):1012-1017.

17. Pellikka PA, Sarano ME, Nishimura RA, et al. Outcome of 622 adults with asymptomatic, hemodynamically significant aortic stenosis during prolonged follow-up. *Circulation.* 2005; 111(24):3290-3295.

18. Blais C, Burwash IG, Mundigler G, et al. Projected valve area at normal flow rate improves the assessment of stenosis severity in patients with low-flow, low-gradient aortic stenosis: the multicenter TOPAS (Truly or Pseudo-Severe Aortic Stenosis) study. *Circulation.* 2006; 113(5):711-721.

19. Burwash IG. Low-flow, low-gradient aortic stenosis: from evaluation to treatment. *Curr Opin Cardiol.* 2007;22(2):84-91.

20. Quere JP, Monin JL, Levy F, et al. Influence of preoperative left ventricular contractile reserve on postoperative ejection fraction in low-gradient aortic stenosis. *Circulation.* 2006; 113(14):1738-1744.

21. deFilippi CR, Willett DL, Brickner ME, et al. Usefulness of dobutamine echocardiography in distinguishing severe from nonsevere valvular aortic stenosis in patients with depressed left ventricular function and low transvalvular gradients. *Am J Cardiol.* 1995;75(2):191-194.

22. Nishimura RA, Grantham JA, Connolly HM, Schaff HV, Higano ST, Holmes DR Jr. Low-output, low-gradient aortic stenosis in patients with depressed left ventricular systolic function: the clinical utility of the dobutamine challenge in the catheterization laboratory. *Circulation*. 2002;106(7):809-813.

23. Burwash IG, Hay KM, Chan KL. Hemodynamic stability of valve area, valve resistance, and stroke work loss in aortic stenosis: a comparative analysis. *J Am Soc Echocardiogr*. 2002; 15(8):814-822.

24. Blais C, Pibarot P, Dumesnil JG, Garcia D, Chen D, Durand LG. Comparison of valve resistance with effective orifice area regarding flow dependence. *Am J Cardiol*. 2001;88(1):45-52.

25. Burwash IG, Thomas DD, Sadahiro M, et al. Dependence of Gorlin formula and continuity equation valve areas on transvalvular volume flow rate in valvular aortic stenosis. *Circulation*. 1994;89(2):827-835.

26. Clavel MA, Fuchs C, Burwash IG, et al. Predictors of outcomes in low-flow, low-gradient aortic stenosis: results of the multicenter TOPAS Study. *Circulation*. 2008;118(14 suppl):S234-S242.

27. Monin JL, Quere JP, Monchi M, et al. Low-gradient aortic stenosis: operative risk stratification and predictors for long-term outcome: a multicenter study using dobutamine stress hemodynamics. *Circulation*. 2003;108(3):319-324.

28. Zuppiroli A, Mori F, Olivotto I, Castelli G, Favilli S, Dolara A. Therapeutic implications of contractile reserve elicited by dobutamine echocardiography in symptomatic, low-gradient aortic stenosis. *Ital Heart J*. 2003;4(4):264-270.

29. Schwammenthal E, Vered Z, Moshkowitz Y, et al. Dobutamine echocardiography in patients with aortic stenosis and left ventricular dysfunction: predicting outcome as a function of management strategy. *Chest*. 2001;119(6):1766-1777.

30. Levy F, Laurent M, Monin JL, et al. Aortic valve replacement for low-flow/low-gradient aortic stenosis operative risk stratification and long-term outcome: a European multicenter study. *J Am Coll Cardiol*. 2008;51(15):1466-1472.

31. Hachicha Z, Dumesnil JG, Bogaty P, Pibarot P. Paradoxical low-flow, low-gradient severe aortic stenosis despite preserved ejection fraction is associated with higher afterload and reduced survival. *Circulation*. 2007;115(22):2856-2864.

32. Otto CM. Valvular aortic stenosis: disease severity and timing of intervention. *J Am Coll Cardiol*. 2006;47(11):2141-2151.

33. Vahanian A, Baumgartner H, Bax J, et al. Guidelines on the management of valvular heart disease: The Task Force on the Management of Valvular Heart Disease of the European Society of Cardiology. *Eur Heart J*. 2007;28(2):230-268.

34. Khot UN, Novaro GM, Popovic ZB, et al. Nitroprusside in critically ill patients with left ventricular dysfunction and aortic stenosis. *N Engl J Med*. 2003;348(18):1756-1763.

35. Cowell SJ, Newby DE, Prescott RJ, et al. A randomized trial of intensive lipid-lowering therapy in calcific aortic stenosis. *N Engl J Med*. 2005;352(23):2389-2397.

36. Moura LM, Ramos SF, Zamorano JL, et al. Rosuvastatin affecting aortic valve endothelium to slow the progression of aortic stenosis. *J Am Coll Cardiol*. 2007;49(5):554-561.

37. Cribier A, Eltchaninoff H, Tron C, et al. Treatment of calcific aortic stenosis with the percutaneous heart valve: mid-term follow-up from the initial feasibility studies: the French experience. *J Am Coll Cardiol*. 2006;47(6):1214-1223.

38. Sharma UC, Barenbrug P, Pokharel S, Dassen WR, Pinto YM, Maessen JG. Systematic review of the outcome of aortic valve replacement in patients with aortic stenosis. *Ann Thorac Surg*. 2004;78(1):90-95.

39. Connolly HM, Oh JK, Schaff HV, et al. Severe aortic stenosis with low transvalvular gradient and severe left ventricular dysfunction:result of aortic valve replacement in 52 patients. *Circulation*. 2000;101(16):1940-1946.

40. Monin JL, Monchi M, Gest V, Duval-Moulin AM, Dubois-Rande JL, Gueret P. Aortic stenosis with severe left ventricular dysfunction and low transvalvular pressure gradients: risk stratification by low-dose dobutamine echocardiography. *J Am Coll Cardiol.* 2001; 37(8):2101-2107.
41. Powell DE, Tunick PA, Rosenzweig BP, et al. Aortic valve replacement in patients with aortic stenosis and severe left ventricular dysfunction. *Arch Intern Med.* 2000;160(9):1337-1341.
42. Blais C, Dumesnil JG, Baillot R, Simard S, Doyle D, Pibarot P. Impact of valve prosthesis-patient mismatch on short-term mortality after aortic valve replacement. *Circulation.* 2003; 108(8):983-988.
43. Kulik A, Burwash IG, Kapila V, Mesana TG, Ruel M. Long-term outcomes after valve replacement for low-gradient aortic stenosis: impact of prosthesis-patient mismatch. *Circulation.* 2006;114(1 suppl):I553-I558.
44. Collinson J, Flather M, Coats AJ, Pepper JR, Henein M. Influence of valve prosthesis type on the recovery of ventricular dysfunction and subendocardial ischaemia following valve replacement for aortic stenosis. *Int J Cardiol.* 2004;97(3):535-541.
45. Cohen G, David TE, Ivanov J, Armstrong S, Feindel CM. The impact of age, coronary artery disease, and cardiac comorbidity on late survival after bioprosthetic aortic valve replacement. *J Thorac Cardiovasc Surg.* 1999;117(2):273-284.
46. Lund O. Preoperative risk evaluation and stratification of long-term survival after valve replacement for aortic stenosis. Reasons for earlier operative intervention. *Circulation.* 1990; 82(1):124-139.
47. Bonow RO. Radionuclide angiography in the management of asymptomatic aortic regurgitation. *Circulation.* 1991;84(3 suppl):I296-I302.
48. Vanky FB, Hakanson E, Tamas E, Svedjeholm R. Risk factors for postoperative heart failure in patients operated on for aortic stenosis. *Ann Thorac Surg.* 2006;81(4):1297-1304.
49. Bonow RO. Aortic regurgitation. In: Zipes D, ed. *Braunwald's Heart Disease: A Textbook of Cardiovascular Medicine. Valvular Heart Disease*, 7 edn, vol 2. Philadelphia: WB Saunders; 2005:1553-1632.
50. Enriquez-Sarano M, Tajik AJ. Clinical practice. Aortic regurgitation. *N Engl J Med.* 2004;351(15):1539-1546.
51. Rigolin VH, Bonow RO. Hemodynamic characteristics and progression to heart failure in regurgitant lesions. *Heart Fail Clin.* 2006;2(4):453-460.
52. Singh JP, Evans JC, Levy D, et al. Prevalence and clinical determinants of mitral, tricuspid, and aortic regurgitation (the Framingham Heart Study). *Am J Cardiol.* 1999;83(6):897-902.
53. Lebowitz NE, Bella JN, Roman MJ, et al. Prevalence and correlates of aortic regurgitation in American Indians: the Strong Heart Study. *J Am Coll Cardiol.* 2000;36(2):461-467.
54. Klodas E, Enriquez-Sarano M, Tajik AJ, Mullany CJ, Bailey KR, Seward JB. Optimizing timing of surgical correction in patients with severe aortic regurgitation: role of symptoms. *J Am Coll Cardiol.* 1997;30(3):746-752.
55. Bonow RO. Chronic aortic regurgitation. Role of medical therapy and optimal timing for surgery. *Cardiol Clin.* 1998;16(3):449-461.
56. Stewart WJ. Optimal timing of surgery in aortic regurgitation. *Heart Fail Clin.* 2006; 2(4):461-471.
57. Borer JS, Hochreiter C, Herrold EM, et al. Prediction of indications for valve replacement among asymptomatic or minimally symptomatic patients with chronic aortic regurgitation and normal left ventricular performance. *Circulation.* 1998;97(6):525-534.
58. Scognamiglio R, Negut C, Palisi M, Fasoli G, Dalla-Volta S. Long-term survival and functional results after aortic valve replacement in asymptomatic patients with chronic severe aortic regurgitation and left ventricular dysfunction. *J Am Coll Cardiol.* 2005; 45(7):1025-1030.

59. Supino PG, Borer JS, Herrold EM, et al. Prognostic impact of systolic hypertension on asymptomatic patients with chronic severe aortic regurgitation and initially normal left ventricular performance at rest. *Am J Cardiol.* 2005;96(7):964-970.

60. Carabello BA. The current therapy for mitral regurgitation. *J Am Coll Cardiol.* 2008;52(5): 319-326.

61. Carabello BA. Progress in mitral and aortic regurgitation. *Prog Cardiovasc Dis.* 2001;43(6): 457-475.

62. Mehta RH, Supiano MA, Grossman PM, et al. Changes in systemic sympathetic nervous system activity after mitral valve surgery and their relationship to changes in left ventricular size and systolic performance in patients with mitral regurgitation. *Am Heart J.* 2004;147(4):729-735.

63. Yoran C, Yellin EL, Becker RM, Gabbay S, Frater RW, Sonnenblick EH. Mechanism of reduction of mitral regurgitation with vasodilator therapy. *Am J Cardiol.* 1979;43(4):773-777.

64. Dujardin KS, Enriquez-Sarano M, Bailey KR, Seward JB, Tajik AJ. Effect of losartan on degree of mitral regurgitation quantified by echocardiography. *Am J Cardiol.* 2001;87(5):570-576.

65. Marcotte F, Honos GN, Walling AD, et al. Effect of angiotensin-converting enzyme inhibitor therapy in mitral regurgitation with normal left ventricular function. *Can J Cardiol.* 1997;13(5):479-485.

66. Tsutsui H, Spinale FG, Nagatsu M, et al. Effects of chronic beta-adrenergic blockade on the left ventricular and cardiocyte abnormalities of chronic canine mitral regurgitation. *J Clin Invest.* 1994;93(6):2639-2648.

67. David TE. Outcomes of mitral valve repair for mitral regurgitation due to degenerative disease. *Semin Thorac Cardiovasc Surg.* 2007 Summer;19(2):116-120.

68. Jokinen JJ, Hippelainen MJ, Pitkanen OA, Hartikainen JE. Mitral valve replacement versus repair: propensity-adjusted survival and quality-of-life analysis. *Ann Thorac Surg.* 2007; 84(2):451-458.

69. Rozich JD, Carabello BA, Usher BW, Kratz JM, Bell AE, Zile MR. Mitral valve replacement with and without chordal preservation in patients with chronic mitral regurgitation. Mechanisms for differences in postoperative ejection performance. *Circulation.* 1992;86(6):1718-1726.

70. Tribouilloy CM, Enriquez-Sarano M, Schaff HV, et al. Impact of preoperative symptoms on survival after surgical correction of organic mitral regurgitation: rationale for optimizing surgical indications. *Circulation.* 1999;99(3):400-405.

71. Matsumura T, Ohtaki E, Tanaka K, et al. Echocardiographic prediction of left ventricular dysfunction after mitral valve repair for mitral regurgitation as an indicator to decide the optimal timing of repair. *J Am Coll Cardiol.* 2003;42(3):458-463.

72. Ling LH, Enriquez-Sarano M, Seward JB, et al. Clinical outcome of mitral regurgitation due to flail leaflet. *N Engl J Med.* 1996;335(19):1417-1423.

73. Trichon BH, Felker GM, Shaw LK, Cabell CH, O'Connor CM. Relation of frequency and severity of mitral regurgitation to survival among patients with left ventricular systolic dysfunction and heart failure. *Am J Cardiol.* 2003;91(5):538-543.

74. Kono T, Sabbah HN, Rosman H, Alam M, Jafri S, Goldstein S. Left ventricular shape is the primary determinant of functional mitral regurgitation in heart failure. *J Am Coll Cardiol.* 1992;20(7):1594-1598.

75. He S, Fontaine AA, Schwammenthal E, Yoganathan AP, Levine RA. Integrated mechanism for functional mitral regurgitation: leaflet restriction versus coapting force: in vitro studies. *Circulation.* 1997;96(6):1826-1834.

76. Mehra MR, Reyes P, Benitez RM, Zimrin D, Gammie JS. Surgery for severe mitral regurgitation and left ventricular failure: what do we really know? *J Card Fail.* 2008;14(2):145-150.

77. Grigioni F, Enriquez-Sarano M, Zehr KJ, Bailey KR, Tajik AJ. Ischemic mitral regurgitation: long-term outcome and prognostic implications with quantitative Doppler assessment. *Circulation.* 2001;103(13):1759-1764.

78. Breithardt OA, Sinha AM, Schwammenthal E, et al. Acute effects of cardiac resynchroniza-
    tion therapy on functional mitral regurgitation in advanced systolic heart failure. *J Am Coll
    Cardiol.* 2003;41(5):765-770.
79. St John Sutton MG, Plappert T, Abraham WT, et al. Effect of cardiac resynchronization ther-
    apy on left ventricular size and function in chronic heart failure. *Circulation.* 2003;
    107(15):1985-1990.
80. Bach DS, Bolling SF. Improvement following correction of secondary mitral regurgitation in
    end-stage cardiomyopathy with mitral annuloplasty. *Am J Cardiol.* 1996;78(8):966-969.
81. Acker MA, Bolling S, Shemin R, et al. Mitral valve surgery in heart failure: insights from the
    Acorn Clinical Trial. *J Thorac Cardiovasc Surg.* 2006;132(3):568-577, 577 e561-e564.
82. Braun J, Bax JJ, Versteegh MI, et al. Preoperative left ventricular dimensions predict reverse
    remodeling following restrictive mitral annuloplasty in ischemic mitral regurgitation. *Eur
    J Cardiothorac Surg.* 2005;27(5):847-853.
83. Mihaljevic T, Lam BK, Rajeswaran J, et al. Impact of mitral valve annuloplasty combined
    with revascularization in patients with functional ischemic mitral regurgitation. *J Am Coll
    Cardiol.* 2007;49(22):2191-2201.
84. Diodato MD, Moon MR, Pasque MK, et al. Repair of ischemic mitral regurgitation does not
    increase mortality or improve long-term survival in patients undergoing coronary artery
    revascularization: a propensity analysis. *Ann Thorac Surg.* 2004;78(3):794-799; discussion
    794-799.
85. Kang DH, Kim MJ, Kang SJ, et al. Mitral valve repair versus revascularization alone in the
    treatment of ischemic mitral regurgitation. *Circulation.* 2006;114(1 suppl):I499-I503.
86. Feldman T, Wasserman HS, Herrmann HC, et al. Percutaneous mitral valve repair using the
    edge-to-edge technique: six-month results of the EVEREST Phase I Clinical Trial. *J Am Coll
    Cardiol.* 2005;46(11):2134-2140.
87. Webb JG, Harnek J, Munt BI, et al. Percutaneous transvenous mitral annuloplasty: initial
    human experience with device implantation in the coronary sinus. *Circulation.* 2006;
    113(6):851-855.
88. Carroll JD, Sutherland JP. *Mitral stenosis in cardiology.* 2nd ed. London: Mosby Int; 2003.
89. Klein AJ, Carroll JD. Left ventricular dysfunction and mitral stenosis. *Heart Fail Clin.*
    2006;2(4):443-452.
90. Lev EI, Sagie A, Vaturi M, Sela N, Battler A, Shapira Y. Value of exercise echocardiography
    in rheumatic mitral stenosis with and without significant mitral regurgitation. *Am J Cardiol.*
    2004;93(8):1060-1063.
91. Halperin Z, Karasik A, Lewis BS, Geft IL, Gotsman MS. Echocardiographic left ventricular
    function in mitral stenosis. *Isr J Med Sci.* 1978;14(8):841-847.
92. Carabello BA. Modern management of mitral stenosis. *Circulation.* 2005;112(3):432-437.
93. Heller SJ, Carleton RA. Abnormal left ventricular contraction in patients with mitral stenosis.
    Circulation. 1970;42(6):1099-1110.
94. Bolen JL, Lopes MG, Harrison DC, Alderman EL. Analysis of left ventricular function
    in response to afterload changes in patients with mitral stenosis. *Circulation.* 1975;
    52(5):894-900.
95. Curry GC, Elliott LP, Ramsey HW. Quantitative left ventricular angiocardiographic findings
    in mitral stenosis. Detailed analysis of the anterolateral wall of the left ventricle. *Am J Cardiol.*
    1972;29(5):621-627.
96. Holzer JA, Karliner JS, O'Rourke RA, Peterson KL. Quantitative angiographic analysis of the left
    ventricle in patients with isolated rheumatic mitral stenosis. *Br Heart J.* 1973;35(5):497-502.
97. Chowdhury UK, Kumar AS, Airan B, et al. Mitral valve replacement with and without chordal
    preservation in a rheumatic population: serial echocardiographic assessment of left ventricular
    size and function. *Ann Thorac Surg.* 2005;79(6):1926-1933.

98. Vahanian A, Iung B, Pierard L, Dion R, Pepper J. Valvular heart disease. In: Camm AJ, Luscher TF, Serruys PW, eds. *The ESC Textbook of Cardiovascular Medicine.* Malden: Blackwell; 2006:625-670.
99. Porter A, Shapira Y, Wurzel M, et al. Tricuspid regurgitation late after mitral valve replacement: clinical and echocardiographic evaluation. *J Heart Valve Dis.* 1999;8(1):57-62.
100. Colombo T, Russo C, Ciliberto GR, et al. Tricuspid regurgitation secondary to mitral valve disease: tricuspid annulus function as guide to tricuspid valve repair. *Cardiovasc Surg.* 2001; 9(4):369-377.
101. Dreyfus GD, Corbi PJ, Chan KM, Bahrami T. Secondary tricuspid regurgitation or dilatation: which should be the criteria for surgical repair? *Ann Thorac Surg.* 2005;79(1):127-132.
102. Soler-Soler J, Galve E. Worldwide perspective of valve disease. *Heart.* 2000;83(6):721-725.
103. Vahanian A, Palacios IF. Percutaneous approaches to valvular disease. *Circulation.* 2004;109(13):1572-1579.
104. Dearani JA, Oleary PW, Danielson GK. Surgical treatment of Ebstein's malformation: state of the art in 2006. *Cardiol Young.* 2006;16(suppl 3):12-20.
105. Brown ML, Dearani JA, Danielson GK, et al. The outcomes of operations for 539 patients with Ebstein anomaly. *J Thorac Cardiovasc Surg.* 2008;135(5):1120-1136, 1136, e1121-1127.
106. Brown ML, Dearani JA, Danielson GK, et al. Functional status after operation for Ebstein anomaly: the Mayo Clinic experience. *J Am Coll Cardiol.* 2008;52(6):460-466.
107. Chaturvedi RR, Redington AN. Pulmonary regurgitation in congenital heart disease. *Heart.* 2007;93(7):880-889.
108. Davlouros PA, Niwa K, Webb G, Gatzoulis MA. The right ventricle in congenital heart disease. *Heart.* 2006;92(suppl 1):i27-i38.

Congenital Heart Disease

4

Konstantinos Dimopoulos, Georgios Giannakoulas,
Wei Li, and Michael A. Gatzoulis

4.1
Heart Failure and Adult Congenital Heart Disease

The American College of Cardiology/American Heart Association (ACC/AHA) and European Society of Cardiology (ESC) define heart failure as a syndrome characterized by symptoms of exercise intolerance in the presence of abnormal cardiac structure and/or function.[1-4] Heart failure is the ultimate expression of the sequelae and complications of adult congenital heart disease (ACHD), even after previous "successful" repair. Surgical or interventional repair may, in fact, appear to restore normal cardiac anatomy, but subtle abnormalities often persist and may have long-term implications.

4.1.1
The Prevalence of Exercise Intolerance in ACHD

Exercise intolerance is common in ACHD, affecting more than a third of patients in the Euro Heart Survey, a large European ACHD registry.[5] Cyanosis, pulmonary hypertension and a univentricular circulation appear to have the highest impact on exercise intolerance.[6-8] Patients with a systemic right ventricle (congenitally corrected transposition of the great arteries (TGA) or those with previous atrial switch operation for complete TGA) also tend to become severely limited in their exercise capacity after the third decade of life.[9-11] However, even "simple" lesions, such as atrial septal defects (ASDs), may cause progressive deterioration of cardiac function and often present with signs and symptoms of heart failure, albeit at a later age.[12]

Wei Li (✉)
Centre for Adult Congenital Heart Disease and Echocardiography Departmnent,
Royal Brompton Hospital, London, UK
e-mail: w.li@rbht.nhs.uk

M.Y. Henein (ed.), *Heart Failure in Clinical Practice*,
DOI: 10.1007/978-1-84996-153-0_4, © Springer-Verlag London Limited 2010

4.2
Quantification and Follow-Up of Exercise Intolerance

4.2.1
Subjective Quantification

Quantification of exercise intolerance is essential in the assessment of ACHD patients. Subjective means of assessment of exercise capacity are routinely used to describe patients' perception of their limitation. The most commonly used classification for quantifying subjective limitation in ACHD is the New York Heart Association (NYHA) or WHO classification. This is preferred by adult cardiologists as it is familiar and easy to apply. When compared to objective measures of exercise capacity, the NYHA classification was reliable to stratify ACHD patients according to their exercise capacity, but appeared to underestimate their degree of impairment.[7,8] In fact, many asymptomatic ACHD patients were found to have significantly reduced exercise capacity on cardiopulmonary exercise testing compared to normal controls.[7]

4.2.2
Objective Quantification

4.2.2.1
Cardiopulmonary Exercise Test

The best method for quantifying exercise tolerance in health and disease is cardiopulmonary exercise testing. It provides accurate objective assessment of the cardiovascular, respiratory and muscular systems and is becoming part of the routine clinical assessment of ACHD patients. Incremental protocols are used to assess indices such as the peak oxygen consumption (peak VO_2), the VE/VCO_2 slope (the slope of the regression line between ventilation and VCO_2), the anaerobic threshold and the heart rate and blood pressure response.

Peak VO_2 is the highest value of oxygen uptake recorded during maximal exercise testing and approximates the maximal aerobic power of an individual, i.e., the upper limit of oxygen utilization by the body. It is expressed in ml/kg/min and reflects the functional state of all mechanisms responsible for the transport of oxygen to the working tissues (muscles). During steady state, oxygen uptake measured at the lungs reflects the amount of oxygen used by the body. Peak VO_2 is the most used exercise parameter because it is simple to interpret and carries prognostic power both in acquired heart failure and ACHD. However, peak VO_2 can only be reliably estimated from maximal exercise tests and is limited by the ability and determination of a patient to exercise to exhaustion.

Cardiopulmonary exercise testing in a large cohort of ACHD patients demonstrated that average peak VO_2 is depressed in all ACHD groups compared to healthy subjects of similar age (Fig. 4.1) and is depressed even in asymptomatic ACHD patients (Fig. 4.2).[7] Patients with cyanotic heart disease and/or pulmonary hypertension and those with complex cardiac anatomy (univentricular hearts with protected pulmonary circulation) had the

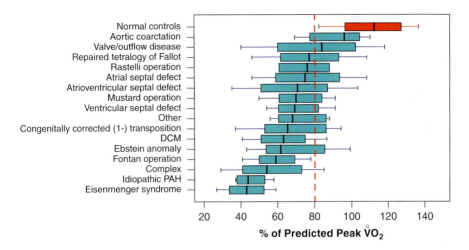

Fig. 4.1 Peak VO$_2$ in various types of ACHD and normal controls. *Boxplots* depict median and interquartile range. *Whiskers* depict range. Exercise capacity is significantly lower compared to normal controls in all ACHD groups and is lowest in patients with Eisenmenger syndrome and or complex/univentricular anatomy. A group of patients with idiopathic pulmonary hypertension is also shown for comparison. Data from Dimopoulos et al[8]

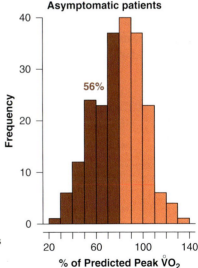

Fig. 4.2 Distribution of peak VO$_2$ in asymptomatic ACHD patients. In this asymptomatic group, 50–60% of patients have an abnormal peak VO$_2$ (less than 80% of predicted), suggesting that patients underestimate their degree of exercise intolerance. Data from Dimopoulos et al[8]

lowest peak VO$_2$ values, well below the threshold for cardiac transplantation in acquired heart disease. Abnormal pulmonary function, arrhythmias and permanent pacing were also associated with lower peak VO$_2$, while there was no relation to ventricular function. A peak VO$_2$ < 15.5 mL/kg/min was associated with a threefold increased risk of death or hospital-ization at a median follow-up of 304 days.[7] Peak circulatory power, expressed as peak exercise oxygen uptake multiplied by mean arterial blood pressure at peak exercise, has also been shown to be a strong predictor of outcome in ACHD.[13]

The anaerobic threshold is the level of VO_2 beyond which aerobic metabolism is substantially supplemented by anaerobic processes.[14,15] Above this threshold, lactate accumulates and is buffered by plasma bicarbonate, resulting in an increase in CO_2 production (VCO_2). Anaerobic threshold can be identified through analysis of the relation between VCO_2 and VO_2 relation, or the ventilation (VE)/VO_2 ratio over time. The anaerobic threshold has an obvious pathophysiologic significance, as it reflects the point after which aerobic metabolism is unable to sustain energy requirement. It also carries significant prognostic information in acquired heart failure and ACHD.[7,16–18]

The VE/VCO_2 slope is used as a measure of ventilatory efficiency. It is a simplification of the complex relationship between ventilation and CO_2 production and is calculated from data throughout exercise. It does not, thus, require maximal exertion. It reflects ventilation/perfusion mismatch and physiological dead space as well as enhanced ventilatory reflex sensitivity. It is easy to calculate, reproducible and a marker of exercise intolerance strongly related to peak VO_2. VE/VCO_2 slope is higher in all major ACHD diagnostic groups compared to normal controls.[8] Eisenmenger patients have disproportionately high VE/VCO_2 slopes, as cyanosis and pulmonary hypertension have a significant impact on ventilation efficiency (Fig. 4.3). The VE/VCO_2 slope was higher in more symptomatic patients (NYHA class 3 or more), suggesting a link between the ventilatory response to exercise and the occurrence of symptoms. Nevertheless, even asymptomatic patients had higher slopes (Fig. 4.4). In noncyanotic ACHD patients, a VE/VCO_2 slope ≥38 above is associated with a tenfold increase in the risk of death within 2 years. Pulmonary valve replacement in patients with tetralogy of Fallot appears to have a beneficial effect on the VE/VCO_2 slope, especially when surgery was performed before 17.5 years of age.[19]

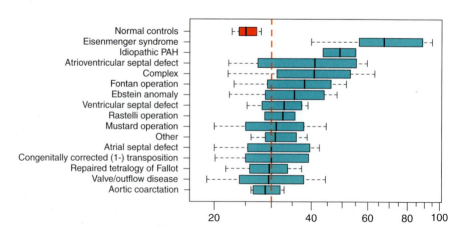

Fig. 4.3 Distribution of VE/VCO_2 slope values in ACHD patients. The VE/VCO_2 slope is significantly higher in most ACHD groups compared to normal controls and highest in the cyanotic population. Data from Dimopoulos et al[8]

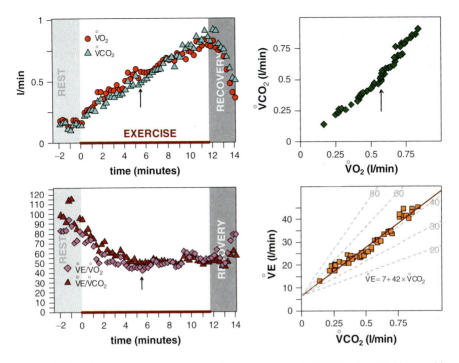

Fig. 4.4 Cardiopulmonary exercise test in a moderately symptomatic (NYHA class III) 29-year-old female patient after Fontan-type operation. The patient exercised for 12.3 min on a modified Bruce protocol and reached a respiratory exchange ratio (ratio of VCO_2/VO_2) at peak exercise of 1.11. She was not cyanotic and no desaturation was recorded during exercise. There was a blunted blood pressure (110/70 to 130/75 mmHg) and heart rate response (90–130 bpm). Peak VO_2 was 810 mL/min (20.5 mL/kg/min), which is 39% of predicted for age, sex, height and weight (*upper left panel*). VE/VCO_2 slope was 42, suggesting significant pulmonary hypoperfusion and ventilation/perfusion mismatch (*lower right panel*). Anaerobic threshold was 590 mL/min (14.8 mL/kg/min, *upper right panel*)

4.2.2.2
The 6-Minute Walk Test

The 6-minute walk test is a simple, submaximal, timed distance exercise test, easy to perform. It reflects ordinary daily activities and its main response variable is the distance covered in 6 min at the patient's own pace. Other parameters measured include oxygen saturations by portable pulse oximetry and the perceived exertion through semiquantitative scales such as the Borg scale. The 6-minute walk test should be prescribed for significantly impaired patients, since in healthy and mildly impaired individuals it is a submaximal test ("ceiling effect") and does not reflect exercise capacity (peak VO_2). A 6-minute walk test distance <450 m equates to a Grade C in the Weber classification for cardiopulmonary exercise testing (peak VO_2 between 10 and 16 mL/min/kg), and brain natriuretic peptide level >100 pg/mL.[20,21]

The 6-minute walk test distance appears to be more sensitive to changes following intervention compared to peak VO_2. It is routinely used to assess the response to advanced therapies in patients with pulmonary hypertension and is the only test approved by the U.S. Food and Drug Administration (FDA) as an endpoint for prospective clinical trials in this population. Adequate standardization of the protocol used is essential for guaranteeing reproducibility and comparability of repeat tests. A significant "learning effect" has also been described and should be kept in mind when comparing the first with subsequent tests.

4.3
Mechanisms of Heart Failure in ACHD

Exercise intolerance and heart failure may occur through a variety of mechanisms in ACHD, both cardiac and extracardiac.

4.3.1
Cardiac Causes of Exercise Intolerance in ACHD

Cardiac output is the product of stroke volume and heart rate. A reduction in cardiac output may occur through a reduction in ventricular function (reduced stroke volume) or through inability to increase heart rate to meet demands. Myocardial dysfunction is common in ACHD and can be caused by ventricular overload, myocardial ischemia and pericardial disease. It can also occur through the effects of medication, permanent pacing, endothelial and neurohormonal activation.

Hemodynamic overload of one or both ventricles is common in ACHD, and can be the result of obstructive or regurgitant lesions, shunting, pulmonary or systemic pulmonary hypertension. Ventricular overload is, by definition in ACHD, long-standing, and often leads to significant ventricular dysfunction. Ventricular dysfunction is encountered in patients after atrial repair of complete TGA, in those with corrected (l-) TGA, and in patients with a Fontan-type operation. Right ventricular systolic dysfunction can also occur in patients with significant volume overload such as those with large ASDs or patients with repaired tetralogy of Fallot and severe pulmonary regurgitation. Left ventricular dysfunction may occur with congenital aortic regurgitation or stenosis, aortic coarctation, and left atrioventricular valve regurgitation in patients with repaired atrioventricular septal defects. Ventricular dysfunction can also be a sequelae of repeated/protracted cardiopulmonary by-pass, especially in previous eras when cardioplegia may have been suboptimal. Repeated ventriculotomies and patch augmentation of the right ventricular outflow tract may also contribute to ventricular dysfunction. Ventricular dysfunction is also encountered in patients with pericardial disease (congenital absence of pericardium or constrictive pericarditis related to previous surgery). Ventricular–ventricular interaction is also seen in conditions such as Ebstein's anomaly, in which left ventricular size and function is affected by the dilated right-sided cavity and reduction in right ventricular output.

Myocardial perfusion abnormalities have been described in ACHD and may also contribute to the development of ventricular dysfunction. Anomalous coronary artery origin and distribution may result in myocardial ischemia, infarction and dysfunction. Reversible and fixed perfusion defects with concordant regional wall motion abnormalities have been reported in patients after atrial or arterial switch repair for (d-) TGA and are thought to affect ventricular function. ACHD patients often present with a coronary circulation which, by conventional criteria, would be classified as anomalous. Whether these abnormalities in the origin and distribution of the coronary circulation seen in ACHD can affect ventricular function remains unknown.

Arrhythmias, permanent pacing, and rate-lowering medication can also cause or exacerbate ventricular dysfunction. ACHD patients are at increased risk of arrhythmias due to intrinsic abnormalities of the conduction system, long-standing hemodynamic overload and scarring from reparative or palliative surgery. Arrhythmias can lead to significant hemodynamic compromise, especially in the presence of myocardial dysfunction, and may become life-threatening when fast or ventricular in origin. However, even relatively slow long-standing supraventricular tachycardias may reduce cardiac output and exercise capacity.

The chronotropic response to exercise is a major component of the increase in cardiac output during exercise. Chronotropic incompetence is the inability to increase heart rate appropriate to metabolic demands. Chronotropic incompetence is common in ACHD, encountered in 62% of ACHD patients in one series. It can be due to intrinsic abnormalities of the conduction system or be iatrogenic.[22] Chronotropic incompetence relates to the severity of exercise intolerance, plasma natriuretic peptide levels and peak VO_2.[23] Chronotropic incompetence is also a prognostic marker in ischemic heart disease and ACHD, particularly in patients with "complex" lesions, Fontan-type surgery and repaired tetralogy of Fallot.[22,24]

Beta-blockers, calcium antagonists and antiarrhythmics can have significant negative inotropic and chronotropic effects and can influence ventricular performance and exercise capacity. ACHD patients on beta-blockers achieved a lower peak heart rate and a lower peak VO_2 during maximal exercise testing in one study.[7] Medication can also help unmask latent conduction system disease and lead to sinus node dysfunction, atrioventricular block or chronotropic incompetence. Permanent pacing causes chronotropic incompetence and ventricular dysfunction. Despite advances in rate-responsive pacemakers, rate responsiveness at higher levels of exercise in young patients may be inadequate to produce a sufficient increase in cardiac output. Right ventricular pacing can also cause ventricular asynchrony, and long-term left ventricular dysfunction and reduced exercise capacity.[25]

4.3.2
Extracardiac Causes of Exercise Intolerance in ACHD

Pulmonary function, both parenchymal and vascular, significantly affects exercise intolerance in ACHD. Subnormal forced vital capacity has been reported in ACHD and affects exercise capacity. Surgery-related lung scarring or atelectasis, chest deformities, diaphragmatic palsy, pulmonary vascular disease with loss of distensibility of peripheral arteries and significant cardiomegaly are possible mechanisms for the abnormal pulmonary function observed in these patients.

Pulmonary vascular disease and cyanosis appear to be the strongest correlates of impaired exercise capacity and ventilatory inefficiency in ACHD. Eisenmenger patients are by far the most symptomatic patients, with 84% complaining of exercise intolerance by age 28. In these patients, cardiac output rises during exercise through an increase in shunting, at the expense of further systemic desaturation and an increase in physiological dead space. Patients with severe pulmonary vascular disease are, in fact, unable to increase pulmonary blood flow during exercise but abruptly increase their ventilation in an attempt to meet oxygen requirements and compensate for right-to-left shunting.[4, 18]

In acquired heart failure, anemia relates to exercise capacity and is a predictor of outcome. Anemia affects exercise capacity by reducing oxygen carrying capacity and causing a premature shift to anaerobic metabolism during exercise. Anemia may affect myocardial function and cause volume overload. In ACHD, anemia may occur as a complication of chronic anticoagulation, surgery or intervention, hemolysis due to prosthetic valves, intracardiac patches or endocarditis or hemoptysis in patients with severe pulmonary hypertension. Moreover, anemia can occur due to chronic renal failure or as the anemia of chronic disease. In cyanotic patients anemia as conventionally defined is rare. However, "relative anemia" i.e., inadequate rise in hemoglobin levels despite chronic cyanosis can occur as a result of iron deficiency and have detrimental effects on exercise capacity and symptomatic status.[26]

4.4
Systemic Effects of the Heart Failure Syndrome in ACHD

Heart failure has important systemic manifestations, which define its natural history and are used as a target for therapy. Neurohormonal activation, chemoreflex and peripheral ergoreflex activation and end-organ failure, such as renal and hepatic dysfunction, are well described complications of acquired heart failure. Neurohormonal and cytokine activation have also been described in ACHD patients even those with "simple" lesions, and relate to worsening NYHA class and ventricular dysfunction.[27, 28] Deranged autonomic nervous activity is also common in ACHD patients late after repair of tetralogy of Fallot and in patients after Fontan-type circulation[29, 30] and appears to play a role in the high incidence of tachyarrhythmias during pregnancy in patients with repaired ACHD.[31, 32] Impaired cardiac autonomic nervous activity was also associated with an increased risk of sudden cardiac death in a small study of 43 ACHD patients.[33] Peripheral metaboreflex (ergoreflex) hypersensitivity and chemoreflex activation has been provided by small studies.[34, 35] Vonder Muhll et al also demonstrated that 1 out of 10 ACHD patients have evidence of cachexia, more prevalent in patients with univentricular circulation and those with cyanosis.[36] Finally, cytokine activation, an important component of the heart failure syndrome and a strong prognostic marker in this setting, has also been described in ACHD patients.[37] Cytokines levels were particularly high in cyanotic patients and those with peripheral edema.

Endothelial dysfunction is thought to play an important role in the pathophysiology of acquired heart failure, by affecting myocardial and skeletal muscle perfusion and function. Evidence of endothelial dysfunction in congenital heart disease (CHD) is available for Fontan patients and for cyanotic ACHD patients, in whom it appears to result from a reduced production or release of nitric oxide despite the hemoconcentration and increase in shear stress.[38, 39]

Renal dysfunction is common in patients with acquired heart failure. The term "cardiorenal syndrome" is nowadays used to define a state of advanced cardiorenal dysregulation.

ACHD patients, despite being younger than those with acquired heart failure, have a high prevalence of impaired renal function with moderate or severe dysfunction present in 1 out of 5 patients.[40] Renal dysfunction in this setting, is likely due to low cardiac output state with decreased kidney perfusion, activation of sympathetic nervous system leading to arterial vasoconstriction and activation of the renin-angiotensin-aldosterone system. Cyanotic patients are at highest risk of renal dysfunction, suggesting an effect of chronic hypoxia, and possibly hyperviscosity, on the kidney. ACHD patients with moderate to severe renal dysfunction were at a threefold increased risk of adverse outcome.

Hypotonic hyponatremia is typical of patients with congestive heart failure, especially those requiring treatment with diuretics, and is a strong prognostic marker in this population and a criterion for transplantation. Hyponatremia has also been described in ACHD patients, affecting 1 out of 7, and is a predictor of outcome independent of renal dysfunction and use of diuretics.[41]

4.5
Controversial Issues in the Care of ACHD Patients: The Heart Failure Perspective

When caring for ACHD patients with evidence of exercise intolerance and/or heart failure, relief of hemodynamic lesions should be the first aim. Surgical or interventional relief of obstructive lesions, repair of valve abnormalities and elimination or reduction of shunts is likely to have a beneficial effect on exercise capacity and possibly outcome.[4,42,43] Improvement in symptoms has been reported after interventions such as Fontan-type operations, tetralogy of Fallot repair, relief of congenital aortic stenosis or pulmonary regurgitation and transcutaneous closure of ASD.[44–48] Other reversible causes of exercise intolerance and ventricular dysfunction, such as ischemic heart disease, anemia and parenchymal pulmonary disease should be sought and treated. Objective means of assessing exercise capacity should, whenever possible, be used to aid in the decision making when considering elective surgery. ACHD patients are, in fact, often unaware of the real degree of exercise limitation and this may impact on the timing and type of therapeutic interventions. A "treat sooner rather than later" approach could be beneficial, especially for patients with right-sided lesions (e.g., severe pulmonary regurgitation after repair of Fallot's tetralogy) who often remain asymptomatic or mildly symptomatic despite significant right ventricular dilatation and dysfunction.[49,50]

Treatment of chronic heart failure is nowadays based on counteracting neurohormonal activation with drugs such as beta-blockers, angiotensin converting enzyme (ACE) inhibitors, angiotensin receptor blockers and spironolactone, which improve hemodynamics and prognosis. Such drugs are increasingly used empirically in ACHD on the basis of similarities in pathophysiology between ACHD and acquired heart failure.[51] This approach is, however, not based evidence-based and ignores important differences between the two conditions and the unique characteristics of individual congenital heart defects, which may influence drug dosage, tolerability and effectiveness.[4,8,26,40,52] Despite numerous trials, no hard evidence of the beneficial effects of such medication is yet available in ACHD (Table 4.1).[53–60] Published trials are usually single-center studies with a small sample size,

Table 4.1 Randomized trials of pharmacological intervention in ACHD

Author	Year	Population	Design	Drug	Sample size	Duration of therapy	Result
Dore et al[53]	2005	TGA post atrial switch and ccTGA	Multicenter, randomized, double-blind, placebo-controlled, crossover	Losartan	29	106 days	No improvement of exercise capacity and no reduction in NT-proBNP levels
Kouatli et al[54]	1997	Fontan	Randomized	Enalapril	18	10 weeks	No benefit in exercise time, cardiac index at echo parameters of diastolic function
Lester et al[55]	2001	TGA post atrial switch	Randomized, controlled, crossover	Losartan	7	8 weeks	Improvement in exercise time, reduction in systemic atrioventricular valve regurgitation
Babu-Narayan et al[56]	2006	Tetralogy of Fallot and pulmonary regurgitation	Randomized, double-blind, placebo controlled	Ramipril	64	6 months	No benefit in right or left ventricular ejection fraction, degree of pulmonary regurgitation, neurohormones, or exercise capacity
Therrien et al[57]	2008	TGA post atrial switch	Randomized, double-blind, placebo controlled	Ramipril	17	1 year	No benefit in right ventricular function
Shaddy et al[58]	2007	Children and adolescents, dilated cardiomyopathy or CHD	Multicenter, randomized, double-blind, placebo controlled	Carvedilol	161	8 months	No clinical improvement
Norozi et al[59]	2007	Tetralogy of Fallot	Randomized, double-blind, placebo controlled	Bisoprolol	33	6 months	No benefit in exercise capacity, natriuretic peptides, right and left ventricular size and function
Galie et al[60], BREATHE-5	2005	Eisenmenger	Multicenter, randomized, double-blind, placebo controlled	Bosentan	54	16 weeks	Decrease in pulmonary vascular resistance, improved 6-minute walking distance and functional class

TGA transposition of the great arteries; *ccTGA* congenitally corrected transposition of the great arteries; *CHD* congenital heart disease

significantly smaller compared to similar trials in acquired heart disease. Two studies in pediatric Fontan patients showed no beneficial effect of ACE inhibitors.[54,61] ACE inhibitors have been used in patients after atrial switch for transposition of great arteries showing no significant improvement in exercise capacity or right ventricular function,[57,62] while losartan, an angiotensin receptor blocker, resulted in a decrease in tricuspid regurgitation and an improvement in exercise time.[55] ACE inhibitors were thought to present a risk to cyanotic patients due to a potential increase in right-to-left shunting caused by the drop in left ventricular afterload. However, a small retrospective report on 10 patients showed no adverse effects of ACE inhibition (captopril and enalapril) on blood pressure and oxygen saturation and an improvement in symptomatic status and quality of life at 1 year.[63] A study of ACE inhibition in patients with repaired tetralogy of Fallot and significant pulmonary regurgitation failed to show any significant effect of ramipril on right ventricular function.[56]

Beta-blockers in infants with heart failure secondary to left-to-right shunting resulted in an improvement in clinical status and neurohormonal levels.[64] Beta-blockers in ACHD patients after aortic valve replacement resulted in a reduction in left ventricular size.[65] A pilot study of 8 patients after atrial repair for complete TGA or corrected TGA and chronic heart failure showed that carvedilol administration may be safe and was associated with positive right ventricular remodeling as well as improved exercise duration.[66] Other reports, however, showed no beneficial effects of bisoprolol on the clinical status and neurohormonal levels of patients with tetralogy of Fallot.[59] A multicenter study in pediatric and adolescents ($n=161$), showed no significant effect of carvedilol on outcome.[58] A small case series of 3 patients with Fontan palliation showed that high-dose spironolactone may be helpful in the remission of protein-losing enteropathy.[67]

In recent years new therapies for the treatment of pulmonary hypertension have become available. Epoprostenol has been shown to improve functional status, systemic saturations and pulmonary hemodynamics in patients with CHD and pulmonary arterial hypertension.[68] Bosentan, an oral dual-receptor endothelin antagonist, improved exercise capacity in patients with Eisenmenger syndrome in several open label intention-to-treat pilot studies and a recent randomized placebo-controlled study.[60] Sildenafil, an oral phospodiasterase-5-inhibitor, improves functional capacity in patients with pulmonary arterial hypertension, including some with CHD. A small randomized trial of sildenafil in 20 patients with pulmonary arterial hypertension found a significant improvement in functional status, exercise capacity and pulmonary pressures in the Eisenmenger subgroup.[69] Oral administration of a single dose of sildenafil acutely improved exercise capacity and hemodynamic response to exercise in 27 patients with Fontan circulation.[70] Other large randomized trials using treprostinil,[71] sildenafil[72] and sitaxsentan[73,74] have included a minority of patients with ACHD in their population. A minority of ACHD patients were also included in the recently published EARLY study assessing the effect of bosentan on patients with pulmonary arterial hypertension in functional class II.[75] None of these studies, however, was powered for formal subgroup analysis, leaving doubts on the applicability of their results to the ACHD population. Moreover, it still remains unclear whether the beneficial effect of these therapies on exercise capacity and clinical status translates into a survival benefit. Finally, it remains unknown whether patients in whom advanced pulmonary arterial hypertension therapies induce a significant improvement in haemodynamics could safely undergo partial or complete repair of the underlying cardiac defect in a "treat-and-repair" fashion.[76]

Ventricular dyssynchrony significantly affects cardiac function and is a target for therapy in patients with left ventricular dysfunction and intraventricular conduction delay.[77–79] While there is mounting evidence that ventricular dyssynchrony is present in patients with CHD, randomized trials of resynchronization in this population are lacking.[80–88] Moreover, implantation of cardiac resynchronization devices in ACHD patients may present significant difficulties due to the varying intracardiac anatomy and should be performed by appropriately trained operators.

Exercise training has established psychological and physical benefits on patients with acquired heart disease.[89] There are limited data on the effects of exercise training in ACHD, with most available studies concluding that exercise training is safe and might be beneficial.[90, 91] The 36th Bethesda conference recommendations for the participation of patients with CHD in sports suggest the use of exercise testing for assessing the impact of exercise on ACHD patients before advising any level of training in the clinical setting.[92] Simple preventive measures such as avoiding excessive dehydration are also recommended. High-impact sport should be discouraged in patients on anticoagulation therapy or carrying a pacemaker as well as patients with Marfan's syndrome. Extreme caution is also recommended in patients at high risk of arrhythmia and sudden death such as those with long QT syndrome, arrhythmogenic right ventricular dysplasia and hypertrophic obstructive cardiomyopathy. All recommendations should be thoroughly discussed with patients.

The role of transplantation, heart and/or lung, remains relatively limited in ACHD. The scarcity of donors, the very slow deterioration with a mortality rate significantly lower to that of end-stage acquired heart failure, the high prevalence of complications such as renal and hepatic dysfunction in severely symptomatic ACHD patients and the often complex cardiovascular anatomy, result in very few actually receiving a transplant.[93]

Randomized controlled trials are urgently needed in ACHD to rationalize treatment in this population.[4] Most randomized trials in this field have been too small to demonstrate a beneficial effect of therapies such as ACE-inhibitors. Despite the exponential increase in the number of ACHD patients followed at specialist centers, the absolute number of patients with individual ACHD diagnoses remains low, with significant within-group heterogeneity (prior interventions, associated lesions etc). Thus, the required sample size for performing a study in ACHD often exceeds the number of available participants in a single center.[94, 95] Moreover, the rate of "hard" endpoints such as mortality is often low in ACHD and surrogate markers of outcome such as ventricular function or exercise capacity may introduce additional noise related to reproducibility of measurements and cost.[96] Careful selection of endpoints to ensure adequate patient participation and compliance to protocol are essential. Education of patients on the importance of trials and the potential benefits to themselves is important.[97, 98] Multicenter studies with longer follow-up could compensate for the lack of power and low event rates, allowing the use of "hard" endpoints.

References

1. Dickstein K, Cohen-Solal A, Filippatos G, et al. ESC Guidelines for the diagnosis and treatment of acute and chronic heart failure 2008: the Task Force for the Diagnosis and Treatment of Acute and Chronic Heart Failure 2008 of the European Society of Cardiology. Developed in collaboration with the Heart Failure Association of the ESC (HFA) and endorsed by the European Society of Intensive Care Medicine (ESICM). *Eur Heart J*. 2008;29:2388-2442.
2. Hunt SA. ACC/AHA 2005 guideline update for the diagnosis and management of chronic heart failure in the adult: a report of the American College of Cardiology/American Heart Association Task Force on Practice Guidelines (Writing Committee to Update the 2001 Guidelines for the Evaluation and Management of Heart Failure). *J Am Coll Cardiol*. 2005;46:e1-e82.
3. Bolger AP, Coats AJ, Gatzoulis MA. Congenital heart disease: the original heart failure syndrome. *Eur Heart J*. 2003;24:970-976.
4. Dimopoulos K, Diller GP, Piepoli MF, Gatzoulis MA. Exercise intolerance in adults with congenital heart disease. *Cardiol Clin*. 2006;24:641-660; vii.
5. Engelfriet P, Tijssen J, Kaemmerer H, et al. Adherence to guidelines in the clinical care for adults with congenital heart disease: the Euro Heart Survey on adult congenital heart disease. *Eur Heart J*. 2006;27:737-745.
6. Veldtman GR, Nishimoto A, Siu S, et al. The Fontan procedure in adults. *Heart*. 2001;86:330-335.
7. Diller GP, Dimopoulos K, Okonko D, et al. Exercise intolerance in adult congenital heart disease: comparative severity, correlates, and prognostic implication. *Circulation*. 2005;112:828-835.
8. Dimopoulos K, Okonko DO, Diller GP, et al. Abnormal ventilatory response to exercise in adults with congenital heart disease relates to cyanosis and predicts survival. *Circulation*. 2006;113:2796-2802.
9. Graham TP Jr, Bernard YD, Mellen BG, et al. Long-term outcome in congenitally corrected transposition of the great arteries: a multi-institutional study. *J Am Coll Cardiol*. 2000;36: 255-261.
10. Puley G, Siu S, Connelly M, et al. Arrhythmia and survival in patients >18 years of age after the mustard procedure for complete transposition of the great arteries. *Am J Cardiol*. 1999;83:1080-1084.
11. Piran S, Veldtman G, Siu S, Webb GD, Liu PP. Heart failure and ventricular dysfunction in patients with single or systemic right ventricles. *Circulation*. 2002;105:1189-1194.
12. Fredriksen PM, Veldtman G, Hechter S, et al. Aerobic capacity in adults with various congenital heart diseases. *Am J Cardiol*. 2001;87:310-314.
13. Giardini A, Specchia S, Berton E, et al. Strong and independent prognostic value of peak circulatory power in adults with congenital heart disease. *Am Heart J*. 2007;154:441-447.
14. Wasserman K. *Principles of Exercise Testing and Interpretation Including Pathophysiology and Clinical Applications*. Philadelphia: Lippincott Williams & Wilkins; 2005.
15. ATS/ACCP. ATS/ACCP statement on cardiopulmonary exercise testing. *Am J Respir Crit Care Med*. 2003;167:211-277.
16. Diller GP, Dimopoulos K, Benson LR, Gatzoulis MA. Ventilatory efficiency and heart rate response are the strongest exercise markers of outcome in noncyanotic adults with congenital heart disease. *J Am Coll Cardiol*. 2007;49:A268.
17. Gitt AK, Wasserman K, Kilkowski C, et al. Exercise anaerobic threshold and ventilatory efficiency identify heart failure patients for high risk of early death. *Circulation*. 2002;106:3079-3084.
18. Glaser S, Opitz CF, Bauer U, et al. Assessment of symptoms and exercise capacity in cyanotic patients with congenital heart disease. *Chest*. 2004;125:368-376.

19. Frigiola A, Tsang V, Bull C, et al. Biventricular response after pulmonary valve replacement for right ventricular outflow tract dysfunction: is age a predictor of outcome? *Circulation*. 2008;118:S182-S190.
20. Niedeggen A, Skobel E, Haager P, Lepper W, Muhler E, Franke A. Comparison of the 6-minute walk test with established parameters for assessment of cardiopulmonary capacity in adults with complex congenital cardiac disease. *Cardiol Young*. 2005;15:385-390.
21. Weber KT, Janicki JS, McElroy PA. Determination of aerobic capacity and the severity of chronic cardiac and circulatory failure. *Circulation*. 1987;76:VI40-VI45.
22. Diller GP, Dimopoulos K, Okonko D, et al. Heart rate response during exercise predicts survival in adults with congenital heart disease. *J Am Coll Cardiol*. 2006;48:1250-1256.
23. Norozi K, Wessel A, Alpers V, et al. Chronotropic incompetence in adolescents and adults with congenital heart disease after cardiac surgery. *J Card Fail*. 2007;13:263-268.
24. Diller GP, Okonko DO, Uebing A, et al. Impaired heart rate response to exercise in adult patients with a systemic right ventricle or univentricular circulation: prevalence, relation to exercise, and potential therapeutic implications. *Int J Cardiol*. 2009;134:59-66.
25. Kaltman JR, Ro PS, Zimmerman F, et al. Managed ventricular pacing in pediatric patients and patients with congenital heart disease. *Am J Cardiol*. 2008;102:875-878.
26. Spence MS, Balaratnam MS, Gatzoulis MA. Clinical update: cyanotic adult congenital heart disease. *Lancet*. 2007;370:1530-1532.
27. Bolger AP, Sharma R, Li W, et al. Neurohormonal activation and the chronic heart failure syndrome in adults with congenital heart disease. *Circulation*. 2002;106:92-99.
28. Hopkins WE, Chen Z, Fukagawa NK, Hall C, Knot HJ, LeWinter MM. Increased atrial and brain natriuretic peptides in adults with cyanotic congenital heart disease: enhanced understanding of the relationship between hypoxia and natriuretic peptide secretion. *Circulation*. 2004;109:2872-2877.
29. Davos CH, Davlouros PA, Wensel R, et al. Global impairment of cardiac autonomic nervous activity late after repair of tetralogy of Fallot. *Circulation*. 2002;106:I69-I75.
30. Davos CH, Francis DP, Leenarts MF, et al. Global impairment of cardiac autonomic nervous activity late after the Fontan operation. *Circulation*. 2003;108(suppl 1):II180-II185.
31. Niwa K, Tateno S, Akagi T, et al. Arrhythmia and reduced heart rate variability during pregnancy in women with congenital heart disease and previous reparative surgery. *Int J Cardiol*. 2007;122:143-148.
32. Tateno S, Niwa K, Nakazawa M, Akagi T, Shinohara T, Yasuda T. Arrhythmia and conduction disturbances in patients with congenital heart disease during pregnancy: multicenter study. *Circ J*. 2003;67:992-997.
33. Lammers A, Kaemmerer H, Hollweck R, et al. Impaired cardiac autonomic nervous activity predicts sudden cardiac death in patients with operated and unoperated congenital cardiac disease. *J Thorac Cardiovasc Surg*. 2006;132:647-655.
34. Brassard P, Poirier P, Martin J, et al. Impact of exercise training on muscle function and ergoreflex in Fontan patients: a pilot study. *Int J Cardiol*. 2006;107:85-94.
35. Georgiadou P, Babu-Narayan SV, Francis DP, Kremastinos DT, Gatzoulis MA. Periodic breathing as a feature of right heart failure in congenital heart disease. *Heart*. 2004;90:1075-1076.
36. Vonder Muhll IF, Cholet A, Stehr K, Bouzas B, Gatzoulis M. Increased metabolic rate as a mechanism for cachexia in adults with congenital heart disease. *J Am Coll Cardiol*. 2004; 43(suppl A):384.
37. Sharma R, Bolger AP, Li W, et al. Elevated circulating levels of inflammatory cytokines and bacterial endotoxin in adults with congenital heart disease. *Am J Cardiol*. 2003;92:188-193.
38. Oechslin E, Kiowski W, Schindler R, Bernheim A, Julius B, Brunner-La Rocca HP. Systemic endothelial dysfunction in adults with cyanotic congenital heart disease. *Circulation*. 2005; 112:1106-1112.
39. Diller GP, van Eijl S, Okonko DO, et al. Circulating endothelial progenitor cells in patients with Eisenmenger syndrome and idiopathic pulmonary arterial hypertension. *Circulation*. 2008;117:3020-3030.

40. Dimopoulos K, Diller GP, Koltsida E, et al. Prevalence, predictors, and prognostic value of renal dysfunction in adults with congenital heart disease. *Circulation*. 2008;117: 2320-2328.

41. Dimopoulos K, Diller JP, Petraco R, et al. Hyponatremia in adults with congenital heart disease: prevalence and relation to outcome. *Eur Heart J*. 2008;29(suppl):744.

42. Dimopoulos K, Peset A, Gatzoulis MA. Evaluating operability in adults with congenital heart disease and the role of pretreatment with targeted pulmonary arterial hypertension therapy. *Int J Cardiol*. 2008;129:163-171.

43. Papadopoulou SA, Dimopoulos K, Gatzoulis MA. Near miss sudden cardiac death on a young patient with repaired atrioventricular septal defect. *Int J Cardiol*. 2008;130:e117-e118.

44. Mott AR, Feltes TF, McKenzie ED, et al. Improved early results with the Fontan operation in adults with functional single ventricle. *Ann Thorac Surg*. 2004;77:1334-1340.

45. Borowski A, Ghodsizad A, Litmathe J, Lawrenz W, Schmidt KG, Gams E. Severe pulmonary regurgitation late after total repair of tetralogy of Fallot: surgical considerations. *Pediatr Cardiol*. 2004;25:466-471.

46. Brown JW, Ruzmetov M, Vijay P, Turrentine MW. Surgical repair of congenital supravalvular aortic stenosis in children. *Eur J Cardiothorac Surg*. 2002;21:50-56.

47. Masetti P, Ussia GP, Gazzolo D, et al. Aortic pulmonary autograft implant: medium-term follow-up with a note on a new right ventricular pulmonary artery conduit. *J Card Surg*. 1998; 13:173-176.

48. Brochu MC, Baril JF, Dore A, Juneau M, De Guise P, Mercier LA. Improvement in exercise capacity in asymptomatic and mildly symptomatic adults after atrial septal defect percutaneous closure. *Circulation*. 2002;106:1821-1826.

49. Bolger AP, Gatzoulis MA. Towards defining heart failure in adults with congenital heart disease. *Int J Cardiol*. 2004;97(suppl 1):15-23.

50. Davlouros PA, Kilner PJ, Hornung TS, et al. Right ventricular function in adults with repaired tetralogy of Fallot assessed with cardiovascular magnetic resonance imaging: detrimental role of right ventricular outflow aneurysms or akinesia and adverse right-to-left ventricular interaction. *J Am Coll Cardiol*. 2002;40:2044-2052.

51. Shaddy RE, Webb G. Applying heart failure guidelines to adult congenital heart disease patients. *Expert Rev Cardiovasc Ther*. 2008;6:165-174.

52. Dimopoulos K. Trials and tribulations in adult congenital heart disease. *Int J Cardiol*. 2008;129:160-162.

53. Dore A, Houde C, Chan KL, et al. Angiotensin receptor blockade and exercise capacity in adults with systemic right ventricles: a multicenter, randomized, placebo-controlled clinical trial. *Circulation*. 2005;112:2411-2416.

54. Kouatli AA, Garcia JA, Zellers TM, Weinstein EM, Mahony L. Enalapril does not enhance exercise capacity in patients after Fontan procedure. *Circulation*. 1997;96:1507-1512.

55. Lester SJ, McElhinney DB, Viloria E, et al. Effects of losartan in patients with a systemically functioning morphologic right ventricle after atrial repair of transposition of the great arteries. *Am J Cardiol*. 2001;88:1314-1316.

56. Babu-Narayan SV, Uebing A, Davlouros PA, et al. ACE inhibitors for potential prevention of the deleterious effects of pulmonary regurgitation in adults with tetralogy of Fallot repair – The APPROPRIATE Study – A Randomised Double-Blinded Placebo-Controlled Trial in adults with congenital heart disease. *Circulation*. 2006;114(suppl II):409.

57. Therrien J, Provost Y, Harrison J, Connelly M, Kaemmerer H, Webb GD. Effect of angiotensin receptor blockade on systemic right ventricular function and size: a small, randomized, placebo-controlled study. *Int J Cardiol*. 2008;129:187-192.

58. Shaddy RE, Boucek MM, Hsu DT, et al. Carvedilol for children and adolescents with heart failure: a randomized controlled trial. *JAMA*. 2007;298:1171-1179.

59. Norozi K, Bahlmann J, Raab B, et al. A prospective, randomized, double-blind, placebo controlled trial of beta-blockade in patients who have undergone surgical correction of tetralogy of Fallot. *Cardiol Young*. 2007;17:372-379.

60. Galie N, Beghetti M, Gatzoulis MA, et al.; for the Bosentan Randomized Trial of Endothelin Antagonist Therapy I. Bosentan therapy in patients with Eisenmenger syndrome: a multi-center, double-blind, randomized, placebo-controlled study. *Circulation*. 2006;114:48-54.

61. Heragu N, Mahony L. Is captopril useful in decreasing pleural drainage in children after modified Fontan operation? *Am J Cardiol*. 1999;84:1109-1112; A1110.

62. Hechter SJ, Fredriksen PM, Liu P, et al. Angiotensin-converting enzyme inhibitors in adults after the Mustard procedure. *Am J Cardiol*. 2001;87:660-663; A611.

63. Hopkins WE, Kelly DP. Angiotensin-converting enzyme inhibitors in adults with cyanotic congenital heart disease. *Am J Cardiol*. 1996;77:439-440.

64. Buchhorn R, Bartmus D, Siekmeyer W, Hulpke-Wette M, Schulz R, Bursch J. Beta-blocker therapy of severe congestive heart failure in infants with left to right shunts. *Am J Cardiol*. 1998;81:1366-1368.

65. Matsuyama K, Ueda Y, Ogino H, et al. beta-blocker therapy in patients after aortic valve replacement for aortic regurgitation. *Int J Cardiol*. 2000;73:49-53.

66. Giardini A, Lovato L, Donti A, et al. A pilot study on the effects of carvedilol on right ventricular remodelling and exercise tolerance in patients with systemic right ventricle. *Int J Cardiol*. 2006.

67. Ringel RE, Peddy SB. Effect of high-dose spironolactone on protein-losing enteropathy in patients with Fontan palliation of complex congenital heart disease. *Am J Cardiol*. 2003; 91:1031-1032; A1039.

68. Rosenzweig EB, Kerstein D, Barst RJ. Long-term prostacyclin for pulmonary hypertension with associated congenital heart defects. *Circulation*. 1999;99:1858-1865.

69. Singh TP, Rohit M, Grover A, Malhotra S, Vijayvergiya R. A randomized, placebo-controlled, double-blind, crossover study to evaluate the efficacy of oral sildenafil therapy in severe pulmonary artery hypertension. *Am Heart J*. 2006;151:851.e1-851.e5.

70. Giardini A, Balducci A, Specchia S, Gargiulo G, Bonvicini M, Picchio FM. Effect of sildenafil on haemodynamic response to exercise and exercise capacity in Fontan patients. *Eur Heart J*. 2008;29:1681-1687.

71. Simonneau G, Barst RJ, Galie N, et al. Continuous subcutaneous infusion of treprostinil, a prostacyclin analogue, in patients with pulmonary arterial hypertension: a double-blind, randomized, placebo-controlled trial. *Am J Respir Crit Care Med*. 2002;165:800-804.

72. Galie N, Ghofrani HA, Torbicki A, et al. Sildenafil citrate therapy for pulmonary arterial hypertension. *N Engl J Med*. 2005;353:2148-2157.

73. Barst RJ, Langleben D, Badesch D, et al. Treatment of pulmonary arterial hypertension with the selective endothelin-A receptor antagonist sitaxsentan. *J Am Coll Cardiol*. 2006;47:2049-2056.

74. Barst RJ, Langleben D, Frost A, et al. Sitaxsentan therapy for pulmonary arterial hypertension. *Am J Respir Crit Care Med*. 2004;169:441-447.

75. Galie N, Rubin L, Hoeper M, et al. Treatment of patients with mildly symptomatic pulmonary arterial hypertension with bosentan (EARLY study): a double-blind, randomised controlled trial. *Lancet*. 2008;371:2093-2100.

76. Giannakoulas G, Dimopoulos K, Gatzoulis MA. Bosentan in mild pulmonary hypertension. *Lancet*. 2008;372:1730-1731; author reply 1731.

77. Bristow MR, Saxon LA, Boehmer J, et al. Cardiac-resynchronization therapy with or without an implantable defibrillator in advanced chronic heart failure. *N Engl J Med*. 2004;350:2140-2150.

78. Young JB, Abraham WT, Smith AL, et al. Combined cardiac resynchronization and implantable cardioversion defibrillation in advanced chronic heart failure: the MIRACLE ICD Trial. *JAMA*. 2003;289:2685-2694.

79. Cazeau S, Leclercq C, Lavergne T, et al. Effects of multisite biventricular pacing in patients with heart failure and intraventricular conduction delay. *N Engl J Med*. 2001;344:873-880.

80. Uebing A, Gibson DG, Babu-Narayan SV, et al. Right ventricular mechanics and QRS duration in patients with repaired tetralogy of Fallot: implications of infundibular disease. *Circulation*. 2007;116:1532-1539.

81. Friedberg MK, Silverman NH, Dubin AM, Rosenthal DN. Right ventricular mechanical dys-synchrony in children with hypoplastic left heart syndrome. *J Am Soc Echocardiogr.* 2007;20:1073-1079.

82. Chow PC, Liang XC, Lam WW, Cheung EW, Wong KT, Cheung YF. Mechanical right ven-tricular dyssynchrony in patients after atrial switch operation for transposition of the great arteries. *Am J Cardiol.* 2008;101:874-881.

83. Janousek J, Vojtovic P, Hucin B, et al. Resynchronization pacing is a useful adjunct to the management of acute heart failure after surgery for congenital heart defects. *Am J Cardiol.* 2001;88:145-152.

84. Zimmerman FJ, Starr JP, Koenig PR, Smith P, Hijazi ZM, Bacha EA. Acute hemodynamic benefit of multisite ventricular pacing after congenital heart surgery. *Ann Thorac Surg.* 2003; 75:1775-1780.

85. Dubin AM, Feinstein JA, Reddy VM, Hanley FL, Van Hare GF, Rosenthal DN. Electrical resyn-chronization: a novel therapy for the failing right ventricle. *Circulation.* 2003;107:2287-2289.

86. Dubin AM, Janousek J, Rhee E, et al. Resynchronization therapy in pediatric and congenital heart disease patients: an international multicenter study. *J Am Coll Cardiol.* 2005;46:2277-2283.

87. Cecchin F, Frangini PA, Brown DW, et al. Cardiac resynchronization therapy (and multisite pacing) in pediatrics and congenital heart disease: five years experience in a single institution. *J Cardiovasc Electrophysiol.* 2009;20:58-65.

88. Saul JP, Epstein AE, Silka MJ, et al. Heart Rhythm Society/Pediatric and Congenital Electrophysiology Society Clinical Competency Statement: training pathways for implanta-tion of cardioverter-defibrillators and cardiac resynchronization therapy devices in pediatric and congenital heart patients. *Heart Rhythm.* 2008;5:926-933.

89. Piepoli MF, Davos C, Francis DP, Coats AJ. Exercise training meta-analysis of trials in patients with chronic heart failure (ExTraMATCH). *BMJ.* 2004;328:189.

90. Therrien J, Fredriksen P, Walker M, Granton J, Reid GJ, Webb G. A pilot study of exercise training in adult patients with repaired tetralogy of Fallot. *Can J Cardiol.* 2003;19:685-689.

91. Thaulow E, Fredriksen PM. Exercise and training in adults with congenital heart disease. *Int J Cardiol.* 2004;97(suppl 1):35-38.

92. Graham TP Jr, Driscoll DJ, Gersony WM, Newburger JW, Rocchini A, Towbin JA. Task Force 2: congenital heart disease. *J Am Coll Cardiol.* 2005;45:1326-1333.

93. Dimopoulos K, Giannakoulas G, Wort SJ, Gatzoulis MA. Pulmonary arterial hypertension in adults with congenital heart disease: distinct differences from other causes of pulmonary arte-rial hypertension and management implications. *Curr Opin Cardiol.* 2008;23:545-554.

94. Schulz KF, Grimes DA. Sample size calculations in randomised trials: mandatory and mystical. *Lancet.* 2005;365:1348-1353.

95. Gatzoulis MA, Webb GD, Daubeney PEF. *Diagnosis and Management of Adult Congenital Heart Disease.* Edinburgh: Churchill Livingstone; 2003.

96. Konstam MA, Udelson JE, Anand IS, Cohn JN. Ventricular remodeling in heart failure: a credible surrogate endpoint. *J Card Fail.* 2003;9:350-353.

97. Gatzoulis MA. Adult congenital heart disease: education, education, education. *Nat Clin Pract Cardiovasc Med.* 2006;3:2-3.

98. Caldwell PH, Murphy SB, Butow PN, Craig JC. Clinical trials in children. *Lancet.* 2004; 364:803-811.

Heart Failure with a Normal Ejection Fraction

5

John E. Sanderson and Yu Ting Tan

It has been increasingly recognized that there are many patients, mainly elderly women, who have symptoms of heart failure but their hearts are not enlarged and echocardiography shows a relatively normal left ventricular ejection fraction. The label "Diastolic heart failure" was coined for this group of patients because it was considered that systolic function was normal in view of the ejection fraction and hence the problem must lie in diastole. However, it has become clear that systolic function is not entirely normal and recent work has demonstrated that in these patients abnormalities exist in left ventricular systolic properties, ventricular-arterial coupling, LV diastolic function, torsion, ventricular–ventricular interaction and pericardial constraint, and other factors such as pulmonary hypertension, impaired chronotropic, vasodilator, and contractile reserves may contribute to the pathophysiology. Thus, the more simple label "heart failure with a normal ejection fraction" or HFNEF is the preferred term to diastolic heart failure (DHF), which implies that the primary or dominant abnormality is in diastole, and as it appears that the problem is not due to diastolic dysfunction only, the label HFNEF is more appropriate, which makes no assumptions about the causation of the condition.[1]

5.1
Epidemiology

Patients with HFNEF typically tend to be older females and to have a history of hypertension and other comorbidities such as obesity, diabetes, mild coronary artery disease, renal failure, anemia, and atrial fibrillation.[2] Bhatia et al found that there was little difference in the symptoms and signs between patients with HFNEF and patients with typical heart failure and reduced ejection fraction (HFREF) or systolic heart failure except that HFREF patients more commonly had a S3 sound whereas ankle edema was more common in the

J.E. Sanderson (✉)
Cardiovascular Medicine, University of Birmingham, Queen Elizabeth Hospital, Birmingham, UK
e-mail: jesanderson@hotmail.com

M.Y. Henein (ed.), *Heart Failure in Clinical Practice*,
DOI: 10.1007/978-1-84996-153-0_5, © Springer-Verlag London Limited 2010

HFNEF group.[3] However, the prognosis of HFNEF is similar to those with HFREF. After 1 year, 22.2% HFNEF patients had died compared to 25.5% of HFREF patients. In a community study from Australia, Abhayaratna et al found that in a cross-sectional survey of 1,275 randomly selected residents of Canberra, aged 60–86 years (mean age 69.4; 50% men), the presence of any diastolic dysfunction was 35% and was associated with higher BNP levels and decreased quality of life even in the absence of overt signs of heart failure.[4] Interestingly, diastolic dysfunction was associated with reduced long axis function and increased LV end-diastolic volumes suggesting the beginning of a remodeling process (see below). LV diastolic dysfunction in this study was assessed by Doppler evaluation of the mitral and pulmonary venous inflow and tissue Doppler imaging of the lateral mitral annulus producing four grades. Aging by itself is associated with increasing degrees of diastolic dysfunction (an abnormal relaxation pattern on the mitral inflow velocity is very common in the elderly and nearly universal in the over 70s) and this makes assessing the prevalence of truly abnormal diastolic function in the elderly difficult.[5] Probably because of the aging population, the prevalence of HFNEF appears to be rising and now maybe the most common type of heart failure in the community.[6] The impression of heart failure prevalence from the hospital environment may be quite misleading as the majority of patients with heart failure are treated in the community by primary care physicians and many of these are elderly ladies with HFNEF who are not referred to hospitals or to cardiologists.

5.2
Diagnosis of HFNEF

According to the recent European Society of Cardiology updated guidelines on the diagnosis of HFNEF[7] four obligatory conditions need to be satisfied for the diagnosis of HFNEF: (1) presence of signs or symptoms of congestive heart failure, (2) a "normal" LVEF>50%, (3) a nondilated LV with LV end-diatolic volume <97 mL/m² and (4) evidence of diastolic LV dysfunction. Two measurement issues arise immediately.

5.2.1
Measurement of LVEF

The LV ejection fraction requires measurement of LV end-diastolic and end-systolic volumes by echocardiography, and this can be performed by measuring LV end-diastolic and end-systolic contours by planimetry of apical images. If these avoid significant foreshortening of the LV and if values are averaged from both four-chamber and two-chamber views, preferably from 2 or 3 beats, then accurate noninvasive measurements can be obtained with fair reproducibility. LV volumes and EF are then calculated by applying the method of discs (Simpson's biplane technique). However, in routine clinical practice and even in many studies of heart failure, EF has unfortunately not been measured but only estimated visually (by "eyeball"). Similarly, the estimation of LV ejection fraction from radial end-diastolic and end-systolic diameters obtained by M-mode echocardiography from a parasternal window, applying the

Teichholz formula, is also not accurate because it involves too many inappropriate and inaccurate assumptions about LV cavity size and shape.[8] Frequently, in many studies, the diagnostic methods have not even been described in detail. Furthermore, although ejection fraction is of some prognostic value, it is affected by preload, afterload, heart rate, dyssynchrony as well as myocardial contractility and is not a true measure of systolic function.[9] It tends to reflect radial more than longitudinal function. McIver and Townsend have demonstrated that in the presence of LV hypertrophy and a normal LV volume, LVEF is mathematically bound to increase, falsely creating the impression of normal systolic function.[10] Using a model, their study illustrates that despite a normal LVEF, there may be significant left ventricular systolic dysfunction as assessed by long axis shortening and stroke volume. The preservation of ejection fraction is directly related to the presence of LVH and the effect of increased muscle mass. Myocardial long axis shortening leads to radial myocardial thickening; increasing myocardial muscle volume leads to an additional increased endocardial displacement and, if myocardial shortening is unchanged, an increased ejection fraction. In the presence of LVH and reduced long axis shortening, the ejection fraction is maintained within the normal range despite a significant reduction in stroke volume.

5.3
Assessment of Diastolic Dysfunction and LV Filling Pressures

Classically, diastolic dysfunction is assessed from pressure–volume loops measured at cardiac catheterisation.[11] The end-diastolic pressure–volume relationship (EDPVR) is thought to represent the passive mechanical properties of the left ventricle. Changes in the LVPVR reflect changes in ventricular capacitance and compliance. Compliance is the slope of the EDPVR. There is little correlation between EDPVR and mitral inflow velocities measured by Doppler echocardiography. Also data from patients with HFNEF have shown that EDPVR curves are highly variable and may be shifted toward lower, normal, and higher volumes. Maurer et al highlighted the heterogeneous results on P–V analysis in patients with HFNEF and that different pathophysiological mechanisms exist in individual patients.[11] As Gibson and Francis stated "in DHF a stiff ventricle is often invoked but seldom documented."[12] The EDPVR is not a measure of stiffness but the extent to which stiffness depends on volume.[12] A normal LV will become "stiff" if volume is increased abnormally, for example, renal failure. In practice therefore EDPVR is not a particularly useful measurement and cannot be considered a "gold" standard as is commonly claimed.

Mitral inflow velocities in contrast are easy to obtain and provide a rough assessment of diastolic function and LV filling pressures. Diastolic function can be graded into broad categories, typically four. However, it is well documented that these are preload and afterload dependent. Also these measurements are highly age-dependent. However, the preload dependence of the peak early mitral inflow velocity (E) can be useful. With high filling pressures E rises and a restrictive filling pattern (high E and reduced peak atrial velocity) is a reliable predictor or a poor outcome, especially if it is persistent.

Tissue Doppler imaging has introduced a number of new indices which can give some help in this difficult area. Since the apex is relatively fixed movement of the mitral valve, annulus is a direct measure of ventricular longitudinal function or the long axis. The same holds true for the tricuspid valve annulus and the right ventricle. Rushmer et al *showed* that the long axis normally shortens by 10–12% with ejection at the same time as the minor axis falls by 25%.[13] Shortening of the long axis begins during the period of isovolumic contraction, causing cavity shape to become more spherical. As pointed out by Henein and Gibson,[14] the fact that this difference can occur demonstrates that motion along the long axis is due to anatomically discrete fibers separate from those supporting the minor axis, rather than the possibility that function in the two directions might merely represent circumferential and longitudinal components of a homogenous set of fibers arranged obliquely. During ejection, the two axes are effectively in phase with each other although peak long axis shortening occurs at aortic valve closure, while minor axis falls by a further 1–2 mm reaching its minimum at the time of mitral valve cusp separation. Mitral ring motion in early diastole correlates with tau.[15] But ring motion starts at the same time as mitral flow, that is, when pressure has fallen, and ring motion is therefore primarily a measure of recoil or ventricular restoring forces. It is however a relatively load-independent measure. In an experimental model of heart failure, the peak early diastolic velocity in the long axis was impaired early and before the anterior–posterior or septal lateral axes velocities.[16] Furthermore, longitudinal peak early diastolic and systolic velocities are powerful predictors of prognosis in a variety of cardiac conditions and heart failure[17–19] and add incremental value to standard clinical and echocardiographic measures. Wang et al[18] found that in heart failure a peak early diastolic velocity (Em) <3 cm/s was the best prognostic index in long-term follow-up and it added incremental value to standard indexes of systolic or diastolic function, including a deceleration time <140 ms and an E/Em>15. Although E/Em>15 improved the prognostic value of a model containing clinical risk factors and mtiral E wave deceleration time (DT) <140 ms, an Em <3 cm/s significantly improved the outcome of a model that contained clinical risk factors, DT<140 ms and E/Em>15. Similar results were found by the same group in hypertensive subjects with left ventricular hypertrophy where again a low Em improved the outcome of a model that contained clinical risk factors, increased septal thickness and either a pseudonormal or restrictive filling pattern.[19] In a group of patients with idiopathic dilated cardiomyopathy, Em was significantly lower in those who recently had pulmonary edema compared to those who were clinically stable.[20] Clinical improvement also paralleled a rise in Em. Decreased Em is one of the earliest markers for diastolic dysfunction and is present in all stages of diastolic dysfunction. Since Em velocity remains reduced and mitral E velocity increases with higher filling pressure, the ratio between transmitral E and Em, E/Em (same as E/E'), correlates well with LV filling pressure or pulmonary capillary wedge pressure (PCWP)[15,21]; PCWP ≥20 mmHg if E/Em ≥15 and normal PCWP if E/Em <10 although this relationship is less sure in those with a reduced LVEF. Thus, the preload dependence of the mitral inflow velocities can be put to good use.

An increased left atrial volume is a good marker of a chronically elevated left atrial pressure. In a population based study, LA volume correlated well with the severity and duration of diastolic dysfunction.[22]

Therefore, using a combination of Em and the ratio E/Em derived from tissue Doppler echocardiography of the mitral annulus or basal myocardial segments (especially if performed during exercise) with LA volume, a reasonable diagnosis of increased filling pressures and probable diastolic dysfunction can be made. However, it must be realized that early diastolic filling is highly dependent on the previous systole. Any reduction in systolic function, coordination or dyssynchrony will have a profound impact on the ability of the ventricle to fill adequately at normal pressures. In practice, the presence of LVH and an enlarged LA volume index on echocardiography in a breathless patient strongly sup-ports a diagnosis of HFNEF.

Exercise echocardiography can be very useful for unmasking any abnormalities of both systolic and diastolic dysfunction. Our recent studies have shown that with even mild exercise there are marked abnormalities of LV rotation, strain, untwisting rate with delay and impaired longitudinal function reserve (see below).

5.4
Pathophysiology of HFNEF

The classical explanations for HFNEF include the following, all of which were based on measurements acquired at rest:

1. An increase in intrinsic myocardial stiffness and impaired relaxation in diastole requires higher left atrial pressures for filling in late diastole, predisposing these patients to pulmonary venous congestion and dyspnea especially on exertion.[23]
2. Increased systolic ventricular and arterial stiffening, that is, deranged ventriculo-arterial coupling, may contribute to the pathophysiology of HFNEF by exaggerating any hyper-tensive response with increased systolic pressure load, and inducing load-dependent diastolic dysfunction especially during exercise or other stresses.[24]
3. Enhanced sensitivity to volume overload from increased LV remodeling and dilation with volume-dependent elevation of filling pressures. This was observed in a small subgroup of hypertensive HFNEF patients who had renal impairment and larger LV volumes but normal systolic ventricular and vascular stiffness.[25] Impaired renal func-tion and associated renal arterial atherosclerosis in the elderly may also be involved in causing rapid rises in blood pressure and excessive fluid retention.

These concepts underestimate the impact of the previous systole on early diastolic filling particularly inco-ordination, dyssynchrony, reduced longitudinal function, and torsion. Furthermore, the orthodox view that systolic function is entirely normal has been chal-lenged in studies using newer echocardiographic techniques which have shown that sys-tolic function does not appear to be entirely normal in all subjects with HFNEF, or those with LV hypertrophy and diabetes which are both common etiologic factors for HFNEF.[1]

5.4.1
Systolic Function in HFNEF

In an early study, Yip et al studied 68 patients with heart failure, 29 with a LVEF>0.45 and 39 with an LVEF<0.45 compared to age-matched controls.[26] They found that the mitral annular peak velocity (Sm) and amplitude in systole were significantly lower in those with HFNEF (4.81 ± 0.23 cm/s) than in the controls (6.10 ± 0.14 cm/s) and were higher than in those with systolic heart failure. A similar pattern was seen with Em. LVEF in the HFNEF group although strictly within normal limit was statistically lower than in age-matched controls. They concluded that there was evidence of abnormal systolic function in many with HFNEF and that true "isolated" diastolic dysfunction is probably rare. These findings have now been confirmed in several studies.[27–32] In a thorough assessment of regional myocardial function, Yu et al[27] studied 339 subjects; 92 were with systolic heart failure (SHF) (EF<50%) and 73 with DHF (EF>50% with diastolic abnormalities on Doppler echocardiography) while 68 had isolated diastolic dysfunction (DD i.e., without symptoms of heart failure) and 106 were normal subjects. Using a 6-basal and 6-mid-segmental model, regional myocardial velocities were constructed off-line. They found that the peak systolic and diastolic velocities were significantly lower in patients with SHF, DHF, and DD than in control subjects in almost all the myocardial segments and that SHF<DHF<DD<controls. Thus despite a normal ejection fraction, systolic function is not normal in HFNEF. This is not surprising as systole is probably affected by left ventricular hypertrophy and the accompanying fibrosis as much as diastole. Shah et al found that peak annular systolic velocity is related to the percentage interstitial fibrosis within the myocardium as was the early diastolic velocity, both being lower with increased fibrosis.[33] Systole and diastole are closely intertwined. In a study of a large number of subjects with a wide range of LVEF, we found a close relationship between systolic and diastolic velocities.[34] Vinereau et al similarly found a strong correlation between the Sm and Em.[30] In reality systole and diastole constitute one cycle and the major determinant of diastolic filling is the strength and coordination of the previous systole. Early diastolic suction is dependent on the force of the previous systolic contraction.[35] In addition, inco-ordinate systolic contraction will prolong isovolumic relaxation and impair diastolic function.[36] This may explain why the peak early diastolic velocity is a powerful predictor of prognosis in a variety of cardiac diseases including heart failure,[19] because the motion of the ventricular base during early diastole is reflecting both systolic and diastolic function of the subendocardial fibers, which because of their position are more susceptible to the effects of fibrosis, hypertrophy and ischemia. All the precursors of HFNEF such as hypertension, left ventricular hypertrophy, aging and diabetes all alter global myocardial architecture and fiber orientation, which will probably have important effects on ventricular torsion and recoil during relaxation.[37]

5.5
Twist, Annular Motion and Myocardial Architecture

The architecture of the heart is engineered to provide both rapid ejection and filling of the heart. This is achieved through the helical structure of the myocardium fibers in opposing layers, which allows the heart to twist.[38] In the normal heart, left ventricular twist during systole stores energy and pulls the mitral annulus toward the apex (which also helps suck blood into the atrium), and the corresponding untwisting process and recoil in early diastole when energy is released generates the negative intraventricular pressure gradient or suction in early diastole, which is vital for rapid filling. This process is followed by recoil of the mitral annulus back toward the base of the heart, which also aids ventricular filling by moving the mitral annulus around the column of the incoming blood. All these aspects of ventricular function increase on exercise, not only to acceler-ate ventricular ejection, but more importantly to enable rapid filling of the ventricle during a shortened diastole while maintaining a low filling pressure.[39] In HFNEF, this close relation between systole and diastole is disrupted, and our recent studies have shown a variety of abnormalities of systolic and diastolic function on exercise: reduced myocardial systolic strain, reduced ventricular systolic rotation at rest (which fails to increase normally on exercise), reduced mitral annular motion in systole and diastole and delayed ventricular untwisting associated with reduced left ventricular suction. Mean mitral annular systolic and diastolic velocities, systolic LV rotation and early dia-stolic untwist on exercise correlated with peak VO$_2$ max.[40] Impaired atrial function on exercise may also contribute to breathlessness.[41] These results confirm again that HFNEF is not an isolated disorder of diastole. Based on these results, a schema for HFNEF pathophysiology is given in Fig. 5.1.

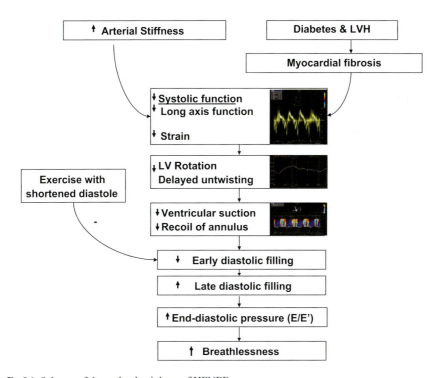

Fig. 5.1 Schema of the pathophysiology of HFNEF

5.6
Other Peripheral Factors

In a model of HFNEF, the time to complete relaxation was significantly prolonged compared to that in controls and this was related to arterial pressure, worsening with higher pressures.[41] End-systolic elastance was also increased in this experimental heart failure model and was closely linked to collagen volume fraction. Afterload affects both systolic and diastolic LV performance prolonging contraction and relaxation. This effect is seen early in the progression of systolic dysfunction and will lead to a shortening of the diastolic filling period. This effect of an increased afterload would be particularly troublesome with faster heart rates such as that on exercise or with atrial fibrillation. Kawaguchi et al found in humans that end-systolic elastance (stiffness) was higher in patients with HFNEF as was effective arterial elastance due to reduced total arterial compliance, and these were higher than that associated with aging and/or hypertension.[24] This ventricular-arterial stiffening, presumably because of abnormal myocardial and arterial collagen, will amplify stress-induced hypertension worsening diastolic dysfunction.[42]

5.7
Dyssynchrony

Two studies have demonstrated that dyssynchrony can occur in both systole and diastole in patients with HFNEF. Wang et al compared 60 patients with DHF (LVEF>50%), 60 with SHF and 35 controls.[43] LV intraventricular delay- the maximum time difference between four basal segments of the time to either peak or *onset* of the systolic myocardial velocity for systolic dyssynchrony and time to *onset* of the peak early diastolic velocity for diastolic dyssynchrony- was abnormal in 58% in diastole and in 33% also in systole. These results were very similar to those with SHF (60% with diastolic dyssynchrony and 40% with dyssynchrony during systole). In a second paper by Yu and colleagues,[44] the prevalence of diastolic and systolic dyssynchrony was similar in 92 patients with HFNEF (56% and 39% respectively). However, they found much higher levels of dyssynchrony in the SHF group in both systole (57%) and diastole (43%) perhaps reflecting the larger numbers ($n=281$) and the technique used to measure dyssynchrony. Yu et al used the technique of standard deviation of time to peak systolic and early diastolic velocities derived from a 6-basal and 6-midsegmental model, i.e., 12 segments which increased the likelihood of detecting dyssynchrony.[45] Twenty-five percent of the DHF patients had isolated systolic dyssynchrony and the relationship between systolic and diastolic dyssynchrony was poor. This is in contrast to the tight curvilinear relationship found between the absolute peak systolic and early diastolic myocardial velocities as discussed above.[34] In both studies the correlation with QRS duration was weak or nonexistent. Thus, the conclusion is that in HFNEF there is evidence of both systolic and diastolic dyssynchrony in a significant number of patients. Systolic dyssynchrony in HFNEF was associated with poorer long axis function (reduced peak basal myocardial velocities), lower stroke work and even lower ejection fraction (although still within the "normal" range) than in those without dyssynchrony. This suggests that systolic dyssynchrony in HFNEF is part of a wider abnormality of systolic function in DHF.[45]

5.7.1
Other Factors

Recent community-based data revealed that pulmonary hypertension is common and often severe in HFNEF[46] and exercise induced pulmonary hypertension is common even in those with a normal LV ejection fraction.[47]

Aging is associated with decreases in the elastic properties of the heart and great vessels, which lead to increased systolic blood pressure and myocardial stiffness. Arterial stiffness is an independent predictor of diastolic dysfunction and linked to impaired coronary flow velocity reserve, which may cause subendocardial ischemia and reduced longitudinal ventricular function.[48] HFNEF patients have attenuated heart rate responses to exercise, similar to HFREF patients.[49] Chronotropic incompetence is associated with more severe exercise intolerance than in those without it. The slower heart rate rise, lower peak heart rate and impaired recovery suggest autonomic (parasympathetic) dysfunction.

5.8
Metabolic Abnormalities in HFNEF

Impairment of cardiac energetic status (assessed by cardiac MR spectroscopy) is well described in HFREF and carries adverse prognostic significance in these patients.[50] It seems likely that increased arterial stiffness (with ventriculoarterial mismatch) combined with cardiac energetic impairment may underlie these dynamic changes in cardiac function on exercise. This opens the possibility of "metabolic modulators" as therapeutic agents.

5.8.1
Remodeling

As noted earlier, the main physiological difference between systolic heart failure and HFNEF is the increase in ventricular volume and change in shape due to remodeling. Myocardial infarctions (and also viral myocarditis) appear to be potent stimulants for the remodeling process which leads to increased ventricular volumes and reduced ejection fraction.[51] In hypertensive heart disease, remodeling is a slower process. Initially left ventricular hypertrophy leads to reduced systolic and diastolic function particularly in the long axis. Compensatory increased radial contraction normalizes the ejection fraction. However, at later stages further remodeling will occur and the left ventricular volumes will increase and the patient will pass from HEFNEF to more obvious systolic heart failure. Thus, from a physiological point it is more sensible to categorize patients with heart failure according to whether remodeling has taken place or not. Remodeling is a very important therapeutic target and reversing remodeling is probably a powerful predictor of improvement.

Table 5.1 summarizes the similarities and differences between HFNEF and HFREF and illustrates that increased ventricular volume, reflecting remodeling, is the main difference between the two. Essentially, there is heart failure with large or small hearts.

Table 5.1 Comparison of clinical features of HFREF and HFNEF

	Heart failure with reduced ejection fraction (HFREF)	Heart failure with normal ejection fraction (HFNEF)
Gender	M>F	F>M
Age	50–70	60–80
Etiology	Myocardial infarction Idiopathic DCM	Hypertension Diabetes Atrial fibrillation Transient ischemia
Clinical progress	Persistent HF	Often episodic HF
Ventricular remodeling (increased volume)	+++	0
LV hypertrophy	±	++
Peak mitral inflow velocity pattern	RFP	ARP
Peak mitral annular velocity	Markedly reduced	Moderately reduced
LA Volume index	Increased	Increased

DCM dilated cardiomyopathy; *HF* heart failure; *RFP* restrictive filling pattern; *ARP* abnormal relaxation pattern

5.9
Evolution of HFNEF into HFREF

There is still debate how often HFNEF can evolve into HFREF.[52] In many parts of the world such as Africa and Asia, it is clear that there are many patients with typical HFREF with large dilated hearts in whom the only etiology appears to be hypertension. It is likely that initially these patients had nondilated ventricles with LVH but that continued poor treatment of hypertension plus perhaps other noxious factors such as alcohol promotes remodeling and ventricular enlargement and the evolution into the typical HFREF or systolic heart failure phenotype. In the Western countries, this happens rarely partly because the typical HFNEF patient is much older and treatment is better. In one study of 159 predominantly middle-aged African American hypertensives with concentric LV hypertrophy and a normal LVEF, 18% developed a reduced LVEF after a follow-up of approximately 4 years.[53]

5.9.1
Treatment

Because all the major therapeutic trials in heart failure required a reduced LV ejection fraction for entry, HFNEF patients were excluded and consequently there is a paucity of evidence on which to base treatment. In the "Effect of candesartan in patients with chronic heart failure and preserved left-ventricular ejection fraction, the CHARM-Preserved Trial" it was found that the angiotensin receptor antagonist (ARB) candesartan modestly reduced hospital admissions for heart failure but did not significantly affect mortality in patients with heart failure with a normal ejection fraction.[54] Another recent study also evaluated the effect of the angiotensin receptor blocker (ARB) irbesartan on mortality and cardiovascular morbidity in patients with heart failure with a normal ejection fraction (I-PRESERVE trial).[55] Four thousand one hundred and twenty eight patients who were at least 60 years of age and had New York Heart Association class II, III, or IV heart failure and an ejection fraction of at least 45% were enrolled and randomly assigned to receive 300 mg of irbesartan or placebo per day. The primary composite outcome was death from any cause or hospitalization for a cardiovascular cause (heart failure, myocardial infarction, unstable angina, arrhythmia or stroke). During a mean follow-up of 49.5 months, the primary outcome occurred in 742 patients in the irbesartan group and 763 in the placebo group. There was no evidence of benefit of irbesartan over placebo in reducing mortality or morbidity from cardiovascular disease in this group of patients. Diuretics remain the mainstay of treatment and in the Hong Kong Diastolic Heart Failure trial which was a small randomized controlled trial, it was found that diuretics alone reduced symptoms and improved quality of life significantly. However, in keeping with the larger trials it was found that adding the angiotensin converting enzyme inhibitor (ACEI) ramipril or the ARB irbesartan was not more efficacious although there was a slight improvement in Em over 1 year.[56] These negative trial results for ACEIs and ARBs are surprising. Fibrosis of the left ventricle is increased with left ventricular hypertrophy and hypertension. ACEIs and ARBs can block the fibrogenic action of angiotensin experimentally and have been shown to reduce fibrosis in patients with hypertension.[57] Fibrosis and altered collagen in left ventricular hypertrophy may have a deleterious effect on overall myocardial architecture, particularly ventricular twist and torsion. Nevertheless, the reduction of fibrosis may be an important therapeutic target, and the ongoing studies of spironolactone in heart failure with a normal ejection fraction will be interesting. In essence, treatment is therefore symptomatic with diuretics for relief of breathlessness and control of blood pressure with usually ACEI or an ARB. A beta-blocker may be helpful by reducing heart rate on exercise to allow more time for filling and will obviously be indicated if there is associated angina. Calcium channel blockers (CCBs) have also be suggested as they may in theory improve myocardial relaxation but there is no good evidence for benefit in HFNEF. Diltiazem may be useful for control of ventricular rate with atrial fibrillation.

5.9.2
Contentious Issues

There are a number of issues which remain unresolved.

1. There is still debate whether HFNEF and HFREF are part of a spectrum of heart failure or whether they are distinct entities. The fact that LVEF is distributed in a unimodel way in large trials and community studies suggests a single syndrome with increasing degrees of remodeling. Supporters of the two syndrome hypothesis point out that

structural, functional, and molecular biological arguments support the theory that clinical heart failure presents and evolves not as a single syndrome but as two syndromes, one with depressed LVEF and other with normal LVEF and specific mechanisms responsible for diastolic LV dysfunction.

2. One way to resolve this question is to demonstrate that patients can evolve from HFNEF to HFREF. Some evidence exists that this can occur but larger studies are needed.

3. There is still debate on how common HFNEF truly is. Many feel that it is over-diagnosed because of inexact diagnostic criteria and difficulties in precisely measuring diastolic function which is complex.

4. The exact pathophysiology is still debated although recent work suggests that there are complex abnormalities of both systolic and diastolic function, myocardial architecture and torsion.

5. Treatment is not evidence based yet. All clinical trials have been disappointing and it is not clear if the traditional therapies for HFREF will work for HFNEF. Most of the successful treatments for HFREF target the remodeled enlarged ventricle which is not part of the mechanism of HFNEF.

In conclusion, HFNEF appears to be a relatively common cause for heart failure especially in the elderly and has a mixture of causes and pathophysiological mechanisms involving both diastole and systole, and probably differing in individual patients. Treatment is still largely empirical.

References

1. Sanderson JE. Heart failure with a normal ejection fraction. *Heart*. 2007;93:155-158.
2. Maeder MT, Kaye DM. Heart failure with normal ejection fraction. *J Am Coll Cardiol*. 2009;53:905-918.
3. Bhatia RS, Tu JV, Lee DS, et al. Outcome of heart failure with preserved ejection fraction in a population based study. *N Engl J Med*. 2006;355:260-269.
4. Abhayaratna WP, Marwick TH, Smith WT, Becker NG. Characteristics of left ventricular diastolic dysfunction in the community: an echocardiographic survey. *Heart*. 2006;92:1259-1264.
5. Henein M, Lindqvist P, Francis D, Morner S, Waldenstrom A, Kazzam E. Tissue Doppler analysis of age-dependency in diastolic ventricular behaviour and filling: a cross-sectional study of healthy hearts (the Umea General Population Heart Study). *Eur Heart J*. 2002;23:162-171.
6. Owan TE, Hodge DO, Herges RM, Jacobsen SJ, Roger VL, Redfield MM. Trends in prevalence and outcome of heart failure with preserved ejection fraction. *N Engl J Med*. 2006; 355:251-259.
7. Paulus WJ, Tschope C, Sanderson JE, et al. How to diagnose diastolic heart failure: a consensus statement on the diagnosis of heart failure with a normal ejection fraction by the Heart failure and Echocardiography associations of the European Society of cardiology. *Eur Heart J*. 2007;28:2539-2550.
8. Lang RM, Bierig M, Devereux RB, et al. American Society of Echocardiography's Nomenclature and Standards Committee; Task Force on Chamber Quantification; American College of Cardiology Echocardiography Committee; American Heart Association; European Association of Echocardiography, European Society of Cardiology. Recommendations for chamber quantification. *Eur J Echocardiogr*. 2006;7:79-108.

9. Mahler F, Ross J Jr, O'Rourke RA, et al. Effects of changes in preload, afterload and inotropic state of ejection and isovolumic phase measures of contractility in the conscious dog. *Am J Cardiol*. 1975;35:625-634.

10. MacIver DH, Townsend M. A novel mechanism of heart failure with normal ejection fraction. *Heart*. 2008;94:446-449.

11. Maurer MS, Kronzon I, Burkhoff D. Ventricular pump function in heart failure with normal ejection fraction: insights from pressure-volume measurements. *Prog Cardiovasc Dis*. 2006;49:182-195.

12. Gibson DG, Francis DP. Clinical assessment of left ventricular diastolic function. *Heart*. 2003;89:231-238.

13. Rushmer RF, Crystal DK, Wagner C. The functional anatomy of the cardiac volume. *Am J Physiol*. 1932;102:559-565.

14. Henein MY, Gibson DG. Normal long axis function. *Heart*. 1999;81:111-113.

15. Ommen SR, Nishimura RA, Appleton CP, et al. Clinical utility of Doppler echocardiography and tissue Doppler imaging in the estimation of left ventricular filling pressures: A comparative simultaneous Doppler-catheterization study. *Circulation*. 2000;102:1788-1794.

16. Hasegawa H, Little WC, Ohno M, et al. Diastolic mitral annular velocity during the development of heart failure. *J Am Coll Cardiol*. 2003;41:1590-1597.

17. Wang M, Yip GWK, Zhang Y, et al. Peak early diastolic annular velocity by tissue Doppler imaging adds independent and incremental prognostic value. *J Am Coll Cardiol*. 2003;41:820-826.

18. Wang M, Yip G, Yu CM, et al. Independent and incremental prognostic value of early mitral annulus velocity in patients with impaired left ventricular systolic function. *J Am Coll Cardiol*. 2005;45:272-277.

19. Wang M, Yip GWK, Wang A, et al. Tissue Doppler Imaging provides incremental prognostic value in patients with hypertension and left ventricular hypertrophy. *J Hypertension*. 2005; 23:183-191.

20. Richartz BM, Werner GS, Ferrari M, Figulla HR. Comparison of left ventricular systolic and diastolic function in patients with idiopathic dilated cardiomyopathy and mild heart failure versus those with severe heart failure. *Am J Cardiol*. 2002;90:390-394.

21. Nagueh SF, Middleton KJ, Kopelen HA, Zoghbi WA, Quinones MA. Doppler tissue imaging: a noninvasive technique for evaluation of left ventricular relaxation and estimation of filling pressures. *J Am Coll Cardiol*. 1997;30:1527-1533.

22. Pritchett AM, Mahoney DW, Jacobsen SJ, Rodeheffer RJ, Karon BL, Redfield MM. Diastolic dysfunction and left atrial volume: a population-based study. *J Am Coll Cardiol*. 2005;45: 87-92.

23. Westermann D, Kasner M, Steendijk P, et al. Role of left ventricular stiffness in heart failure with normal ejection fraction. *Circulation*. 2008;117:2051-2060.

24. Kawaguchi M, Hay I, Fetics B, Kass DA. Combined ventricular systolic and arterial stiffening in patients with heart failure and preserved ejection fraction: implications for systolic and diastolic reserve limitations. *Circulation*. 2003;107:714-720.

25. Maurer MS, King DL, El-Khoury Rumbarger L, Packer M, Burkhoff D. Left heart failure with a normal ejection fraction: identification of different pathophysiologic mechanisms. *J Card Fail*. 2005;11:177-187.

26. Yip G, Wang M, Zhang Y, Fung JWH. Ho P Sanderson JE Left ventricular long axis function in diastolic heart failure is reduced in both diastole and systole: time for a redefinition? *Heart*. 2002;87:121-125.

27. Yu CM, Lin H, Yang H, Kong SL, Zhang Q, Lee SW. Progression of systolic abnormalities in patients with "isolated" diastolic heart failure and diastolic dysfunction. *Circulation*. 2002;105:1195-1201.

28. Petrie MC, Caruana L, Berry C, McMurray JJ. "Diastolic heart failure" or heart failure caused by subtle left ventricular systolic dysfunction. *Heart*. 2002;87:29-31.

29. Nikitin NP, Witte KK, Clark AL, Cleland JG. Color tissue Doppler-derived long-axis left ventricular function in heart failure with preserved global systolic function. *Am J Cardiol.* 2002;90:1174-1177.

30. Vinereanu D, Nicolaides E, Tweddel AC, Fraser AG. "Pure" diastolic dysfunction is associated with long-axis systolic dysfunction. Implications for the diagnosis and classification of heart failure. *Eur J Heart Fail.* 2005;7:820-828.

31. Garcia EH, Perna FR, Farias EF, et al. Reduced systolic performance by tissue Doppler in patients with preserved and abnormal ejection fraction: new insights into chronic heart failure. *Int J Cardiol.* 2006;108:181-188.

32. Bruch C, Gradaus R, Gunia S, Breithardt G, Wichter T. Doppler tissue analysis of mitral annular velcoties: evidence for systolic abnormalities in patients with diastolic heart failure. *J Am Soc Echocardiogr.* 2003;16:1031-1036.

33. Shan K, Bick RJ, Poindexter BJ, et al. Relation of tissue Doppler derived myocardial velocities to myocardial structure and beta-adrenergic receptor density in humans. *J Am Coll Cardiol.* 2000;36:891-896.

34. Yip GW, Zhang Y, Tan PYH, et al. Left ventricular long-axis changes in early diastole and systole: impact of systolic function on diastole. *Clin Sci (London).* 2002;102:515-522.

35. Steine K, Stugaard M, Smiseth OA. Mechanisms of retarded apical filling in acute ischemic left ventricular failure. *Circulation.* 1999;99:2048-2054.

36. Gibson DG, Brown DJ. Relation between diastolic left ventricular wall stress and strain in man. *Br Heart J.* 1974;36:1066-1077.

37. Ashikaga H, Criscione JC, Omens JH, Covell JW, Ingels NB. Transmural left ventricular mechanics underlying torsional recoil during relaxation. *Am J Physiol Heart Circ Physio.* 2004;286:H640-H647.

38. Torrent-Guasp F, Kocica MJ, Corno AF, et al. Towards new understanding of the heart structure and function. *Eur J Cardiothoracic Surg.* 2005;27:191-201.

39. Notomi Y, Popovic ZB, Yamada H, et al. Ventricular untwisting: a temporal link between left ventricular relaxation and suction. *Am J Physiol Heart Circ Physiol.* 2008;294:H505-H513.

40. Tan YT, Wenzelburger F, Li E, et al. The patho-physiology of heart failure with normal ejection fraction: exercise echocardiography reveals complex abnormalities of both systolic and diastolic ventricular function involving torsion, untwist and longitudinal motion. *J Am Coll Cardiol.* 2009;54:36-46.

41. Munagala VK, Hart CYT, Burnett JC, Meyer DM, Redfield MM. Ventricular structure and function in aged dogs with renal hypertension. A model of experimental diastolic heart failure. *Circulation.* 2005;111:1128-1135.

42. Frenneaux M, Williams L. Ventricular-arterial and ventricular-ventricular interactions and their relevance to diastolic filling. *Progr Cardiovasc Dis.* 2007;49:252-262.

43. Wang J, Kurrelmeyer KM, Torre-Amione G, Nagueh SF. Systolic and diastolic dyssynchrony in patients with diastolic heart failure and the effects of medical treatment. *J Am Coll Cardiol.* 2007;49:88-96.

44. Yu C-M, Zhang Q, Yip GWK, et al. Diastolic and systolic asynchrony in patients with diastolic heart failure: a common but ignored condition. *J Am Coll Cardiol.* 2007;49:97-105.

45. Sanderson JE. Systolic and diastolic dyssynchrony in systolic and diastolic heart failure. *J Am Coll Cardiol.* 2007;49:106-108.

46. Lam CS, Roger VL, Rodeheffer RJ, Borlaug BA, Enders FT, Redfield MM. Pulmonary hypertension in heart failure with preserved ejection fraction: a community-based study. *J Am Coll Cardiol.* 2009;53:1119-1126.

47. Ha JW, Choi D, Park S, et al. Determinants of exercise-induced pulmonary hypertension in patients with normal left ventricular ejection fraction. *Heart.* 2009;95:490-494.

48. Saito M, Okayama H, Nishimura K, et al. Possible link between large artery stiffness and coronary flow velocity reserve. *Heart.* 2008;94:e20.

49. Borlaug BA, Melenovsky V, Russell SD, et al. Impaired chronotropic and vasodilator reserves limit exercise capacity in patients with heart failure and a preserved ejection fraction. *Circulation*. 2006;114:2138-2147.
50. Neubauer S, Horn M, Cramer M, et al. Myocardial phosphocreatine-to-ATP ratio is a predictor of mortality in patients with dilated cardiomyopathy. *Circulation*. 1997;96(7):2190-2196.
51. Mann DL, Bristow MR. Mechanisms and models in heart failure: the biomechanical model and beyond. *Circulation*. 2005;111:2837-2849.
52. Drazner MH. The transition from hypertrophy to failure: how certain are we? *Circulation*. 2005;112:936-938.
53. Rame JE, Ramilo M, Spencer N, et al. Development of a depressed left ventricular ejection fraction in patients with left ventricular hypertrophy and a normal ejection fraction. *Am J Cardiol*. 2004;93:234-237.
54. Yusuf S, Pfeffer MA, Swedberg K, et al.; for the CHARM investigators and committees. Effect of candesartan in patients with chronic heart failure and preserved left-ventricular ejection fraction: the CHARM-Preserved Trial. *Lancet*. 2003;363:777-781.
55. Massie BM, Carson PE, McMurray JJ, et al. Irbesartan in patients with heart failure and preserved ejection fraction. *N Engl J Med*. 2008;359:2456-2467.
56. Yip GW, Wang M, Wang T, et al. The Hong Kong diastolic heart failure study: a randomized controlled trial of diuretics, irbesartan and ramipril on quality of life, exercise capacity, left ventricular global and regional function in heart failure with a normal ejection fraction. *Heart*. 2008;94:573-580.
57. Weber KT. Targeting pathological remodeling. Concepts of cardioprotection and reparation. *Circulation*. 2000;102:1342-1345.

Right Heart Failure

6

Per Lindqvist and Michael Y. Henein

Cardiac output is determined by the efficient left and right ventricular performance; therefore, one should always see the right ventricle as an important integral part of the overall cardiac pump function. A strong evidence supporting the role of the right ventricle in determining exercise tolerance as well as clinical outcome in patients with heart failure exists.[1-3]

Historically, the old belief considered the right heart much less important than the left heart. A possible explanation for this might be the 1943 experimental study by Starr, which showed severe right ventricular damage that affected neither the central venous pressure nor the cardiac output, so long as the pulmonary vascular resistance was maintained.[4] In 1982, Goldstein et al. corrected this understanding by clearly demonstrating a fall in left ventricular size, cardiac output and systemic pressure as a result of acute increase of right ventricular size, and end-diastolic pressure as a consequence of right coronary artery occlusion. These abnormal pressure and cavity size changes normalized only when the pericardium was opened.[5]

6.1
Right Ventricular Anatomy and Physiology

In order to clearly understand the role the right heart plays in the syndrome of heart failure, one should be familiar with the normal right ventricular anatomy and physiology. The right ventricle is structurally made of three components: inflow, apical and outflow tract. The inflow axis of the right ventricle is at a significantly wider angle with the outflow axis, compared to the left ventricle. Such anatomical differences in shape between the two pumps result in significant functional variations. While systolic left ventricular function is mono-cavity, that of the right ventricle is peristaltic controlled by its three compartments, showing a clearly distinguished contraction of the inflow tract compartment 25–30 ms before the outflow tract.[6] The myocardial fiber architecture of the right

P. Lindqvist (✉)
Heart Centre, Public Health and Clinical Medicine, Umeå University Hospital, Umeå, Sweden
e-mail: per.lindqvist@medicin.umu.se

M.Y. Henein (ed.), *Heart Failure in Clinical Practice*,
DOI: 10.1007/978-1-84996-153-0_6, © Springer-Verlag London Limited 2010

ventricle also supports this design. The inflow tract myocardial fibers are predominantly longitudinal, thus behaving as a piston, but those of the outflow tract are mainly circumferential, exhibiting contraction force mainly across the outflow tract radial axis, and hence adding to the competence of the pulmonary valve, in systole. Furthermore, the outflow tract systolic function is the one that determines ejection time relations of the right ventricle.[7] The apical part of the right ventricle is heavily trabeculated and is the least contributor to its overall systolic function. Probably, the major role of the apical component of the right ventricle is to support the stroke volume pumped by the inlet compartment while being diverted to the outflow tract. The relationship between the two ventricles and the circulations they support is also different. The right ventricular inflow and outflow tract walls are significantly thinner than the left ventricle, despite filling by and ejecting the same stroke volume. This could be explained by the known features of the pulmonary circulation; lower vascular resistance, higher distensibility, no progressive stiffness between central and peripheral arteries, and low pulse amplitude compared to the properties of the systemic circulation. This results in the right ventricle having to pump the same stroke volume of the left ventricle, but with only 25% of the stroke work since it is required to produce only 25% the respective systolic pressure produced by the left ventricle. Such fundamental structural and functional differences between the right and left ventricles explain the difference in response between the two pumps to severe rise in afterload. While with mild and moderate rise in afterload, the two ventricles similarly hypertrophy, with progressive increase in afterload, the left ventricle continues to hypertrophy, but the right ventricle dilates. This highlights again, the effect of the baseline muscle thickness on individual cavity response to afterload. Finally, the contribution of septal motion to the right ventricular normal systolic function is only modest compared to its role in the left ventricle.[8]

6.2
Ventricular Interaction

Despite the well-established differences between the right and left ventricular structure and function, the two pumps are in close interaction. Under control conditions, the ventricular interaction is consequential in nature with each of the two ventricles following the other. Few pathological conditions dictate the two ventricles to interact simultaneously in a reciprocal fashion either with respect to different phases of the cardiac cycle or the respiratory cycle. Raised left ventricular systolic pressure caused by increased afterload e.g., systemic hypertension, aortic valve stenosis or outflow tract obstruction does not usually affect the right ventricle. However, significant rise in early diastolic left ventricular pressure gradient, as is the case in patients with restrictive physiology, can cause transmitted high tension across the ventricular septum and suppress the reciprocal right ventricular filling component and compromises its stroke volume.[9] This situation could be reversed by successful left atrial pressure offloading therapy with vasodilators.[10] The opposite occurs in patients with raised right ventricular systolic pressures by increased afterload e.g., in pulmonary hypertension when the right ventricle hypertrophies then dilates and the septum

Fig. 6.1 Abnormal septal motion in pulmonary hypertension

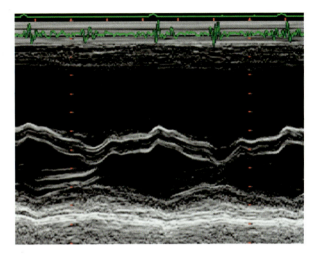

becomes significantly asynchronous (Fig. 6.1). This pattern of cavity dysfunction and raised early diastolic right ventricular pressure with respect to that of the left ventricle suppresses early diastolic left ventricular filling. Isolated diastolic right ventricular pressure changes do not affect left ventricular function because of the natural pressure difference between the two chambers. The second example of ventricular interaction is across the pericardial space e.g., cardiac tamponade. The increased intrapericardial pressure above right ventricular pressure makes its filling and ejection very sensitive to respiration and changes in intrathoracic pressures, and they occur predominantly during inspiration. If this condition is ignored, it eventually affects left ventricular filling and ejection, and the two become mainly expiratory and hence the clinical description of pulsus paradoxus.[11] Similar disturbances can be seen with massive left pleural effusion as well as severe entrapped air in the chest cage e.g., cystic fibrosis.

6.3
Right Ventricular Dysfunction in Left Ventricular Failure

Right ventricular function is usually quite maintained in patients with mild and moderate left ventricular dysfunction. It is only when left atrial pressure rises as a result of increased left ventricular stiffness, irrespective of its etiology, the right ventricular function is affected.[12,13] Even at this stage, the increased left atrial pressure may take time until its effect on the right ventricle becomes obvious as shown by the noninvasive measurements e.g., Doppler echocardiographic features of restrictive filling. Patients with fluctuating left atrial pressure (described as pseudonormal left ventricular filling pattern), in whom E/E′ (early diastolic filling velocity divided by early diastolic myocardial velocity) is usually inconclusive,[14] may continue to have a well-preserved right ventricular function and pressures for long time. Those with well-established raised left atrial pressure (restrictive left ventricular filling pattern) commonly present with raised right ventricular systolic pressure as assessed by the retrograde pressure drop across the tricuspid valve (tricuspid regurgitation) using the modified Bernoulli equation $p = 4V^2$, with values exceeding 40 mmHg.[10,13] In such patients, long-standing pulmonary venous hypertension, particularly in the presence of mitral valve disease, may result in irreversibly raised pulmonary vascular resistance and stiff pulmonary circulation, which may devalue a successful surgical or interventional repair of the structural valve problem (persistent raised pulmonary vascular resistance after mitral valve surgery). Likewise, irreversibly raised left atrial pressure in patients with severe left ventricular myocardial disease may result in established pulmonary venous, then arterial hypertension and its drastic consequences of right ventricular dysfunction. Doubling of right ventricular afterload (from 25 to 50 mmHg) has been shown to affect its systolic function and reduce its ejection fraction by approximately 10%. The tricuspid annulus eventually dilates and secondary tricuspid regurgitation develops which itself, if significant, adds to the clinical deterioration with further drop of right ventricular stroke volume and intractable fluid retention. Eventually, such patients develop liver and kidney dysfunction with their known effects on the overall clinical condition and outcome. The end result is significant drop in right ventricular systolic function and cavity compliance.

6.4
Assessment of Right Ventricular Dysfunction

Right ventricular ejection fraction can be accurately measured by cardiac magnetic resonance (CMR) and values are usually quite reproducible.[15] Having established right ventricular anatomical features, more detailed assessment of its various compartments can be obtained using echocardiography. Systolic right ventricular outflow tract function is assessed by measuring its fractional shortening, as the relative fall in its dimension in systole with respect to that in diastole.[16] Systolic function of the inflow compartment of the right ventricle is easily studied from the systolic excursion of the tricuspid valve annulus towards the apex, i.e., long axis.[17] Values less than 20 mm suggest some degree of dysfunction, and values less than 15 mm are consistent with an overall ejection fraction of less than 45%.[15] Right ventricular systolic myocardial velocities and time relations can also be measured using other echo techniques, myocardial tissue Doppler, strain and strain rate and speckle tracking.[18, 19] In view of the multi compartmental right ventricular anatomy, the ideal echocardiographic means of assessing its function is the 3-dimensional technique. The currently fast development of this echocardiographic modality holds good promises.[15] Assessment of diastolic right ventricular function, particularly in patients with fluid retention, is very important. Doppler echocardiography is the mainstay in this scenario. Functional markers are generally very similar to those conventionally used in the left side of the heart. Myocardial diastolic velocities, particularly those of the inlet compartment of the right ventricle, are easy to measure and are highly reproducible. Signs of right ventricular asynchrony are also similar to those of the left. Delayed onset of right ventricular long-axis systolic or diastolic movement reflect respective asynchrony. The same could be applied to myocardial velocity–time relations. Finally, spectral Doppler assessment of right atrial and right ventricular filling pattern reflects phasic pressure changes and hence provides an accurate diagnosis, particularly in patients with significant right ventricular dysfunction. A dominant transtricuspid "A" wave, commonly seen in pulmonary hypertension, reflects asynchronous right ventricle, while a dominant "E" wave with short deceleration time, along with an early diastolic right atrial filling component, is consistent with restrictive right ventricular physiology[20] (Fig. 6.2). A more than 25% increase in right ventricular filling and ejection velocity during inspiration in a patient with fluid retention reflects raised intrathoracic pressure, irrespective of its cause. Secondary tricuspid and pulmonary valve dysfunction are common in right heart disease. While CMR is very accurate in assessing pulmonary valve regurgitation severity,[21] continuous and pulsed wave Doppler techniques are irreplaceable in quantifying tricuspid regurgitation severity and its consequences.[22, 23] It must be mentioned that although transtricuspid retrograde pressure drop (tricuspid regurgitation) is currently the most accurate measure of peak systolic pulmonary artery pressure it has its known limitations. It tends to underestimate the severity of pulmonary hypertension in patients[24] with raised right atrial pressure e.g., because of a stiff right ventricle and raised end-diastolic pressure. Also, it underestimates pulmonary artery pressure in patients with significant tricuspid regurgitation, even in the absence of obvious organic tricuspid valve disease. Finally, transtricuspid retrograde pressure drop can be accurately recorded in approximately 70% of patients, hence the need for a similar accurate marker for pulmonary hypertension.[25] A prolonged right ventricular isovolumic relaxation time more than 50 ms and 65 ms (corrected for heart rate) measured by traditional trans tricuspid forward flow and pulsed tissue Doppler are consistent with systolic pulmonary artery pressure of >40 mmHg.[26] A short forward pulmonary flow acceleration time of less than 100 ms

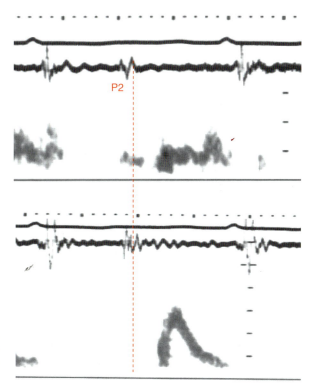

Fig. 6.2 Dominant A velocity in pulmonary hypertension (*upper*) and dominant E wave velocity in restrictive filling pattern (*lower*)

signifies raised pulmonary vascular resistance.[27] Pulmonary regurgitation early diastolic pressure drop reflects mean pulmonary artery systolic pressure[28] (Fig. 6.3).

6.5
Treatment of Right Ventricular Dysfunction in Patients with Left Ventricular Disease

This involves treatment of the underlying cause of pulmonary venous hypertension as early as possible before it becomes well established. Left-sided valve diseases are dealt with surgically or interventionally.[29, 30] Left ventricular outflow tract obstructive myocardial diseases are treated with heart rate controlling medications,[31] myoectomy or nonsurgical myocardial

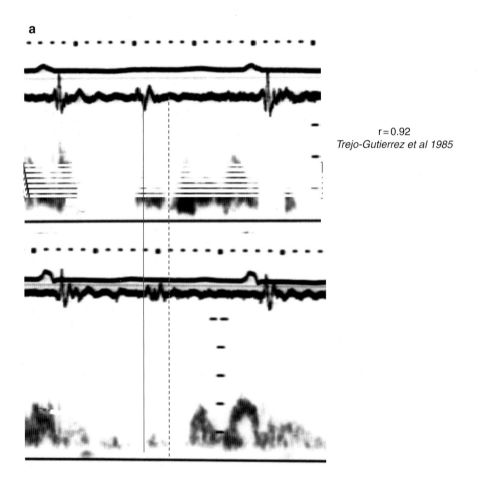

r = 0.92
Trejo-Gutierrez et al 1985

Fig. 6.3 (**a**) Dominant A wave velocity from transtricuspid forward flow and with increased isovolumic relaxation time indicating pulmonary hypertension. (**b**) Normal isovolumic relaxation time (IVRTm) in myocardium (*upper*) and increased IVRTm indicating pulmonary hypertension (*lower left* and *right*)

b

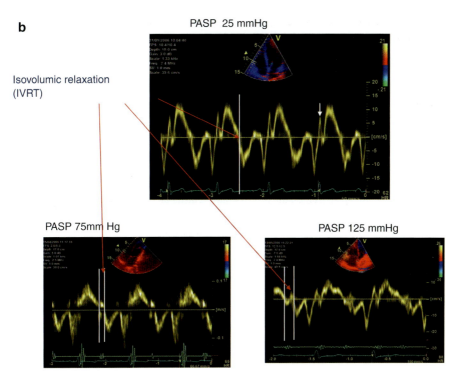

Isovolumic relaxation
(IVRT)

Fig. 6.3 (continued)

reduction procedure.[32] Patients with restrictive or dilated cardiomyopathy and raised left atrial pressure are treated with vasodilators e.g., ACE-Inhibitors, A2 blockers or long-acting nitrates particularly in those with impaired kidney function.[33] As left atrial pressure drops, the early diastolic left ventricular pressure gradient falls and its filling becomes predominantly of the late diastolic pattern.[9] This results in restoration of right ventricular normal diastolic filling pattern.[10] Secondary right heart complications are treated individually. For instance, severe tricuspid regurgitation is treated with diuretics and vasodilators while keeping a sensitive balance between them and the minimum right atrial pressure, needed to maintain adequate right ventricular filling. It should be remembered that patients with significant functional tricuspid regurgitation have some degree of inherent right ventricular dysfunction. Excessive diuretics use in such patients may result in compromised stroke volume and cardiac output.

Most patients with severe left ventricular dysfunction who fulfill the clinical criteria for potential benefit from cardiac resynchronization therapy (CRT) have some degree of right ventricular dysfunction. The available evidence for the effect of CRT on right ventricular function in these patients is limited. However, a number of studies have already shown significant improvement of right ventricular function following CRT. This effect was almost acute[34] and remained for months afterwards.[35, 36] Markers of improvement in right ventricular function were prolongation of filling time, increased systolic velocities and fractional area change as well as reduced Tei index and tricuspid regurgitation.[34, 36] In contrast, patients with asynchronous right ventricular function that causes limited filling time are not recommended for the same electrical treatment, particularly those with raised left atrial pressure. In fact, the latter group have already been shown to have limited response to cardiac resynchronization therapy.[37, 38]

6.6
Cardiopulmonary Bypass Circulation and the Right Ventricle

The right ventricle plays a pivotal role in any cardiac surgery procedure, particularly coronary artery bypass graft surgery and aortic valve surgery. Most patients undergoing such operations end up with significant fall of right ventricular free wall systolic function.[39] Despite the remaining unclear cause of such surgical consequence, the overall right ventricular function seems to remain preserved as a result of septal reversed motion.[40, 41] A successful coronary or valve surgery may be undervalued because of a missed poorly functioning right ventricle preoperatively which fails to support the circulation postoperatively, either immediately after surgery or during the early perioperative period.[42] It is, therefore, a serious responsibility to critically assess right ventricular function preoperatively, particularly in patients with additional pathologies e.g., chronic obstructive pulmonary diseases (COPD) or raised pulmonary vascular resistance. Noteworthy, the response of right ventricular function to left cardiac surgery seems to be irrespective of on-pump or off-pump technique.[43] Finally, patients with severe left ventricular failure needing assist device support (LVAD) may suffer right ventricular complications as a result.[44] With LVAD, right ventricular afterload falls, but preload increases, which results in increased right ventricular diastolic volume and myocardial contractile activity. However, patients with prior right ventricular myocardial disease may behave differently. It is worth remembering that right ventricular failure occurs in up to 25% of patients receiving LVAD and is always associated with poor outcome[44] (Fig. 6.4).

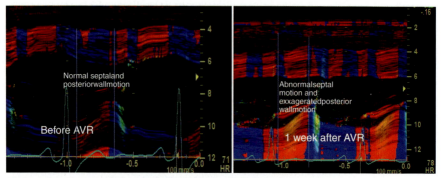

Fig. 6.4 Septal motion before and 1 week after aortic valve replacement

6.7
Right Ventricular Dysfunction Secondary to Pulmonary Disease

The commonest cause of right ventricular dysfunction in these patients is COPD. Long-standing COPD may result in various degrees of right ventricular systolic and diastolic dysfunction, but it rarely causes pulmonary hypertension at rest.[45] Other left-sided pathologies e.g., moderate aortic stenosis or coronary artery disease may mask the symptoms caused by COPD. Stress echocardiography provides an ideal tool for discriminating between these conditions when the pressure gradient significantly increases with stress at the time of symptom development, suggesting a primary valve problem.[46] Systemic sclerosis (scleroderma) is another parenchymal disease which has been proposed to cause subendocardial fibrosis and dysfunction.[47] Severe cases may present with significant pulmonary hypertension which could be quite limiting and associated with poor clinical outcome.[48] Finally, other parenchymal fibrotic disease e.g., cystic fibrosis may also involve right ventricular myocardium and cause significant systolic and diastolic dysfunction, even in the absence of pulmonary hypertension. Patients with end-stage cystic fibrosis may present with a picture similar to cardiac tamponade, as a result of the increased intrathoracic pressure. Although right ventricular function in most pulmonary conditions may look normal at rest, its behavior at fast heart rate remains to be determined.

The commonest pulmonary vascular disease that affects the right ventricle is pulmonary embolism, which represents acute increase in afterload. Like the left side of the heart, acute changes in the circulation at any level are poorly tolerated. Small pulmonary embolism may be compensated for, but a massive one could be fatal.[49] The right ventricle acutely dilates and its systolic function falls.[50] Also, right ventricular systolic pressure will acutely increase as a result of the vascular obstruction. Even if the effect of pulmonary embolism on the right ventricle is not direct, it may be through the drastic effect of the reflected waves, as is the case in acute aortic clamping that causes left ventricular dysfunction.[51] Pulmonary embolectomy, in addition to thrombolysis and supportive therapy, may save the right ventricle irreversible damage and improve its function.[52]

6.8
Primary Right Ventricular Dysfunction

The commonest cause of primary dysfunction is right ventricular infarction. It occurs in approximately 30% of patients presenting with acute inferior infarction and may result in severe hemodynamic compromise with a variable clinical outcome.[5] Acute right coronary artery occlusion proximal to the right ventricular branch often causes free wall dysfunction. Patients presenting with right ventricular infarction have low cardiac output and fluid retention during the acute presentation. As right ventricular myocardial perfusion occurs during both diastole and systole, the systolic flow component diminishes as a result of the elevated chamber pressure[53, 54] during the acute attack. Therefore, maintaining coronary flow is crucial when right ventricular systolic pressure is elevated. Patients with right ventricular infarction often respond positively to fluid treatment (Frank Starling mechanism) and early myocardial reperfusion enhances the recovery of right ventricular performance and significantly improves clinical outcome.[5] Fine adjustment and monitoring of cardiac hemodynamics, fluid retention and conventional diuretics and vasodilation treatment should be adhered to.

6.9
Prognostic Value of Right Ventricular Function

Despite often ignored during management planning, right ventricular dysfunction has been shown to carry significant prognostic value in various cardiac conditions; ischemic[55] and nonischemic cardiomyopathy,[56] acute myocardial infarction[57] and myocarditis.[58] Right ventricular ejection fraction <35% carries poor prognosis, and patients with values above 35% usually have satisfactory oxygen uptake levels with exercise.[2] In fact, right ventricular ejection fraction has been found to better correlate with MVO_2 than that of the left ventricle.[1] Furthermore, right ventricular long-axis amplitude of >14 mm has been shown to be associated with better survival than values <14 mm.[59] This applies not only to patients with various myocardial pathologies but also to those receiving cardiac resynchronization therapy who do not demonstrate significant functional improvement[60] (Fig. 6.5).

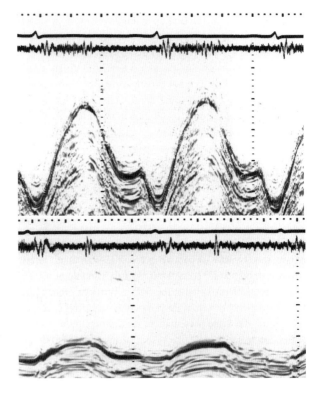

Fig. 6.5 Normal (*upper*) and reduced (*lower*) right ventricular long axis amplitude

References

1. Baker BJ, Wilen MM, Boyd CM, Dinh H, Franciosa JA. Relation of right ventricular ejection fraction to exercise capacity in chronic left ventricular failure. *Am J Cardiol*. 1984;54(6):596-599.
2. Di Salvo TG, Mathier M, Semigran MJ, Dec GW. Preserved right ventricular ejection fraction predicts exercise capacity and survival in advanced heart failure. *J Am Coll Cardiol*. 1995; 25(5):1143-1153.
3. Ghio S, Gavazzi A, Campana C, et al. Independent and additive prognostic value of right ventricular systolic function and pulmonary artery pressure in patients with chronic heart failure. *J Am Coll Cardiol*. 2001;37(1):183-188.
4. Starr I, Jeffers WA, Meade RH. The absence of conspicuous increments of venous pressure after severe damage of the right ventricle in dog, with discussion of the relation between clinical congestive heart failure and heart disease. *Am Heart J*. 1943;26:291-301.
5. Goldstein JA. Right heart ischemia: pathophysiology, natural history, and clinical management. *Prog Cardiovasc Dis*. 1998;40(4):325-341.
6. Armour JA, Randall WC. Structural basis for cardiac function. *Am J Physiol*. 1970;218(6): 1517-1523.
7. Calcuteea A, Maras D, Lei W, Hodson M, Henein M. Myocardial determinants of right ventricular ejection in pulmonary hypertension: 2D strain rate and spectral doppler study. *Eur J Echocardiogr*. 2008;9(suppl 1):S53.
8. Kaul S. The interventricular septum in health and disease. *Am Heart J*. 1986;112(3):568-581.
9. Henein MY, Gibson DG. Suppression of left ventricular early diastolic filling by long axis asynchrony. *Br Heart J*. 1995;73(2):151-157.
10. Henein MY, O'Sullivan CA, Coats AJ, Gibson DG. Angiotensin-converting enzyme (ACE) inhibitors revert abnormal right ventricular filling in patients with restrictive left ventricular disease. *J Am Coll Cardiol*. 1998;32(5):1187-1193.
11. Guntheroth WG. Sensitivity and specificity of echocardiographic evidence of tamponade: implications for ventricular interdependence and pulsus paradoxus. *Pediatr Cardiol*. 2007; 28(5):358-362.
12. Grose R, Strain J, Yipintosoi T. Right ventricular function in valvular heart disease: relation to pulmonary artery pressure. *J Am Coll Cardiol*. 1983;2(2):225-232.
13. Enriquez-Sarano M, Rossi A, Seward JB, Bailey KR, Tajik AJ. Determinants of pulmonary hypertension in left ventricular dysfunction. *J Am Coll Cardiol*. 1997;29(1):153-159.
14. Ommen SR, Nishimura RA, Appleton CP, et al. Clinical utility of Doppler echocardiography and tissue Doppler imaging in the estimation of left ventricular filling pressures: a comparative simultaneous Doppler-catheterization study. *Circulation*. 2000;102(15):1788-1794.
15. Kjaergaard J, Petersen CL, Kjaer A, Schaadt BK, Oh JK, Hassager C. Evaluation of right ventricular volume and function by 2D and 3D echocardiography compared to MRI. *Eur J Echocardiogr*. 2006;7:430-438.
16. Lindqvist P, Henein M, Kazzam E. Right ventricular outflow-tract fractional shortening: an applicable measure of right ventricular systolic function. *Eur J Echocardiogr*. 2003;4(1):29-35.
17. Kaul S, Tei C, Hopkins JM, Shah PM. Assessment of right ventricular function using two-dimensional echocardiography. *Am Heart J*. 1984;107(3):526-531.
18. Hoffmann R, Hanrath P. Tricuspid annular velocity measurement. Simple and accurate solution for a delicate problem? *Eur Heart J*. 2001;22(4):280-282.
19. Lindqvist P, Calcuteea A, Henein M. Echocardiography in the assessment of right heart function. *Eur J Echocardiogr*. 2008;9(2):225-234.
20. Lam YY, Kaya MG, Goktekin O, Gatzoulis MA, Li W, Henein MY. Restrictive right ventricular physiology: its presence and symptomatic contribution in patients with pulmonary valvular stenosis. *J Am Coll Cardiol*. 2007;50(15):1491-1497.

21. Puchalski MD, Askovich B, Sower CT, Williams RV, Minich LL, Tani LY. Pulmonary regurgitation: determining severity by echocardiography and magnetic resonance imaging. *Congenit Heart Dis*. 2008;3(3):168-175.
22. Currie PJ, Seward JB, Chan KL, et al. Continuous wave Doppler determination of right ventricular pressure: a simultaneous Doppler-catheterization study in 127 patients. *J Am Coll Cardiol*. 1985;6(4):750-756.
23. Zoghbi WA, Enriquez-Sarano M, Foster E, et al. Recommendations for evaluation of the severity of native valvular regurgitation with two-dimensional and Doppler echocardiography. *J Am Soc Echocardiogr*. 2003;16(7):777-802.
24. Brecker SJ, Gibbs JS, Fox KM, Yacoub MH, Gibson DG. Comparison of Doppler derived haemodynamic variables and simultaneous high fidelity pressure measurements in severe pulmonary hypertension. *Br Heart J*. 1994;72(4):384-389.
25. Barst RJ, McGoon M, Torbicki A, et al. Diagnosis and differential assessment of pulmonary arterial hypertension. *J Am Coll Cardiol*. 2004;43(12 suppl S):40S-47S.
26. Lindqvist P, Henein MY, Wikstrom G. Right ventricular myocardial velocities and timing estimate pulmonary artery systolic pressure. *Int J Cardiol*. 2009;137:130-136.
27. Dabestani A, Mahan G, Gardin JM, et al. Evaluation of pulmonary artery pressure and resistance by pulsed Doppler echocardiography. *Am J Cardiol*. 1987;59(6):662-668.
28. Posteraro A, Salustri A, Trambaiolo P, Amici E, Gambelli G. Echocardiographic estimation of pulmonary pressures. *J Cardiovasc Med*. 2006;7(7):545-554.
29. Cohn WE. Percutaneous valve interventions: where we are and where we are headed. *Am Heart Hosp J*. 2006 Summer;4(3):186-191.
30. Vahanian A, Baumgartner H, Bax J, et al. Guidelines on the management of valvular heart disease. *Rev Esp Cardiol*. 2007;60(6):1e-50e.
31. Seggewiss H. Medical therapy versus interventional therapy in hypertropic obstructive cardiomyopathy. *Curr Controlled Trials Cardiovasc Med*. 2000;1(2):115-119.
32. Henein MY, O'Sullivan CA, Ramzy IS, Sigwart U, Gibson DG. Electromechanical left ventricular behavior after nonsurgical septal reduction in patients with hypertrophic obstructive cardiomyopathy. *J Am Coll Cardiol*. 1999;34(4):1117-1122.
33. Henein MY, Amadi A, O'Sullivan C, Coats A, Gibson DG. ACE inhibitors unmask incoordinate diastolic wall motion in restrictive left ventricular disease. *Heart*. 1996;76(4):326-331.
34. Donal E, Vignat N, De Place C, et al. Acute effects of biventricular pacing on right ventricular function assessed by tissue Doppler imaging. *Europace*. 2007;9(2):108-112.
35. Bleeker GB, Schalij MJ, Nihoyannopoulos P, et al. Left ventricular dyssynchrony predicts right ventricular remodeling after cardiac resynchronization therapy. *J Am Coll Cardiol*. 2005;46(12):2264-2269.
36. Rajagopalan N, Suffoletto MS, Tanabe M, et al. Right ventricular function following cardiac resynchronization therapy. *Am J Cardiol*. 2007;100(9):1434-1436.
37. Gradaus R, Stuckenborg V, Loher A, et al. Diastolic filling pattern and left ventricular diameter predict response and prognosis after cardiac resynchronisation therapy. *Heart*. 2008; 94(8):1026-1031.
38. Salukhe TV, Francis DP, Clague JR, Sutton R, Poole-Wilson P, Henein MY. Chronic heart failure patients with restrictive LV filling pattern have significantly less benefit from cardiac resynchronization therapy than patients with late LV filling pattern. *Int J Cardiol*. 2005;100(1):5-12.
39. Wranne B, Pinto FJ, Hammarstrom E, StGoar FG, Puryear J, Popp RL. Abnormal right heart filling after cardiac surgery: time course and mechanisms. *Br Heart J*. 1991; 66(6):435-442.
40. Tamborini G, Muratori M, Brusoni D, et al. Is right ventricular systolic function reduced after cardiac surgery? A two- and three-dimensional echocardiographic study. *Eur J Echocardiogr*. 2009;10(5):630-634.
41. Joshi SB, Salah AK, Mendoza DD, Goldstein SA, Fuisz AR, Lindsay J. Mechanism of paradoxical ventricular septal motion after coronary artery bypass grafting. *Am J Cardiol*. 2009;103(2):212-215.

42. Vlahakes GJ. Right ventricular failure following cardiac surgery. *Coron Artery Dis*. 2005; 16(1):27-30.

43. Pegg TJ, Selvanayagam JB, Karamitsos TD, et al. Effects of off-pump versus on-pump coronary artery bypass grafting on early and late right ventricular function. *Circulation*. 2008; 117(17):2202-2210.

44. Santambrogio L, Bianchi T, Fuardo M, et al. Right ventricular failure after left ventricular assist device insertion: preoperative risk factors. *Interact Cardiovasc Thorac Surg*. 2006;5(4):379-382.

45. Arcasoy SM, Christie JD, Ferrari VA, et al. Echocardiographic assessment of pulmonary hypertension in patients with advanced lung disease. *Am J Respir Crit Care Med*. 2003;167(5):735-740.

46. Nishimura RA, Carabello BA, Faxon DP, et al. ACC/AHA 2008 Guideline update on valvular heart disease: focused update on infective endocarditis: a report of the American College of Cardiology/American Heart Association Task Force on Practice Guidelines endorsed by the Society of Cardiovascular Anesthesiologists, Society for Cardiovascular Angiography and Interventions, and Society of Thoracic Surgeons. *J Am Coll Cardiol*. 2008;52(8):676-685.

47. Henein MY, Cailes J, O'Sullivan C, du Bois RM, Gibson DG. Abnormal ventricular long-axis function in systemic sclerosis. *Chest*. 1995;108(6):1533-1540.

48. Proudman SM, Stevens WM, Sahhar J, Celermajer D. Pulmonary arterial hypertension in systemic sclerosis: the need for early detection and treatment. *Intern Med J*. 2007;37(7):485-494.

49. Kjaergaard J, Schaadt BK, Lund JO, Hassager C. Prognostic importance of quantitative echocardiographic evaluation in patients suspected of first non-massive pulmonary embolism. *Eur J Echocardiogr*. 2009;10(1):89-95.

50. Kjaergaard J, Schaadt BK, Lund JO, Hassager C. Quantitative measures of right ventricular dysfunction by echocardiography in the diagnosis of acute nonmassive pulmonary embolism. *J Am Soc Echocardiogr*. 2006;19(10):1264-1271.

51. Henein MY, Das SK, O'Sullivan C, Kakkar VV, Gillbe CE, Gibson DG. Effect of acute alterations in afterload on left ventricular function in patients with combined coronary artery and peripheral vascular disease. *Heart*. 1996;75(2):151-158.

52. Mahmud E, Raisinghani A, Hassankhani A, et al. Correlation of left ventricular diastolic filling characteristics with right ventricular overload and pulmonary artery pressure in chronic thromboembolic pulmonary hypertension. *J Am Coll Cardiol*. 2002;40(2):318-324.

53. Ribeiro A, Lindmarker P, Johnsson H, Juhlin-Dannfelt A, Jorfeldt L. Pulmonary embolism: a follow-up study of the relation between the degree of right ventricle overload and the extent of perfusion defects. *J Intern Med*. 1999;245(6):601-610.

54. Gomez A, Bialostozky D, Zajarias A, et al. Right ventricular ischemia in patients with primary pulmonary hypertension. *J Am Coll Cardiol*. 2001;38(4):1137-1142.

55. Polak JF, Holman BL, Wynne J, Colucci WS. Right ventricular ejection fraction: an indicator of increased mortality in patients with congestive heart failure associated with coronary artery disease. *J Am Coll Cardiol*. 1983;2(2):217-224.

56. Juilliere Y, Barbier G, Feldmann L, Grentzinger A, Danchin N, Cherrier F. Additional predictive value of both left and right ventricular ejection fractions on long-term survival in idiopathic dilated cardiomyopathy. *Eur Heart J*. 1997;18(2):276-280.

57. Shah PK, Maddahi J, Staniloff HM, et al. Variable spectrum and prognostic implications of left and right ventricular ejection fractions in patients with and without clinical heart failure after acute myocardial infarction. *Am J Cardiol*. 1986;58(6):387-393.

58. Mendes LA, Dec GW, Picard MH, Palacios IF, Newell J, Davidoff R. Right ventricular dysfunction: an independent predictor of adverse outcome in patients with myocarditis. *Am Heart J*. 1994;128(2):301-307.

59. Kjaergaard J, Akkan D, Iversen KK, Kober L, Torp-Pedersen C, Hassager C. Right ventricular dysfunction as an independent predictor of short- and long-term mortality in patients with heart failure. *Eur J Heart Fail*. 2007;9(6-7):610-616.

60. Ghio S, Freemantle N, Scelsi L, et al. Long-term left ventricular reverse remodelling with cardiac resynchronization therapy: results from the CARE-HF trial. *Eur J Heart Fail*. 2009; 11(5):480-488.

Pulmonary Arterial Hypertension

7

Stefan Söderberg and Michael Y. Henein

Pulmonary arterial hypertension (PAH) is a syndrome resulting from restricted flow of blood through the pulmonary arterial circulation due to increased pulmonary vascular resistance and is complicated ultimately by right heart failure. A number of pathological pathways are involved in the development of PAH, including those at the genetic and molecular levels, and arterial smooth muscle, endothelial cells and adventitia. The imbalance in the vasoconstrictor/vasodilator milieu represents the basis for current medical therapies, although PAH also involves an imbalance of proliferation and apoptosis. The present classification of pulmonary hypertension (PH) was established in 1998 at the World Congress of PH in Evian, and was later revised in Dana Point in 2008 (Table 7.1).[1]

7.1
Classification

Idiopathic pulmonary hypertension (IPAH) was previously considered a rare disease that affected mainly young women (formerly labeled primary PH). However, recent data from a French registry suggests that the disorder is more common and affects not only young women but also middle aged and elderly women. The female dominance is seen in all age groups with approximately doubled prevalence compared to men. Familial PAH (FPAH) often results from a mutation in the bone morphogenic protein receptor-2 (BMRP2) and is inherited as an autosomal dominant disease with incomplete penetrance. PAH is also associated with connective tissue diseases, in particular with scleroderma and systemic lupus erytematosis, congenital heart disease with systemic-to-pulmonary shunts, portal hypertension, HIV infection, drugs and toxins, and haemolytic anemias. These groups together compromise the World Health Organization (WHO) Group I PAH. Group II is associated with left heart disease, Group III with lung disease and/or hypoxemia, Group IV with chronic thrombotic and/or embolic disease (CTEPH), and Group V is caused by other miscellaneous pathologies.

S. Söderberg (✉)
Heart Centre, Umeå University Hospital, Umeå, Sweden
e-mail: stefan.soderberg@medicin.umu.se

M.Y. Henein (ed.), *Heart Failure in Clinical Practice*,
DOI: 10.1007/978-1-84996-153-0_7, © Springer-Verlag London Limited 2010

Table 7.1 Updated clinical classification of pulmonary hypertension (Dana Point, 2008[1])

1 Pulmonary arterial hypertension (PAH)

  1.1 Idiopathic

  1.2 Heritable

      1.2.1 BMPR2
      1.2.2 ALK1, endoglin (with or without hereditary haemorrhagic telangiectasia)
      1.2.3 Unknown

  1.3 Drugs and toxins induced

  1.4 Associated with (APAH)

      1.4.1 Connective tissue diseases
      1.4.2 HIV infection
      1.4.3 Portal hypertension
      1.4.4 Congenital heart disease
      1.4.5 Schistosomiasis
      1.4.6 Chronic haemolytic anaemia

  1.5 Persistent pulmonary hypertension of the newborn

1′ Pulmonary veno-occlusive disease and/or pulmonary capillary haemangiomatosis

2 Pulmonary hypertension due to left heart disease

  2.1 Systolic dysfunction
  2.2 Diastolic dysfunction
  2.3 Valvular disease

3 Pulmonary hypertension due to lung diseases and/or hypoxaemia

  3.1 Chronic obstructive pulmonary disease
  3.2 Interstitial lung disease
  3.3 Other pulmonary diseases with mixed restrictive and obstructive pattern
  3.4 Sleep-disordered breathing
  3.5 Alveolar hypoventilation disorders
  3.6 Chronic exposure to high altitude
  3.7 Developmental abnormalities

4 Chronic thromboembolic pulmonary hypertension

5 PH with unclear and/or multifactorial mechanisms

  5.1 Haematological disorders: myeloproliferative disorders, splenectomy.
  5.2 Systemic disorders: sarcoidosis, pulmonary Langerhans cell histiocytosis, lymphangi-oleiomyomatosis, neurofibromatosis, vasculitis
  5.3 Metabolic disorders: glycogen storage disease, Gaucher disease, thyroid disorders
  5.4 Others: tumoural obstruction, fibrosing mediastinitis, chronic renal failure on dialysis

ALK-1 = activin receptor-like kinase 1 gene; APAH = associated pulmonary arterial hypertension; BMPR2 = bone morphogenetic protein receptor, type 2; HIV = human immunodeficiency virus; PAH = pulmonary arterial hypertension.

It must be remembered that IPAH is only a small proportion of all causes of PH, the commonest of which are diseases of the left side of the heart and pulmonary disorders. These conditions are not the focus for this chapter but are important to consider whenever PH is investigated.

7.2
Definition and Pathophysiology

The hemodynamic definition of PH is a mean pulmonary artery pressure of 25 mmHg or higher at rest. Notably, the definition is based on mean pressures, obtained by right heart catherization (RHC). The definition of PAH also requires a normal wedge pressure (or normal end diastolic pressure in the left ventricle) ($\leq$15 mmHg), and pulmonary vascular resistance of more than three Wood units. Our understanding of the pathophysiology of PAH has improved over the last decades. Three basic mechanisms seem to contribute to the increased pulmonary vascular resistance; vasoconstriction, proliferation of the components of the wall of the small pulmonary arteries, and local thrombus formation, which create an increased work load for the right ventricle (RV) and ultimately, cavity failure. Endothelial dysfunction is a central process with marked alterations in the balance between nitric oxide (NO), prostacyclin and entothelin. These alterations are thus the foundation for the modern medical treatment of PAH.

7.3
Pulmonary Hypertension and the Right Heart

PH represents increased afterload on the RV. Mild degree of PAH is well tolerated by the RV as it develops mild degree of hypertrophy, which may be difficult to notice. With moderate degree of PH and peak PA pressure exceeding 60 mmHg right ventricular hypertrophy becomes more apparent and its cavity shape changes, showing a flat interventricular septum which is reflected on left ventricular sphericity index with leftward shift.[2] Up till this stage the right ventricular response to pressure overload is almost similar to that of the left ventricle. However, with further increase in PA pressures the RV dilates at its outflow tract as well as inflow tract compartments. Clinicians rely on this picture for diagnosing PH in a breathless patient. This picture, in the presence of normal left atrial pressure, is suggestive of PAH pathology (Group 1). It is difficult to exclude with certainty chronic thromboembolic pathology as a possible etiology, using transthoracic echocardiography. However, echocardiography is the most accurate noninvasive investigation for identifying the exact primary left sided lesion and determining the best management policy. The commonest cause of PH, in the west, is hypertensive left ventricular disease with or without diabetes. In these patients, the left ventricular cavity is normal in size and systolic function is preserved but the left atrium is enlarged in the absence of any detectable mitral valve disease. The reason behind the left atrial dilatation is the rise in its pressure as a result of a stiff left ventricle with raised end-diastolic pressure. Furthermore, a significant number of patients presenting with this pattern have either established or paroxysmal atrial arrhythmia, as additional cause of their breathlessness. The raised left atrial pressure is transferred to the pulmonary veins and hence the development of pulmonary venous hypertension as a precursor to PAH. Similar pathophysiology is seen in patients with dilated left ventricle and stiff myocardium irrespective of its etiology. Finally, long standing aortic valve disease, particularly stenosis may cause left ventricular disease and raised left atrial pressure. Mitral valve disease results primarily into pulmonary venous hypertension and its consequences. Mitral regurgitation however, if ignored, may cause irreversible left ventricular myocardial dysfunction and pulmonary venous hypertension, which may persist, even after successful valve repair surgery.

7.3.1
Estimating Systolic Pulmonary Artery Pressure

The conventional echocardiographic evaluation of systolic PA pressure is made from the sum of the retrograde pressure drop across the tricuspid valve and right atrial pressure.[2] Values for systolic PA pressure exceeding 60 mmHg are consistent with severe PH. A parallel finding is the prolongation of isovolemic relaxation time, measured from spectral Doppler filling or myocardial tissue Doppler velocities of the RV.[3] Recently, equations combining isovolumic time and velocities have been proposed as a sensitive means for estimating catheter-based measurements of peak systolic PA pressure.[4] Even in the absence of significantly raised quantified systolic PA pressure, Doppler recordings of PA proximal velocities accurately reflect the rise in pulmonary vascular resistance, an acceleration time of 100 ms or less is consistent with raised pulmonary vascular resistance.[5] Finally, peak early diastolic pressure drop between the PA and the RV, from the pulmonary regurgitation continuous wave Doppler velocity display, reflects mean PA pressure.[2]

7.3.2
Right Ventricular Function Response to PH

Increases in PA pressures are reflected on right ventricular structure and function. The first response is an increase in wall thickness followed by rapid unpredicted increase in cavity size and change in its shape. The increase in right ventricular systolic pressure abducts the interventricular septum to function as part of the RV rather than the left ventricle. This results in flattening of the interventricular septum and diversion of the septal direction of power generation to become right ventricular. Of course, this affects left ventricular cavity shape and functional efficiency, with the septum being asynchronous in motion. Although the effect of the progressive increase in PA pressure on the right ventricular trabecular apex is very little, it does have significance consequences on the outflow tract. The latter is made of circumferential fibers, the function of which has been shown to determine ejection time relations of the RV. In patients with significant PAH the outflow tract compartment of the RV becomes dilated and its systolic function significantly reduced as assessed by the fractional shortening equation.[6] Furthermore, the outflow tract loses its function as the determinant of right ventricular ejection time relations.[7] This function becomes transferred to the mid-cavity region of the RV. It must be remembered that with chronic long standing PAH significant right ventricular shape change occurs. The well distinct inflow an doutflow tract at a wide angle become an almost cylindrical cavity, with less efficient function.

Long-standing severe PAH perpetually deteriorates right heart function, and changes may become irreversible. Noncompliant cavity results in increased end-diastolic pressure, which is reflected on the known clinical signs, dominant "a" wave and deep "Y" descent in the jugular venous pulse along with respective Doppler flow velocities in SVC and IVC. Stiff RVs also fill with a typical restrictive pattern, the features of which are dominant early diastolic filling component followed by only a modest end-diastolic filling component and hence the respective flow reversal in venae cavae and hepatic veins. The combination of long standing right ventricular disease and raised right atrial pressure may cause tricuspid annulus dilatation and significant tricuspid regurgitation. When happens it alters the jugular venous pulse pattern, demonstrating a large "V" wave followed by deep "Y" descent with corresponding systolic flow reversal and dominant early diastolic flow in the systemic venous system. This pattern of right ventricular physiology can easily be demonstrated by pulsed and color flow Doppler. Finally, progressive enlargement of the right atrium as a result of the pressure or volume overload may lay the foundation for unstable atrial mechanical function and arrhythmia.

In view of the above, early identification of patients with or prone to develop PAH is of significant importance. This can easily be achieved by stress echocardiography, with its noninvasive objective and highly reproducible measurements of changes in pulmonary vascular resistance and PA pressure at fast heart rate, at the time of symptom development. Aggressive treatment of such patients with combined medication may prove a great future investment for disease prevention.[8]

7.3.3
Incidence and Natural History

The actual incidence of IPAH is unclear; approximately between 2 and 10 new cases per million and year. The prevalence is also unclear, from the above-mentioned French registry, a prevalence of 15 cases per million was reported, with significant regional differences. Half of the prevalence was attributed to IPAH. Twenty percent of scleroderma patients develop PAH and scleroderma itself is the underlying cause of the PAH in 20% of the PAH population. The natural history of IPAH has been well characterized, with a median survival of 2.8 years in a cohort followed during the eighties. Prognosis is also influenced by the underlying etiology, as patients with scleroderma related PAH having shorter survival compared to those with congenital heart disease. Despite modern therapy, the prognosis is still poor, with annual mortality of approximately 15%. Predictors of poor prognosis include: advanced functional class (FC), poor exercise capacity measured by 6-minute walk test (6MWT) or cardiopulmonary exercise test, high right atrial pressure, RV dysfunction, RV failure, low cardiac index, elevated brain natriuretic peptide, and underlying diagnosis of scleroderma.

7.3.4
Clinical Assessment

The clinical presentation of PAH is not specific with symptoms like dyspnea, tiredness and reduced physical ability. Chest pain and syncope develop with advanced disease. The symptoms are slowly progressive and often patients report a long prediagnostic phase of symptoms that have been misinterpreted. With our current knowledge of the disease this diagnostic delay should not be allowed hence the need for serious proactive approach towards early patient identification. Furthermore, regular screening for PH is recommended for patients with all other conditions known to be related to PAH e.g., scleroderma. At each clinical examination, critical evaluation of symptoms, quality of life and degree of exercise intolerance should be undertaken, and FC ascertained, I for no symptoms, II for symptoms at more than ordinary physical activity, III for symptoms with ordinary activities, and IV for symptoms at rest or slightest activity. This classification is important as FC is related to prognosis and is essential in guiding towards best treatment option.

7.3.5
Investigations

A suggested algorithm for necessary diagnostic investigations is presented in Fig. 7.1. A breathless patient should be investigated with a chest-X-ray, a spirometry, an electrocardiogram, and an echocardiogram. In most cases, a diagnosis related to Group II or III is reached based on these tests and appropriate treatment is commenced. If the diagnosis remains uncertain objective assessment of exercise capacity and pulmonary embolism should be undertaken. If these investigations raise the possibility of PH related to Group I, IV or V, a right heart catheter with provocation should be performed at a centre with experience in PAH.

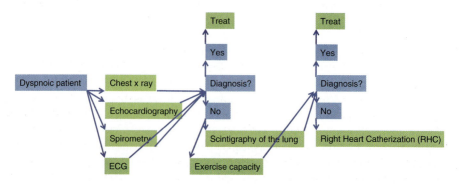

Fig. 7.1 PAH diagnostic strategy

The RHC should provide the following measurements:

Right atrial pressure and ventricular systolic and end-diastolic pressure

PA systolic, diastolic and mean pressure

PA wedge pressure (or left ventricular end-diastolic pressure)

Cardiac output and index using thermodilution except with significant tricuspid regurgitation or significant intracardiac shunt when Fick's method is required.

Pulmonary vascular resistance, calculated as the ratio between the transpulmonary gradient (mean PA pressure – mean wedge pressure) and the cardiac output and is expressed in Wood units.

A vasoreactive test is done with inhaled NO or infused epoprostenol. A positive response (reduction of mean PA pressure by $\geq$10 mmHg to an absolute level of 40 mmHg or less without a decrease in cardiac output) is seen in 10% of IPAH cases. This test has prognostic significance and should guide physicians towards best treatment choice.

Several other investigations may be needed to differentiate between Group 1 subgroups e.g., history of anorexinogenic drugs and serum markers for rheumatologic disease. Also, portal circulation Doppler studies, for portal hypertension, transesophageal echocardiography and magnetic resonance imaging for detection of shunts can all be used to achieve definitive diagnosis. All efforts must be made to exclude chronic thromboembolic status as a cause of PH (CTEPH), which may require scintegraphy, CT angio and pulmonary angiography, as this is a potentially curable condition.

7.3.6
Treatment

The development of therapeutic options for PAH over the last 20 years has been very favorable to the introduction of new pharmaceutical principles that are currently investigated. Despite PAH being rare, of diversified etiology, a number of clinical trials have already been completed and reported. Several of these studies are small and the majority included patients in FC III and IV. Also, most studies included various etiologies within Group I, although some have included Group IV subjects. Different outcomes have been studied; hemodynamic parameters e.g., cardiac index, mean PA pressure, pulmonary vascular resistance, exercise capacity using 6MWT, and clinical parameters like time to clinical worsening e.g., death, lung transplantation, hospitalization, atrial septostomy, or the need for additional PAH medications. Twenty-three randomized controlled trials (RCT) including 3,140 patients focusing on the above principles have been published. A recent meta-analysis demonstrated a clear effect on mortality, with a 43% reduction in patients on active treatment compared to placebo.[9]

General treatment measures include warfarin, particularly in patients with IPAH. The objective is to limit thrombus formation in the small pulmonary arterioles. Diuretics and spironolactone are given to patients with right heart failure. Oxygen should be generously given, keeping oxygen saturation above 90% if hypoxemia develops, as restored oxygen levels can reduce the pulmonary vascular resistance. Low grade aerobic exercise such as walking should be encouraged, and more intensive training has also contributed to better quality of life and clinical outcome. Exposure to high altitude should be avoided and some patients may need oxygen on commercial aircrafts. Pregnancy should be avoided, as the hemodynamic changes are potentially devastating with a high maternal mortality

(30–50%). If the vasoreactive test is positive, calcium channel blockers may be tried, but should never be given without a detailed RHC, for the fear of inducing low cardiac output on top of an impaired right ventricular function, and potential death. In contrast, IPAH patients with positive test (5–10%), preserved cardiac output and normal right ventricular function should be given a calcium channel blocker e.g., nifedipin, deltiazem, or amlodipine, as their prognosis is excellent in responding patients.

7.3.7
New Pharmacologiocal Therapies

Recent treatment algorithms have been developed and resulted in halting disease progress in many cases, improved quality of life and FC (Fig. 7.2). Directions for the use of these drugs have been included in international guidelines, the latest by the American Heart Association in 2009.[10] These drugs interfere with endothelin, NO and prostacyclin pathways in the vessel wall.

7.4
Endothelin Receptors Blockers

Endothelin-1 is a strong vasoconstrictor and a smooth muscle mitogen, and its effects are mediated through ETA and ETB receptors in endothelial and smooth muscle cells. In PAH, plasma levels of endothelin-1 are increased as its active expression in the PA wall. Three

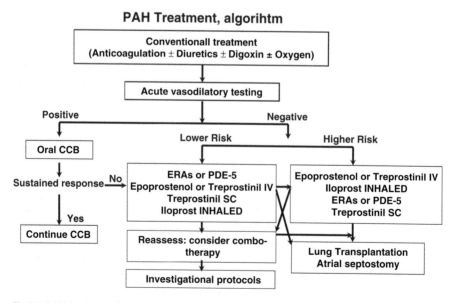

Fig. 7.2 PAH treatment algorithm

endothelin receptor blocking agents are available, bosentan blocking both ETA and ETB, and sitaxentan and ambrisentan blocking selectively the ETA receptor. The most common side effect of these drugs is abnormal liver function, which occurs more frequently with bosentan at any time after initiation, and hence the need for continuous monitoring of liver enzymes. Theoretically there are pros and cons for blocking one or both receptors, but there is no available evidence suggesting superiority of one or the other. However, the profile of side effects may differ with less abnormal liver function reported with ambrisentan and sitaxentan therapy. The longest and most extensive experience is with bosentan, which has been evaluated in IPAH, FPAH, APAH (scleroderma, congenital heart disease with Eisenmenger), and with CTEPH. Most studies have included patients in FC III, but effect has also been shown in FC II. Sitaxentan and ambrisentan have been tried in FC III and FC II , respectively.

7.5
Phosphodiesterase-5 Inhibitors

The mediator of the vasodilatory effects of NO is cGMP, and by blocking the enzyme Phosfodiesterase-5 (PDE5), the content of cGMP is augmented in the vascular smooth muscle. Sildanefil and tadafil are PDE5 inhibitors. The SUPER-1 study has shown clear and sustained effects of sildanefil 20 mg three times daily on hemodynamic parameters, FC and exercise capacity.

7.6
Prostanoids

Prostacyclin synthase is reduced in PAH, resulting in inadequate production of prostacyclin I_2, a vasodilator with antiproliferative effects. Administering prostanoids has been the mainstay for PAH therapy for more than a decade. Three prostanoids are commercially available: epoprostenol, treprostinil and iloprost. Epoprostenol is still used for patients in FC IV who are in late stage disease and right heart failure. Practical constraints for its use include continuous intravenous infusion through a central venous catheter with risk of septicemia, short half life and risk for life-threatening rebound effects in case of infusion interruption. This treatment option should thus be prescribed and followed by highly dedicated PAH centers, and as a rule, a lung transplantation should be considered if the patient needs epoprostenol. However, epoprostenol may postpone the need for lung transplantation and may even be replaced with an oral therapy with an endothelin receptor blockade if consistent clinical improvement occurs.

Due to the practical problems related to epoprostenol, other options for prostacyclin delivery have been investigated. In Europe, iloprost is approved for treatment of FC III and is given as inhalation. Theoretically, this is an optimal therapy as the drug is given directly into the diseased lung vasculature. The delivery is however cumbersome, as iloprost must be given 6–9 times per day through a specific inhalation device. Treprostinil is the latest development in the prostanoid group. It can be given with a micro-pump as a continuous infusion subcutaneously at room temperature. Treprostinil has been tried in IPAH and APAH associated with scleroderma and congenital heart disease. The main problem is local pain at the infusion site, which can be intractable hence limit its use. Treprostinil can also be given intravenously as an alternative to epoprostenol, and as an inhalation with hopefully longer duration than iloprost.

Assessment of satisfactory response to therapy has been performed using 6MWT, FC, echocardiography, right heart catheterization and BNP. Walking distance of more than 400 m and FC II suggest a favorable prognosis. In many patients, it has become obvious that a single drug treatment is not sufficient and various combinations are currently used and tested in clinical trials. Usually, an endothelin receptor antagonist is combined with sildanefil. The unanswered question remains as if whether the combination should be used from the start of the treatment or commenced later after a single drug has been tried. Critically ill patients with PH present a particular challenge as volume resuscitation and mechanical ventilation can worsen the hemodynamics.[11] Patients with decompensated PH, require therapy for right ventricular failure. Very few human studies have addressed the use of vaopressors and pulmonary vasodilators in these patients, but the use of dobutamine, milrinone, inhaled NO, and intravenous prostacyclin have the greatest support in the literature.

7.7
Thromboendarterectomy

Chronic thromboembolic PH (CTEPH) merits specific attention.[12] The incidence of acute pulmonary embolism is up to 1 per 1,000, but most likely is much higher, as many cases are never diagnosed. The early mortality is 10–12%, and for those who survive, the hemodynamic changes in the pulmonary circulation slowly resolve.[13] The thrombotic material does not disappear and chronic changes include narrowing and obliteration of both proximal and distal arteries, which develop and result in PH. These developments cause progressive symptoms and reduced survival. These patients should be carefully looked for, as there is a potential for cure, through pulmonary thromboendarterectomy, when the diseased intima is removed from diseased larger vessels.[14] With this procedure, a remarkable improvement with normalized hemodynamics can be achieved. The risks are however not negligible and a careful preoperative investigation and patient selection must be considered. For patients with changes in the periphery and those with remaining PH after surgery, medical treatment is an option and studies have shown positive hemodynamic changes for all three principles described above. To identify patients who may benefit from this thromboendarterctomy, the follow up of acute pulmonary embolism should be more stringent with active search for residual symptoms e.g., dyspnea. Breathless patients should be thoroughly assessed by echocardiography and pulmonary scintegraphy, and if signs of PH are confirmed, a pulmonary angiogram and right heart catheter should be performed.

The achievements in understanding PAH over the last years have been remarkable and today we have options that halt and reverse this malignant disease, and more options and combinations will be presented in the near future. As the evaluation can be very difficult, it is important that these patients are handled at specialized PAH centers. Furthermore, the medical treatment is extremely expensive and it is important that the right patient gets the correct treatment, and national registers are properly established.

References

1. Galie N, Hoeper MM, Humbert M, Torbicki A, et al. Guidelines for the diagnosis and treatment of pulmonary hypertension: The Task Force for the Diagnosis and Treatment of Pulmonary Hypertension of the European Society of Cardiology (ESC) and the European Respiratory Society (ERS), endorsed by the International Society of Heart and Lung Transplantation (ISHLT). *Eur Heart J*. 2009;30:2493-2537.
2. Celermajer DS, Marwick T. Echocardiographic and right heart catheterization techniques in patients with pulmonary arterial hypertension. *Int J Cardiol*. 2008;125:294-303.
3. Lindqvist P, Waldenstrom A, Wikstrom G, Kazzam E. Right ventricular myocardial isovolumic relaxation time and pulmonary pressure. *Clin Physiol Funct Imaging*. 2006;26:1-8.
4. Lindqvist P, Henein MY, Wikstrom G. Right ventricular myocardial velocities and timing estimate pulmonary artery systolic pressure. *Int J Cardiol*. 2008;137:130-136.
5. Dabestani A, Mahan G, Gardin JM, et al. Evaluation of pulmonary artery pressure and resistance by pulsed Doppler echocardiography. *Am J Cardiol*. 1987;59:662-668.
6. Lindqvist P, Henein M, Kazzam E. Right ventricular outflow-tract fractional shortening: an applicable measure of right ventricular systolic function. *Eur J Echocardiogr*. 2003;4:29-35.
7. Calcuteea A, LP, Maras D, Lei W, Hodson M, Henein M. Myocardial determinants of right ventricular ejection in pulmonary hypertension: 2D strain rate and spectral doppler study. *Eur J Echocardiogr*. 2008;9:S53.
8. Menzel T, Wagner S, Kramm T, et al. Pathophysiology of impaired right and left ventricular function in chronic embolic pulmonary hypertension: changes after pulmonary thromboendarterectomy. *Chest*. 2000;118:897-903.
9. Galie N, Manes A, Negro L, Palazzini M, Bacchi-Reggiani ML, Branzi A. A meta-analysis of randomized controlled trials in pulmonary arterial hypertension. *Eur Heart J*. 2009;30:394-403.
10. McLaughlin VV, Archer SL, Badesch DB, et al. ACCF/AHA 2009 expert consensus document on pulmonary hypertension: a report of the American College of Cardiology Foundation Task Force on Expert Consensus Documents and the American Heart Association: developed in collaboration with the American College of Chest Physicians, American Thoracic Society, Inc., and the Pulmonary Hypertension Association. *Circulation*. 2009;119:2250-2294.
11. Zamanian RT, Haddad F, Doyle RL, Weinacker AB. Management strategies for patients with pulmonary hypertension in the intensive care unit. *Crit Care Med*. 2007;35:2037-2050.
12. Hoeper MM, Mayer E, Simonneau G, Rubin LJ. Chronic thromboembolic pulmonary hypertension. *Circulation*. 2006;113:2011-2020.
13. Pengo V, Lensing AW, Prins MH, et al. Incidence of chronic thromboembolic pulmonary hypertension after pulmonary embolism. *N Engl J Med*. 2004;350:2257-2264.
14. Jamieson SW, Kapelanski DP, Sakakibara N, et al. Pulmonary endarterectomy: experience and lessons learned in 1,500 cases. *Ann Thorac Surg*. 2003;76:1457-1462; discussion 1462-1464.

Cardiac Cachexia in Chronic Heart Failure: The Metabolic Facet of CHF

8

Wolfram Doehner and Stefan D. Anker

8.1
Introduction

Our understanding of the pathophysiology of chronic heart failure (CHF) has significantly advanced over the last 15 years from the historic haemodynamic model of mere pumping failure to a much more complex approach including multiple body systems. The concept of neuroendocrine activation is the cornerstone of the current pathophysiological understanding as well as of the therapeutic approaches that are available today. On this basis, the treatment of CHF has made significant advances over the last two decades. Moreover, treatments for acute cardiac events have improved considerably. As a consequence of effective acute and chronic therapy and a steadily growing population of the aged, a growing number of patients live for prolonged periods in a state of compensated cardiac failure. As a result not only a significant increase in prevalence numbers of CHF can be observed giving rise to the word of an epidemic proportion in the development on heart failure. Also clinical features and complications of a long-term disease progression are increasingly coming to the fore in the clinical presentation of patients. With growing understanding of the complexity of CHF pathophysiology and modern therapy starting to adopt to tailored treatment strategies of specific aspects in patients subgroups a broader and more differentiated perspective on the patients might be required with.

Beyond neuroendocrine activation, systemic immunologic and metabolic impairment emerged recently as characteristic features inherent to CHF. Changes in hormonal signalling and metabolic balance may occur as an early response to the impaired hemodynamics. This adaptive response to injury will, however, in the prolonged course of the disease lead to maladaptive changes in metabolic regulation and substrate flux. The emerging catabolic/ anabolic imbalance leads to increased tissue degradation. Weight loss and the development of cachexia in the long-term course of heart failure have been recognized as a severe complication of CHF with further deterioration of clinical symptoms

W. Doehner (✉)
Center for Stroke Research, Charité - Universitätsmedizin Berlin, Berlin, Germany
e-mail: Wolfram.doehner@charite.de

M.Y. Henein (ed.), *Heart Failure in Clinical Practice*,
DOI: 10.1007/978-1-84996-153-0_8, © Springer-Verlag London Limited 2010

and a particular grave prognosis. CHF mortality remains high and, about half of the patients with CHF die within 4 years of diagnosis.[1] The situation is even worse once cardiac cachexia is present. In unselected patients with CHF, mortality rates were as high as 50% in the cachectic subset compared to 17% in the noncachectic subset at 18 months of follow-up.[2]

Cachexia is not only associated with poor outcome, but also with advanced symptomatic status, poor quality of life and an unfavourable response to drug treatment. We are only beginning to understand the complex and interrelated pathways that are involved in the abnormal regulation of body composition and metabolic in balance in cardiac cachexia. Cachexia is of course seen in advanced stages of a range of chronic illnesses, including cancer, chronic kidney and liver disease, rheumatoid arthritis, acquired immunodeficiency syndrome (AIDS), and others. Based on observed similarities in signalling and regulatory processes in cachectic patients of varying origin a common final pathway of weight loss in chronic disease has been hypothesized.[3] In this chapter an overview of the current knowledge of metabolic imbalance, weight loss and the significance of cardiac cachexia in CHF is presented.

8.2
Body Composition in Chronic Heart Failure: The Obesity Paradox

Body weight is a dynamic parameter showing in healthy conditions a certain rhythm over the lifespan.[4] Public appreciation of body weight and body composition has a fairly unidirectional perspective concerned with overweight and weight gain, and therefore most of the programs in adults are aiming at the reduction of body size.[5] In fact the aim to lose weight has been thoroughly implemented in the public consciousness as surrogates for physical and mental well-being. This makes it hard to establish a more differential view on the association between body composition and morbidity and mortality. It is important to differentiate between principles that have been proven for healthy populations and those for patients suffering from chronic diseases, where the former truths may have limited applicability. In fact, convincing evidence has been accumulated that the WHO criteria of normal body mass index (18.5–25 kg/m^2) may not be transferable to patients with CHF with regard to optimum survival. Data from a range of different large scale and multicenter heart failure studies over a broad spectrum of varying disease severity and different clinical settings have been gathered including a total of more than 30,000 patients. In these analyses it has consistently been shown that in CHF overweight and mild obesity is associated with decreased mortality.[6–9] This applies not only to patients with *chronic* HF. Data from the ADHERE database including more than 100,000 patients admitted to A&E for acutely decompensated HF have shown that higher BMI is associated with lower in-hospital mortality.[10]

The effect of body weight on all cause mortality was also evaluated in a meta-analysis of nine observational trials in CHF populations with a total of 28,209 patients.[9] Looking at a mean follow-up period of 2.7 years, it has been shown uniformly for all studies included, that overweight and obesity were associated with lower all-cause mortality and cardiovascular mortality rates. Based on repeatedly confirmed observations of higher BMI not being associated with increased mortality in CHF patients – but rather the opposite – the term "obesity paradox" has being introduced. Further studies in a range of chronic and acute diseases resulted in similar findings, extending the obesity paradox to an increasingly broader picture of chronic and acute disease conditions.[11]

An important conclusion from these findings is that metabolic balance and body composition needs to be viewed from a different perspective in patients with a chronic disease such as CHF as compared to healthy subjects. Weight management recommendations should therefore be given to CHF patients with great care and on individually adjusted grounds as general rules from a primary prevention perspective may not apply to these patients.

8.3
Definition of Cachexia

Cachexia has long been recognized by physicians as a signum mali ominis in many illnesses indicating advanced disease stage and an impaired prognosis. However, beyond this mere observation detailed investigations into the clinical implications and the underlying mechanisms have only recently been gathering momentum. Surprisingly, until recently a specific uniform definition of cachexia was missing which is of course essential to identify and categorize the problem and institute corrective measures to treat cachexia. Several definitions of cardiac cachexia have been put forward in different settings using a range of clinical tests such as skin fold thickness, fat tissue content, BMI and others. Only in 2006, a consensus meeting held by clinicians and scientists in Washington, DC, defined a consensus on the constellation of abnormalities that have been grouped under the name cachexia (Fig. 8.1a).[3] According to this definition cachexia results from adaptation not only to an underlying illness such as CHF but also cancer, COPD, CKD, HIV, and others. In the course of the disease an environment establishes that may be characterized by inflammation, loss of appetite (anorexia), low levels of anabolic hormones such as testosterone, insulin, growth hormone, and others. Decreased food intake and anorexia result in loss of body and muscle mass. In addition, inflammation, insulin resistance, and low levels of anabolic hormones result in global tissue wasting of muscle but also fat and bone tissue.

The consensus statement also proposed a set of diagnostic criteria that support the diagnosis of cachexia with at least three out of five clinical or laboratory criteria that need to be present for the diagnosis of cachexia (Fig. 8.1b). Notable, however, the foremost clinical feature of cachexia in adult patients is weight loss. This needs correction of course for fluid balance as weight change merely due to fluid retention or mobilization has to be taken into account. In cardiac cachexia, the presence of oedema complicates the assessment of weight loss over time, which highlights the importance of a non-oedematous state for the adequate assessment of body weight changes in this context.

a Definition of cachexia

"Wasting disease (i.e. cachexia) is a complex metabolic syndrome associated with underlying illness and characterized by loss of muscle with or without loss of fat mass.

The prominent clinical feature of cachexia is weight loss in adults (corrected for fluid retention) or growth failure in children (excluding endocrine disorders).

Anorexia, inflammation, insulin resistance and increased muscle protein breakdown are frequently associated with wasting disease.

Wasting disease is distinct from starvation, age-related loss of muscle mass, primary depression, malabsorption and hyperthyroidism and is associated with increased morbidity

b Diagnostic criteria for cachexia

Weight loss of at least 5% in 12 months or less in the presence of underlying illness

Plus three of the following:

- Decreased muscle strength
- Anorexia
- Fatigue
- Low fat-free mass index
- Abnormal biochemistry
  a) increased inflammatory markers (e.g. CrP, sTNFR's, TNF, IL-6),
  b) anaemia (<12 g/dL),
  c) low serum albumin (<32g/L)

Fig. 8.1 (**a**) Consensus definition of cachexia. (**b**) Diagnostic criteria for cachexia[3]

It is important to differentiate cachexia from anorexia and starvation, were weight loss is the result of mostly fat mass being consumed for energy yield and muscle mass is mostly spared.[4, 10] In cachectic CHF patients in turn, not only a loss of muscle mass is observed but also other compartments are involved as fat mass and bones are affected by the tissue degradational processes (see below).

8.4
Mechanisms of Altered Body Composition

Cardiac cachexia as a clinical entity presenting with the overt observation of weight loss is, however, appreciated as a complex syndrome with multiple and mutually interrelated factors. Patients usually experience complex body composition alterations and disturbed homeostasis of several body systems. Beside the activation of neuroendocrine signalling pathways, activation of inflammatory systems may contribute as well as intestinal malabsorption and disturbed regulation of appetite.[12,13] Weight loss in the cachectic patient predominantly affects muscle protein, however, bone and fat tissue are likewise involved later in the course of the disease. The timelines differ widely between patients. We are only beginning to understand the factors that trigger the progression from clinically and weight stable, ambulatory CHF to cardiac cachexia. The importance of individual pathways and their exact interplay are still incompletely understood.

8.4.1
Nutrition and Appetite

Loss of appetite and inadequate food intake are important components contributing to the development of weight loss and cachexia in CHF. This anorexia may occur as a consequence of symptomatic disablement of the patients from weakness, dyspnea, fatigue, or lethargy.[14] Often a change in eating behavior may be observed from a normal and regular food intake toward an irregular pattern of nibbling of smaller amounts of food. Also intestinal edema leading to nausea and diminished absorption and protein-loosing enteropathy has been described in this context.[15] Notably, iatrogenic factors may unfavorably contribute to the decreased appetite and food intake of patients as a consequence of multiple daily drug regimens. Also imposed dietary restrictions may have a role, which, in view of the above mentioned, need to be viewed with great care on an individual basis.

   Impaired regulation of appetite as the central stimulus of feeding may occur as the result from impaired balance within the fine tuned satiety-hunger homeostasis. The hypothalamus is the central regulating site of appetite with a lateral "feeding area" and a medial "satiety center".[16] Numerous mediators take part in controlling these centres in the hypothalamus. Orexigenic factors such as neuropeptide Y, agouti-related protein (AgRP), and anti orexigenic factors such as melanocortins are in turn not only regulated by a multitude of mediators including leptin, insulin, ghrelin, adiponection, but also cytokines, GIP, metabolic intermediates and others. In normal conditions, a balanced equilibrium between signals for hunger and satiety results in an individually defined "set point" of fairly stable body weight and composition.

   Although anorexia is certainly a common characteristic in HF and a contributing factor to the development of cachexia, this feature alone cannot explain the metabolic changes observed during this perturbation. It is among the common misconceptions that feeding and enhanced nutritional and caloric supplementation alone may be sufficient to adequately reverse the process of losing weight in patients with cachexia.

8.4.2
Impaired Gastrointestinal Function

Intestinal absorption may be reduced due to impaired gastrointestinal function in CHF thereby contributing to cardiac cachexia. As peripheral blood flow and vascular resistance in significantly impaired in patients with cardiac cachexia[17] nonocclusive ischaemia may likewise occur in the mesenteric vascular area and disturbed intestinal microcirculation in CHF may lead to tissue hypoxia and latent bowl wall oedema. In accordance with this concept, we have shown that bowel wall thickness in the terminal ileum, ascending colon, transverse colon, descending colon and sigmoid are increased in CHF patients.[18] Both, intestinal oedema and impaired integrity of the mucosal transporters may account for reduced absorption of nutrients from the food ingested.

In fact, decreased intestinal uptake of both fat,[19] and proteins[20] has been observed in advanced stages of CHF. Notably, loss of nutrients was highest in cachectic CHF patients with 24% loss of fat and 19% loss of protein via stool compared to patients without cachexia.[20] Nutritional deficits are also apparent from hypoalbuminaemia observed in 20–30% of patients with CHF).[21] This hypoalbuminaemia has been shown to be associated with a twofold increase in mortality in outpatients with CHF.[22]

Further, impaired microcirculation and bowl wall oedema will compromise the intestinal barrier function that separates the intraluminal bacterial milieu from the inner body compartments. Increased immune activation may result from interaction of gut bacteria with the host due to translocation of bacterial products such as lipopolysaccharides (LPS).[23]

8.4.3
Immune Activation

Inflammatory activation is a commonly observed characteristic in CHF that may contribute to impaired metabolic efficiency and energy balance. TNF-α is the dominant cytokines reported in this context but other proinflammatory cytokines including interleukin (IL)-1 and IL-6 are also activated. Since the initial reports on immune activation and increased cytokine levels in CHF[24] a number of different hypotheses have been suggested to explain the origin of immune activation in this disease. Increased secretion of proinflammatory cytokines by mononuclear cells has been discussed. The myocardium seems to be another important source of increased cytokine release, although it appears that only the *failing* myocardium is capable of TNF-α production.[25] Some evidence suggests that catecholamines augment myocardial cytokine release. Other concepts suggest a response to myocardial injury[26] and under-perfusion of peripheral tissues[27] as underlying mechanisms. It has also been proposed that increased bowel wall oedema may cause impairment of bowl wall barrier function. As outlined above, this may result in increased translocation of LPS from bacterial colonization of the intestine.[18] LPS, a cell wall component from Gram-negative bacteria, is one of the strongest inducers of proinflammatory cytokines and especially of TNF-α.[23] Indeed, it has been shown that very small (pathophysiological) amounts of this substance are capable of inducing TNF-α secretion.[28] Notably, LPS levels are particularly elevated in the bloodstream of patients with CHF during oedematous decompensation, i.e., when clinical signs of severe tissue congestion are present.[29]

It is well possible that the aforementioned hypotheses rather complement than exclude one another, but it is certainly true that inflammatory activation is much more than an epiphenomenon in CHF.

The activation TNF-α (formerly known as cachectin) is one of most important factors associated with the development of tissue wasting and cachexia via several signalling pathways. TNF-α induces apoptosis via specific receptors on the cell surface and activates proteasome-dependent protein breakdown in striate muscle and other tissues thus maintaining the wasting process. It has been observed that the ceramide second messenger system is up-regulated in CHF being highest in cachectic patients.[30] Ceramide has recently been shown to be the key downstream messenger for cytokine-induced impairment of muscle protein synthesis by blocking IGF-1 receptor dependent signalling.[31] TNF-α increases the expression of the adipocyte-derived catabolic hormone leptin, which again inhibits food intake.[32] Further, TNF-α contributes to endothelial dysfunction and hence to impaired blood supply to skeletal muscles.[33] This, in turn, yields reduced exercise endurance and lack of nutrient supply. In CHF it has been shown that plasma levels of soluble TNF-α receptors are associated with impaired long- and short-term prognosis.[34,35] However, direct antagonism of TNF-α in patients with CHF has largely failed in clinical trials (see below)[36] and further studies are needed to test the potential role of anti-inflammatory therapy in CHF.

8.4.4
Anabolic Failure

Increasing evidence emerged recently that metabolic failure contributes significantly to symptomatic status and prognosis in CHF. These data suggest that impaired metabolic capacity is an important aspect within CHF pathophysiology. The metabolic derangements in CHF can globally be described as an overall catabolic/anabolic imbalance with decreased anabolic capacity and a dominating catabolic drive (Fig. 8.2). Several of the major anabolic pathways are impaired in CHF.

8.4.5
GH Resistance

CHF has been observed as a state of acquired GH resistance with the typical pattern of high GH and low IGF-1 levels.[37,38] This pattern is shared with a range of catabolic diseases including surgery, trauma, sepsis, cancer, uremia, chronic obstructive pulmonary disease, and chronic liver disease.[39] A threefold increase in GH levels has been noted in cachectic patients with CHF compared to noncachectic patients with CHF and healthy subjects.[14] IGF-1 levels, on the other hand, are reduced, in particular in patients with cachexia.[37] The concept of acquired GH resistance may provide an explanation of the disappointing results of several studies that tested the therapeutic approach of GH administration in patients with CHF.[40-42]

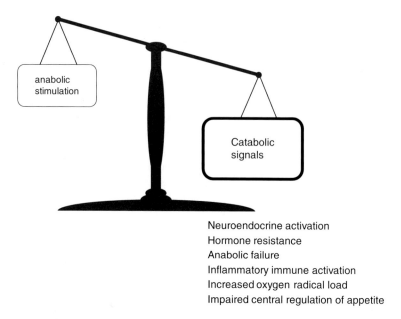

Neuroendocrine activation
Hormone resistance
Anabolic failure
Inflammatory immune activation
Increased oxygen radical load
Impaired central regulation of appetite

Fig. 8.2 Catabolic anabolic Imbalance

8.4.6
Insulin Resistance

Also insulin resistance is a common feature in CHF. Notably, beside the central function in regulating glucose homeostasis in general, insulin is the strongest anabolic hormone in human physiology. It is long known that there is a tight interrelation between diabetes mellitus (DM) and CHF with mutual augmentation of both comorbidities. The Euro Heart Failure Survey reported an incidence of DM as high as 27% among the CHF population.[43] As insulin and glucose metabolism are impaired long before the clinical diagnosis of DM becomes apparent, the true incidence of insulin resistance may be much higher. Indeed, subclinical impairment of glucose metabolism has been reported for 43% of patients with CHF.[44]

Importantly, insulin resistance may occur secondary to CHF, independently and on top of the metabolic syndrome, that is a well known risk factor for ischemic type heart failure. Insulin resistance in CHF correlates directly with the symptomatic status.[45] Moreover, a recent study identified insulin resistance as a prognosticator in non-DM patients with CHF independently of previously established prognosticators.[46] Mechanisms that cause insulin resistance in patients with CHF are not entirely understood. It seems that neurohormonal activation, over-activity of the immune system, metabolic disturbances, oxidative stress, haemodynamic impairment and tissue hypo perfusion, and others all play a contributing role (Fig. 8.3). Muscle specific alterations in insulin signaling and glucose transport capacity such as reduced GLUT4 transport protein have been observed in CHF.[47] Medication for heart failure, dietary changes and skeletal muscle adaptation to a sedentary life style may also contribute to impair the glucose regulatory- and anabolic efficacy of insulin.

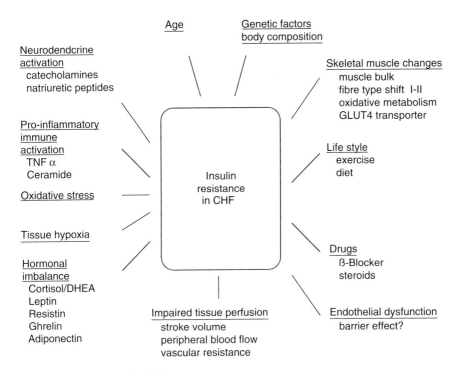

Fig. 8.3 Insulin resistance in CHF

Pathophysiological mechanisms suggest insulin resistance as a potential treatment target, in particular when body wasting and cachexia are involved. On these grounds insulin sensitizers might be an intriguing option. Selective agonists for the peroxisome proliferators activated receptor-γ or thiazolidinediones (TZD) modulate genes involved in glucose and lipid metabolism and improved insulin resistance. In a retrospective survey of 1,868 diabetic patients and 1,868 matched controls, pioglitazone treatment was associated with 50% less risk (hazard ratio 0.50, 95% confidence interval 0.33–0.76) to develop CHF.[48] There are recent studies reporting promising data in favor of this concept with regard to prognostic benefit,[48,49] as well as myocardial functional assessment.[50] The use of TZD in CHF is, however, limited by their marked characteristic to increase fluid retention and edema commonly interpreted as progression of heart failure[51] and leading to increased hospitalization.[52] Moreover, given the heated and ongoing controversy on increased cardiovascular risk following TZD therapy, their use in CHF patients is currently not recommended.[53] Future research will show whether there is a role for TZD in the therapy of CHF patients, particular in those with cardiac cachexia.

8.4.7
Testosterone and Others

Further data emerged recently on the complex interplay of anabolic deficiency in CHF as it has been shown that also signalling via dehydroepiandrosterone sulfate (DHEAS) and testosterone are compromised in CHF patients.[54] It was observed in this study that deficiencies in circulating total testosterone (total and free testosterone), DHEAS, and IGF-1 are common in men with CHF. Each of these anabolic hormone deficits independently predicted poor prognosis. Deficiency of more than one of these hormones resulted in an additive effect on mortality.[54]

Using testosterone deficit as a novel therapeutic target a randomized controlled trial has shown that testosterone replacement improves exercise capacity and symptomatic status in men with CHF.[55] Also indirect effects via hormonal metabolic interaction towards improved insulin sensitivity have been observed after testosterone therapy.[56] The combined improvement in anabolic stimulation in this pilot interventional study resulted in increased body mass. Whether testosterone replacement therapy may indeed become applicable in general clinical practice for CHF needs to be seen from future studies. The known cardio-toxic effects of anabolic steroids and the substantial number of skin reactions (seen in 55% of cases in the above study) and other side effects may negatively impact on the wider acceptance of this therapeutic option.

While these mechanisms are investigated in some details in CHF, there are more candidates and potential contributing factors that add to the overall network of metabolic imbalance. The detailed pathophysiologic mechanisms and the complex interplay between hormonal, immunologic and metabolic signaling pathways are still incompletely understood. Mediators such as ghrelin,[57] leptin,[58] resistin,[59] adiponectin,[60] natriuretic peptides,[61] and others are investigated. The emerging data provide increasing evidence of the importance of the metabolic involvement in the pathophysiology of CHF. Association with both symptomatic status (i.e., morbidity) and mortality of these patients suggest metabolic pathways as intriguing targets for novel therapeutic options to be tested.

8.5
Tissue Degradation

Weight loss is the key and most overt clinical feature of cachexia. Investigations of specific tissue compartments reveal, however, detailed characteristics of body wasting with regard to different compartments. Lean body mass depletion is a dominant feature of cardiac cachexia. Muscle atrophy is observed in up to 68% of patients with CHF.[62] Reduction in muscle tissue is of utmost importance for the progression of symptomatic status of the patients. Interestingly, the process of skeletal muscle degradation starts early in the course of the disease and can be observed already in CHF patients with stable body weight (Fig. 8.4).[63] The lack of a weight difference between CHF and healthy controls despite lower muscle mass suggests replacement of muscle with nonfunctional tissue. The reduced exercise capacity in CHF patients results largely from muscle wasting[64] adding to the impaired metabolic and functional capacity. In fact, skeletal muscle quantitative and qualitative changes might explain some of the major symptoms such as early fatigue, exercise limitation and exertional dyspnea better than abnormalities of central haemodynamic parameters.[65,66] On this basis the muscle hypothesis has been proposed as further pathophysiologic concept of CHF (Fig. 8.5).[67]

Fig. 8.4 Muscle loss in CHF with stable weight and with cardiac cachexia

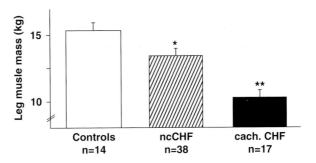

Fig. 8.5 Muscle hypothesis

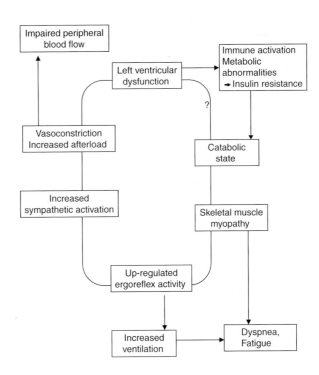

According to this hypothesis peripheral skeletal muscle metabolic and functional abnormalities develop in response to impaired tissue perfusion, impaired neuroendocrine, immune and metabolic signalling. Adaptation of feedback signalling loops such as ergo reflex over-activity may enter a vicious cycle of self-maintained augmentation and may thus contribute to the progression of the disease.[68]

It has been shown that beyond muscle tissue degradation, fat tissue and bone tissue are also decreas later in the course of the disease, all adding to the observed net weight loss of the patients. Lipolysis has been shown to be up-regulated in CHF. Catecholamines, via β-adrenoceptors are major determinants of lipolysis. This is in accordance with the observation that the weight gain effect of beta-blocker therapy (see below) appears to be largely determined by an increase in body fat mass.[69] Recently natriuretic peptides (atrial, B-type and C-type natriuretic peptides) were identified to be involved in fat-cell metabolism.[61,70] The natriuretic peptides control lipid mobilization and lipid oxidation by increasing intracellular cGMP.[71]

Further, also bone tissue undergoes accelerated remodeling in CHF. Genuine osteoporosis has been observed in advanced stages of the diseases.[72] In fact reduced 1,25(OH)(2) D levels (Vit D3) in inverse relation to increased osteoporosis and frailty score were reported in CHF patients.[73] Also calcium levels were observed lower in CHF patients with bone mineral content and bone mineral density being lower in cachectic, but not in non-cachectic patients compared to healthy controls.[74] In an earlier study markers of bone turnover were investigated in 101 patients with advanced CHF (NYHA class III–IV).[75] Osteoporosis was present in 7–19%, osteopenia in 42–47% of patients with higher percentages in women compared to men. Notably, low serum vitamin D metabolites were associated with biochemical evidence of increased bone turnover.[75] Much of the details of the underlying mechanisms of bone wasting in cardiac cachexia still need to be elucidated.

8.6
Therapeutic Options

Despite the emerging evidence as outlined above there is currently no approved therapeutic option to specifically target metabolic failure, weight loss or cachexia in CHF. In the evaluation of metabolically targeted interventions in CHF three different approaches may need separate examination: (a) The impact of current state of the art medical therapy in CHF on metabolic regulation and balance, (b) specific nutritional considerations with regard to cardiac cachexia and (c) potential novel therapies with specific metabolically targeted intervention. Retrospective analyses are available for some of these; others have even shown their efficacy in clinical pilot studies. New therapies are in the developmental pipeline based on intriguing theoretical concepts and have yet to prove their therapeutic benefit.

8.7
Metabolic Effects of State of the Art CHF Medical Therapies

8.7.1
Beta-Blockers

Cardio-selective beta-blockers without intrinsic sympatho-mimetik activity have convincingly shown their benefit in CHF therapy on both morbidity and mortality. In addition beta-blockers are also known to exert effects on weight development. This effect might be explained by the inhibition of catecholamine-induced lipolysis[76] and decreased resting energy expenditure.[77] A small (+1.1 kg) significant increase in weight following carvedilol therapy has been shown in the COPERNICUS population (Carvedilol Prospective Randomized Cumulative Survival).[78] Bisoprolol prevented or delayed the risk of weight loss in patients with CHF as reported from the CIBIS II-study (Cardiac Insufficiency Bisoprolol Study).[79] Interestingly, 6 months of beta-blocker therapy yielded a significantly greater weight gain in patients classified as cachectic than in the noncachectic patients ($+5.2 \pm 9.6$ vs. $+0.8 \pm 5.0$ kg, $p = 0.027$).[80] Whether this weight gain should be viewed as an unwanted side effect or rather as reflection of effective therapeutic interaction needs to be clarified.[81]

The heterogeneity between beta-blockers may not allow a common conclusion with regard to insulin sensitivity as negative and positive impact of beta blockers has been reported. It has been shown that β_1-selective blockers have no important adverse effect on glucose metabolism[82,83] and do not prolong hypoglycemia or mask hypoglycemic symptoms.[84]

Beneficial effects of metoprolol and atenolol on insulin sensitivity have been observed in subjects with impaired glucose tolerance,[85] but also conflicting results have also been reported.[86] Further analyses are needed to clarify individual and/or common effects of beta-blockers on glucose metabolism in CHF patients.

8.7.2
Angiotensin-Converting Enzyme Inhibitors and Angiotensin Receptor Antagonists

The neurohormonal inhibition is the main effect of angiotensin converting enzyme (ACE) inhibitors and angiotensin receptor blockers (ARB). However a range of additional effects of these compounds have been identified that add to the favorable properties. Retrospective analyses from the SOLVD database have shown that ACE inhibitors may prevent or delay the risk of weight loss in patients with CHF.[87] Additionally, ACE inhibitors may exert beneficial effects towards improvement of insulin resistance.[88] A delay of new-onset of diabetes with the use of ramipril in high-risk patients with vascular comorbidity was observed in a substudy of the HOPE trial (heart outcomes prevention evaluation).[89] A meta-analysis from 22 clinical trials including 143,153 patients free of diabetes at randomization concluded a significant reduced risk for development of diabetes with ARB or ACE inhibitor.[90]

8.7.3
Statins

Statins are well established to significantly reduce plasma cholesterol and hence cardiovascular risk.[91,92] Multiple regulatory effects beyond the cholesterol reduction, and the so-called pleiotropic effects of statins are intensely discussed and have been in the focus of research for several years. Statins have been found to improve endothelial function by induction of endothelial nitric oxide synthase (eNOS),[93] increase in nitric oxide release,[94] and reduced oxidative stress.[95] Statins are also able to mobilize endothelial progenitor cells from the bone marrow[96,97] and possess anti-inflammatory properties.[98,99]

Favorable findings in retrospective observations and meta-analyses suggested a significant effect of statin therapy in CHF patients. The prospective CORONA (Controlled Rosuvastatin Multinational Trial in Heart Failure) study surprisingly failed, however, to show a significant effect for the primary outcome (composite of death from cardiovascular causes, nonfatal myocardial infarction, or nonfatal stroke). The interpretation of the data is ongoing but also the GISSI-HF trial (Gruppo Italiano per lo Studio della Sopravvivenza nell'Insufficienza Cardiaca) failed to show a beneficial effect of statin therapy on all cause mortality or admission to hospital for cardiovascular reasons in CHF. On the basis of these two large trials, it seems unlikely that unselective statin therapy will translate into clinical benefit in CHF.

8.8
Specific Nutritional Considerations in Cardiac Cachexia

Nutritional recommendations for CHF patients are mainly considered with limited fluid administration and a sodium restricted diet. Energy and substrate input are naturally major determinants of the bodies' metabolic balance. Nutritional supply, hence contributes significantly to the prevention of tissue wasting. Patients with CHF are prone to reduced appetite and reduced food intake.[100] As outlined above, impaired regulation of hunger and satiety, derangements in bowel perfusion, altered intestinal barrier and absorptive capacity may all contribute to reduced nutritional uptake of the body including both deficiencies in micronutrients and macronutrients.

Optimized food intake may therefore take into account both macronutrient and micronutrient supplementation as well as eating patterns of the patients. A multitude of nutritional recommendations in general are available to adjust for specific nutritional factors such as vitamins, microelements including zinc, selenium, copper, magnesium and others, branched-chain amino acids, polyunsaturated fatty acids, etc. Also mere high caloric enteral support has been tested in a small randomized placebo controlled study in cardiac cachexia showing significant weight gain after 12 weeks of follow up.[101]

It is important to understand, however, that merely increased food intake may eventually not be sufficient to overcome the overall catabolic process underlying the development of weight loss and cachexia. The complex pathophysiology of tissue wasting includes impairment of resorption, assimilation, storage, and utilization of energy and substrates. Increased nutritional supply needs to be accompanied by improved metabolic efficiency of the body's tissues and boosted anabolic drive in order to prevent or reverse a continued catabolic spiral towards cachexia.

8.9
Potential Novel Therapies with Specific Metabolically Targeted Intervention

With the emerging evidence of weight loss and metabolic failure significantly contributing to morbidity and mortality on CHF, it is surprising that there is currently no approved therapy available to prevent, reduce or reverse the tissue wasting in these patients. A range of compounds is in use for other conditions. Their value for the setting in CHF, however, is unclear if not controversial. Others are under development but need to be tested in clinical settings to show the efficacy in cardiac cachexia.

- Appetite stimulating compounds such as progesterone derivates have shown in a number of randomized controlled trials their efficacy in stimulating appetite in cachectic patients.[102,103]
- Cannabinoids are well known to stimulate appetite and have been studied in AIDS[104] and cancer related cachexia[105,106] but may be problematic in CHF due to substantial cardiac side effects such as tachycardia, hypotension and decreased cardiac function.[107]
- Anabolic steroids are an obvious consideration in cachectic patients. As outlined above, testosterone replacement was shown to improve functional capacity and symptoms in general heart failure patients.[55,108] Weight gaining effects have been observed in cachexia due to chronic obstructive pulmonary disease and in HIV patients[109] but no study has been performed in patients with cardiac cachexia.
- Anti-inflammatory approaches have an intriguing pathophysiological concept, to suppress inflammation, especially the production or the action of proinflammatory cytokines.[110] Several approaches such as therapies with etanercept[36] and Infliximab[111] showed, however, disappointing results.
- Thalidomide has been observed to exert a potent anti-inflammatory capacity.[112] After the historic tragedy of this compound in recent medical history to induce characteristic phocomelia and other teratogenic effects[113] it could be that the immune-modulatory effects yield a revival of thalidomide as therapeutic compound.
- Pentoxifylline has been investigated recent studies observing inhibition of TNF-α formation.[114] Studies in patients with CHF showed improved LVEF in parallel to reduced TNF-α plasma levels[115,116] and increased NYHA classes.[117] Other studies were, however, unable to confirm the former findings in CHF.[118] Future studies need to define the role of pentoxifylline in the setting of cachexia.

8.10
Conclusion

Metabolic failure is increasingly recognized as intrinsic part of CHF pathophysiology contributing to morbidity and mortality of CHF. In contrast to healthy subjects were overweight and obesity indicate an increased risk for cardiovascular and metabolic diseases, a survival benefit has been observed for CHF patients that are overweight and an obesity paradox has been proposed to explain this unexpected finding. Notably, different metabolic rules may apply in these chronic patients and translation of data from healthy physiology may not reflect the full picture. The complex interplay of imbalanced metabolic regulation, neuroendocrine and immunologic over-activation results in a net catabolic/ anabolic imbalance. Weight loss and tissue degradation of all compartments are the key clinical features of cardiac cachexia indication accelerated disease progression and a particular grave prognosis. The emerging pathophysiology of cardiac cachexia is exceedingly complex, and we still do not understand when and how CHF progresses into this syndrome. Despite convincing concepts on pathophysiological ground, several approaches failed to translate into clinical benefit.

No studies are currently available that have specifically targeted cardiac cachexia using a pharmacological approach. Nutritional recommendations to prevent or reverse cardiac cachexia remain largely speculative, and no large-scale randomized, controlled trials have been performed. Novel compounds and therapeutic concepts are being tested and future research will show whether those approaches may translate into clinical improvement of patients with cardiac cachexia.

References

1. Remme WJ, Swedberg K. Guidelines for the diagnosis and treatment of chronic heart failure. *Eur Heart J*. 2001;22:1527-1560.
2. Anker SD, Ponikowski P, Varney S, et al. Wasting as independent risk factor for mortality in chronic heart failure. *Lancet*. 1997;349:1050-1053.
3. Evans WJ, Morley JE, Argilés J, et al. Cachexia: a new definition. *Clin Nutr*. 2008;27:793-799.
4. Wallace JI, Schwartz RS. Epidemiology of weight loss in humans with special reference to wasting in the elderly. *Int J Cardiol*. 2002;85:15-21.
5. Dansinger ML, Tatsioni A, Wong JB, Chung M, Balk EM. Meta-analysis: the effect of dietary counseling for weight loss. *Ann Intern Med*. 2007;147:41-50.
6. Horwich TB, Fonarow GC, Hamilton MA, MacLellan WR, Woo MA, Tillisch JH. The relationship between obesity and mortality in patients with heart failure. *J Am Coll Cardiol*. 2001;38:789-795.
7. Curtis JP, Selter JG, Wang Y, et al. The obesity paradox: body mass index and outcomes in patients with heart failure. *Arch Intern Med*. 2005;165:55-61.
8. Kenchaiah S, Pocock SJ, Wang D, et al.; CHARM Investigators. Body mass index and prognosis in patients with chronic heart failure: insights from the Candesartan in heart failure: assessment of reduction in mortality and morbidity (CHARM) program. *Circulation*. 2007; 116:627-636.
9. Oreopoulos A, Padwal R, Kalantar-Zadeh K, Fonarow GC, Norris CM, McAlister FA. Body mass index and mortality in heart failure: a meta-analysis. *Am Heart J*. 2008;156:13-22.
10. Fonarow GC, Srikanthan P, Costanzo MR, Cintron GB, Lopatin M; ADHERE Scientific Advisory Committee and Investigators. An obesity paradox in acute heart failure: analysis of body mass index and inhospital mortality for 108,927 patients in the Acute Decompensated Heart Failure National Registry. *Am Heart J*. 2007;153:74-81.
11. Doehner W, Clark A, Anker SD. Obesity paradox, weighing the benefit. *Eur Heart J*. 2009; 31:146-148.
12. von Haehling S, Doehner W, Anker SD. Nutrition, metabolism and the complex pathophysiology of cachexia in chronic heart failure. *Cardiovasc Res*. 2007;73:298-309.
13. Strassburg S, Springer J, Anker SD. Muscle wasting in cardiac cachexia. *Int J Biochem Cell Biol*. 2005;37:1938-1947.
14. Akashi YJ, Springer J, Anker SD. Cachexia in chronic heart failure: prognostic implications and novel therapeutic approaches. *Curr Heart Fail Rep*. 2005;2:198-203.
15. Schwengel RH, Gottlieb SS, Fisher ML. Protein-energy malnutrition in patients with ischemic and nonischemic dilated cardiomyopathy and congestive heart failure. *Am J Cardiol*. 1994;73:908-910.

16. Ganong WF. Central regulation of visceral function. In: *Review of Medical Physiology*. Norwalk: Appleton & Lange; 1999.

17. Doehner W, Rauchhaus M, Florea VG, et al. Uric acid in cachectic and non-cachectic CHF patients - relation to leg vascular resistance. *Am Heart J*. 2001;141:792-799.

18. Sandek A, Bauditz J, Swidsinski A, et al. Altered intestinal function in patients with chronic heart failure. *J Am Coll Cardiol*. 2007;50:1561-1569.

19. King D, Smith ML, Chapman TJ, et al. Fat malabsorption in elderly patients with cardiac cachexia. *Age Ageing*. 1996;25:144-149.

20. Arutyunov GP, Kostyukevich OI, Serov RA, et al. Collagen accumulation and dysfunctional mucosal barrier of the small intestine in patients with chronic heart failure. *Int J Cardiol*. 2008;125:240-245.

21. Kalantar-Zadeh K, Anker SD, Horwich TB, Fonarow GC. Nutritional and anti-inflammatory interventions in chronic heart failure. *Am J Cardiol*. 2008;101:89E-103E.

22. Horwich TB, Kalantar-Zadeh K, MacLellan RW, Fonarow GC. Albumin levels predict survival in patients with systolic heart failure. *Am Heart J*. 2008;155:883-889.

23. Anker SD, Egerer KR, Volk HD, Kox WJ, Poole-Wilson PA, Coats AJ. Elevated soluble CD14 receptors and altered cytokines in chronic heart failure. *Am J Cardiol*. 1997;79:1426-1430.

24. Levine B, Kalman J, Mayer L, Fillit HM, Packer M. Elevated circulating levels of tumor necrosis factor in severe chronic heart failure. *N Engl J Med*. 1990;323:236-241.

25. Mann DL. Recent insights into the role of tumor necrosis factor in the failing heart. *Heart Fail Rev*. 2001;6:71-80.

26. Matsumori A, Yamada T, Suzuki H, Matoba Y, Sasayama S. Increased circulating cytokines in patients with myocarditis and cardiomyopathy. *Br Heart J*. 1994;72:561-566.

27. Tsutamoto T, Hisanaga T, Wada A, et al. Interleukin-6 spillover in the peripheral circulation increases with the severity of heart failure, and the high plasma level of interleukin-6 is an important prognostic predictor in patients with congestive heart failure. *J Am Coll Cardiol*. 1998;31:391-398.

28. Genth-Zotz S, von Haehling S, Bolger AP, et al. Pathophysiologic quantities of endotoxin-induced tumor necrosis factor-alpha release in whole blood from patients with chronic heart failure. *Am J Cardiol*. 2002;90:1226-1230.

29. Niebauer J, Volk HD, Kemp M, et al. Endotoxin and immune activation in chronic heart failure: a prospective cohort study. *Lancet*. 1999;353:1838-1842.

30. Doehner W, Bunck AC, Rauchhaus M, et al. Secretory sphingomyelinase is upregulated in chronic heart failure: a second messenger system of immune activation relates to body composition, muscular functional capacity, and peripheral blood flow. *Eur Heart J*. 2007;28:821-828.

31. Strle K, Broussard SR, McCusker RH, et al. Proinflammatory cytokine impairment of insulin-like growth factor I- induced protein synthesis in skeletal muscle myoblasts requires ceramide. *Endocrinology*. 2004;145:4592-4602.

32. Kirchgessner TG, Uysal KT, Wiesbrock SM, et al. Tumor necrosis factor-alpha contributes to obesity-related hyperleptinemia by regulating leptin release from adipocytes. *J Clin Invest*. 1997;100:2777-2782.

33. Anker SD, von Haehling S. Inflammatory mediators in chronic heart failure: an overview. *Heart*. 2004;90:464-470.

34. Ferrari R, Bachetti T, Confortini R, et al. Tumor necrosis factor soluble receptors in patients with various degrees of congestive heart failure. *Circulation*. 1995;92:1479-1786.

35. Rauchhaus M, Doehner W, Francis DP, et al. Plasma cytokine parameters and mortality in patients with chronic heart failure. *Circulation*. 2000;102:3060-3067.

36. Mann DL, McMurray JJ, Packer M, et al. Targeted anticytokine therapy in patients with chronic heart failure: results of the Randomized Etanercept Worldwide Evaluation (RENEWAL). *Circulation*. 2004;109:1594-1602.

37. Anker SD, Volterrani M, Pflaum CD, et al. Acquired growth hormone resistance in patients with chronic heart failure: implications for therapy with growth hormone. *J Am Coll Cardiol*. 2001;38:443-452.

38. Doehner W, Pflaum CD, Rauchhaus M, et al. Leptin, insulin sensitivity and growth hormone binding protein in chronic heart failure with and without cardiac cachexia. *Eur J Endocrinol.* 2001;145:727-735.

39. Cicoira M, Kalra PR, Anker SD. Growth hormone resistance in chronic heart failure and its therapeutic implications. *J Card Fail.* 2003;9:219-226.

40. Osterziel KJ, Strohm O, Schuler J, et al. Randomised, double blind, placebo-controlled trial of human recombinant growth hormone in patients with chronic heart failure due to dilated cardiomyopathy. *Lancet.* 1998;351:1233-1237.

41. Frustaci A, Gentiloni N, Russo MA. Growth hormone in the treatment of dilated cardiomyopathy. *N Engl J Med.* 1996;335:672-673.

42. Isgaard J, Bergh CH, Caidahl K, Lomsky M, Hjalmarson A, Bengtsson BA. A placebo-controlled study of growth hormone in patients with congestive heart failure. *Eur Heart J.* 1998;19:1704-1711.

43. Cleland JG, Swedberg K, Follath F, et al.; Study Group on Diagnosis of the Working Group on Heart Failure of the European Society of Cardiology. The EuroHeart Failure survey programme – a survey on the quality of care among patients with heart failure in Europe. Part 1: patient characteristics and diagnosis. *Eur Heart J.* 2003;24:442-463.

44. Suskin N, McKelvie RS, Burns RJ, et al. Glucose and insulin abnormalities relate to functional capacity in patients with congestive heart failure. *Eur Heart J.* 2000;21:1368-1375.

45. Swan JW, Anker SD, Walton C, et al. Insulin resistance in chronic heart failure: relation to severity and etiology of heart failure. *J Am Coll Cardiol.* 1997;30:527-532.

46. Doehner W, Rauchhaus M, Ponikowski P, et al. Impaired insulin sensitivity as an independent risk factor for mortality in patients with stable chronic heart failure. *J Am Coll Cardiol.* 2005;46:1019-1026.

47. Doehner W, Gathercole D, Cicoira M, et al. Reduced glucose transporter GLUT4 in skeletal muscle predicts insulin resistance in non-diabetic chronic heart failure patients independently of body composition. *Int J Cardiol.* 2010;138:19-24.

48. Rajagopalan R, Rosenson RS, Fernandes AW, Khan M, Murray FT. Association between congestive heart failure and hospitalization in patients with type 2 diabetes mellitus receiving treatment with insulin or pioglitazone: a retrospective data analysis. *Clin Ther.* 2004;26:1400-1410.

49. Masoudi FA, Inzucchi SE, Wang Y, Havranek EP, Foody JM, Krumholz HM. Thiazolidinediones, metformin, and outcomes in older patients with diabetes and heart failure: an observational study. *Circulation.* 2005;111:583-590.

50. Dargie HJ, Hildebrandt PR, Riegger GA, et al. A randomized, placebo-controlled trial assessing the effects of rosiglitazone on echocardiographic function and cardiac status in type 2 diabetic patients with New York Heart Association Functional Class I or II Heart Failure. *J Am Coll Cardiol.* 2007;49:1696-1704.

51. Lipscombe LL, Gomes T, Lévesque LE, Hux JE, Juurlink DN, Alter DA. Thiazolidinediones and cardiovascular outcomes in older patients with diabetes. *JAMA.* 2007;298(22):2634-2643.

52. Giles TD, Miller AB, Elkayam U, Bhattacharya M, Perez A. Pioglitazone and heart failure: results from a controlled study in patients with type 2 diabetes mellitus and systolic dysfunction. *J Card Fail.* 2008;14:445-452.

53. Nissen SE, Wolski K. Effect of rosiglitazone on the risk of myocardial infarction and death from cardiovascular causes. *N Engl J Med.* 2007;356:2457-2471.

54. Jankowska EA, Biel B, Majda J, et al. Anabolic deficiency in men with chronic heart failure: prevalence and detrimental impact on survival. *Circulation.* 2006;114:1829-1837.

55. Malkin CJ, Pugh PJ, West JN, van Beek EJ, Jones TH, Channer KS. Testosterone therapy in men with moderate severity heart failure: a double-blind randomized placebo controlled trial. *Eur Heart J.* 2006;27:57-64.

56. Malkin CJ, Jones TH, Channer KS. The effect of testosterone on insulin sensitivity in men with heart failure. *Eur J Heart Fail.* 2007;9:44-50.

57. Nagaya N, Uematsu M, Kojima M, et al. Elevated circulating level of ghrelin in cachexia associated with chronic heart failure: relationships between ghrelin and anabolic/catabolic factors. *Circulation.* 2001;104:2034-2038.

58. Doehner W, Rauchhaus M, Godsland IF, et al. Insulin resistance in moderate chronic heart failure is related to hyperleptinaemia, but not to norepinephrine or TNF-alpha. *Int J Cardiol.* 2002;83:73-81.
59. Frankel DS, Vasan RS, D'Agostino RB Sr, et al. Resistin, adiponectin, and risk of heart failure the Framingham offspring study. *J Am Coll Cardiol.* 2009;53:754-762.
60. Tsukamoto O, Fujita M, Kato M, et al. Natriuretic peptides enhance the production of adiponectin in human adipocytes and in patients with chronic heart failure. *J Am Coll Cardiol.* 2009;53:2070-2077.
61. Birkenfeld AL, Boschmann M, Moro C, et al. Lipid mobilization with physiological atrial natriuretic peptide concentrations in humans. *J Clin Endocrinol Metab.* 2005;90:3622-3628.
62. Mancini DM, Walter G, Reichek N, et al. Contribution of skeletal muscle atrophy to exercise intolerance and altered muscle metabolism in heart failure. *Circulation.* 1992;85:1364-1373.
63. Anker SD, Ponikowski PP, Clark AL, et al. Cytokines and neurohormones relating to body composition alterations in the wasting syndrome of chronic heart failure. *Eur Heart J.* 1999; 20:683-693.
64. Anker SD, Swan JW, Volterrani M, et al. The influence of muscle mass, strength, fatigability and blood flow on exercise capacity in cachectic and non-cachectic patients with chronic heart failure. *Eur Heart J.* 1997;18(2):259-269.
65. Franciosa JA, Park M, Levine TB. Lack of correlation between exercise capacity and indexes of resting left ventricular performance in heart failure. *Am J Cardiol.* 1981;47:33-39.
66. Harrington D, Anker SD, Chua TP, et al. Skeletal muscle function and its relation to exercise tolerance in chronic heart failure. *J Am Coll Cardiol.* 1997;30:1758-1764.
67. Coats AJ, Clark AL, Piepoli M, Volterrani M, Poole-Wilson PA. Symptoms and quality of life in heart failure: the muscle hypothesis. *Br Heart J.* 1994;72(suppl):S36-S39.
68. Piepoli M, Ponikowski P, Clark AL, Banasiak W, Capucci A, Coats AJ. A neural link to explain the "muscle hypothesis" of exercise Intolerance in chronic heart failure. *Am Heart J.* 1999;137:1050-1056.
69. Lainscak M, Keber I, Anker SD. Body composition changes in patients with systolic heart failure treated with beta blockers: a pilot study. *Int J Cardiol.* 2006;106:319-322.
70. Sengenès C, Berlan M, De Glisezinski I, Lafontan M, Galitzky J. Natriuretic peptides: a new lipolytic pathway in human adipocytes. *FASEB J.* 2000;14:1345-1351.
71. Lafontan M, Moro C, Berlan M, Crampes F, Sengenes C, Galitzky J. Control of lipolysis by natriuretic peptides and cyclic GMP. *Trends Endocrinol Metab.* 2008;19:130-137.
72. Lee AH, Mull RL, Keenan GF, et al. Osteoporosis and bone morbidity in cardiac transplant recipients. *Am J Med.* 1994;96:35-41.
73. Abou-Raya S, Abou-Raya A. Osteoporosis and congestive heart failure (CHF) in the elderly patient: Double disease burden. *Arch Gerontol Geriatr.* 2008;49:250-254.
74. Anker SD, Clark AL, Teixeira MM, Hellewell PG, Coats AJ. Loss of bone mineral in patients with cachexia due to chronic heart failure. *Am J Cardiol.* 1999;83:612-615.
75. Shane E, Mancini D, Aaronson K, et al. Bone mass, vitamin D deficiency, and hyperparathyroidism in congestive heart failure. *Am J Med.* 1997;103:197-207.
76. Langin D. Adipose tissue lipolysis as a metabolic pathway to define pharmacological strategies against obesity and the metabolic syndrome. *Pharmacol Res.* 2006;53:482-491.
77. Lamont LS, Brown T, Riebe D, Caldwell M. The major components of human energy balance during chronic beta-adrenergic blockade. *J Cardiopulm Rehabil.* 2000;20:247-250.
78. Anker SD, Coats AJ, Roecker EB, Scherhag A, Packer M. Does carvedilol prevent and reverse cardiac cachexia in patients with severe heart failure? Results of the COPERNICUS study. *Eur Heart J.* 2002;23:394 [abstract].
79. Anker SD, Lechat P, Dargie HJ. Prevention and reversal of cachexia in patients with chronic heart failure by bisoprolol: results from the CIBIS II-study. *J Am Coll Cardiol.* 2003;41:156A-157A [abstract].
80. Hryniewicz K, Androne AS, Hudaihed A, Katz SD. Partial reversal of cachexia by beta-adrenergic receptor blocker therapy in patients with chronic heart failure. *J Card Fail.* 2003; 9:464-468.

81. Szabó T, von Haehling S, Doehner W. Weight change with beta-blocker use – a side effect put into perspective. *Am J Med*. 2008;121:e15.
82. Ekberg G, Hansson BG. Glucose tolerance and insulin release in hypertensive patients treated with the cardioselective beta-receptor blocking agent metoprolol. *Acta Med Scand*. 1977;202:393-397.
83. William-Olsson T, Fellenius E, Bjorntorp P, Smith U. Differences in metabolic responses to beta-adrenergic stimulation after propranolol or metoprolol administration. *Acta Med Scand*. 1979;205:201-206.
84. Sawicki PT, Siebenhofer A. Betablocker treatment in diabetes mellitus. *J Intern Med*. 2001; 250:11-17.
85. Fagerberg B, Berglund A, Holme E, Wilhelmsen L, Elmfeldt D. Metabolic effects of controlled-release metoprolol in hypertensive men with impaired or diabetic glucose tolerance: a comparison with atenolol. *J Intern Med*. 1990;227:37-43.
86. Pollare T, Lithell H, Selinus I, Berne C. Sensitivity to insulin during treatment with atenolol and metoprolol: a randomised, double blind study of effects on carbohydrate and lipoprotein metabolism in hypertensive patients. *BMJ*. 1989;298:1152-1157.
87. Anker SD, Negassa A, Coats AJ, et al. Prognostic importance of weight loss in chronic heart failure and the effect of treatment with angiotensin-converting-enzyme inhibitors: an observational study. *Lancet*. 2003;361:1077-1083.
88. Paolisso G, Balbi V, Gambardella A, et al. Lisinopril administration improves insulin action in aged patients with hypertension. *J Hum Hypertens*. 1995;9:541-546.
89. Yusuf S, Gerstein H, Hoogwerf B, et al.; for the HOPE Study Investigators. Ramipril and the development of diabetes. *JAMA*. 2001;286:1882-1885.
90. Elliott WJ, Meyer PM. Incident diabetes in clinical trials of antihypertensive drugs: a network meta-analysis. *Lancet*. 2007;369:201-207.
91. Shepherd J, Cobbe SM, Ford I, et al. Prevention of coronary heart disease with pravastatin in men with hypercholesterolemia. West of Scotland Coronary Prevention Study Group. *N Engl J Med*. 1995;333:1301-1307.
92. The Long-Term Intervention with Pravastatin in Ischaemic Disease (LIPID) Study Group. Prevention of cardiovascular events and death with pravastatin in patients with coronary heart disease and a broad range of initial cholesterol levels. *N Engl J Med*. 1998;339:1349-1357.
93. Laufs U, La Fata V, Plutzky J, Liao JK. Upregulation of endothelial nitric oxide synthase by HMG CoA reductase inhibitors. *Circulation*. 1998;97:1129-1135.
94. Feron O, Dessy C, Desager JP, Balligand JL. Hydroxy-methylglutaryl-coenzyme A reductase inhibition promotes endothelial nitric oxide synthase activation through a decrease in caveolin abundance. *Circulation*. 2001;103:113-118.
95. Wassmann S, Laufs U, Baumer AT, et al. HMG-CoA reductase inhibitors improve endothelial dysfunction in normocholesterolemic hypertension via reduced production of reactive oxygen species. *Hypertension*. 2001;37:1450-1457.
96. Condorelli G, Borello U, De Angelis L, et al. Cardiomyocytes induce endothelial cells to trans-differentiate into cardiac muscle: implications for myocardium regeneration. *Proc Natl Acad Sci USA*. 2001;98:10733-10738.
97. Vasa M, Fichtlscherer S, Adler K, et al. Increase in circulating endothelial progenitor cells by statin therapy in patients with stable coronary artery disease. *Circulation*. 2001;103:2885-2890.
98. Albert MA, Danielson E, Rifai N, Ridker PM; for the PRINCE Investigators. Effect of statin therapy on C-reactive protein levels: the pravastatin inflammation/CRP evaluation (PRINCE): a randomized trial and cohort study. *JAMA*. 2001;286:64-70.
99. Ridker PM, Cannon CP, Morrow D, et al.; for the Pravastatin or Atorvastatin Evaluation and Infection Therapy-Thrombolysis in Myocardial Infarction 22 (PROVE IT-TIMI 22) Investigators. C-reactive protein levels and outcomes after statin therapy. *N Engl J Med*. 2005;352:20-28.

100. Gibbs CR, Jackson G, Lip GY. ABC of heart failure. Non-drug management. *BMJ.* 2000;320:366-369.
101. Rozentryt P, Michalak A, Nowak JU, Brachowska A, Polonski L, Anker SD. The effects of enteral supplementation in patients with cardiac cachexia – a prospective, randomised, double-blind, placebo controlled trial. Third Cachexia Conference Abstract Book, Rome, Italy, 2005:82.
102. Yavuzsen T, Davis MP, Walsh D, LeGrand S, Lagman R. Systematic review of the treatment of cancer-associated anorexia and weight loss. *J Clin Oncol.* 2005;23:8500-8511.
103. Neri B, Garosi VL, Intini C. Effect of medroxyprogesterone acetate on the quality of life of the oncologic patient: a multicentric cooperative study. *Anticancer Drugs.* 1997;8:459-465.
104. Beal JE, Olson R, Laubenstein L, et al. Dronabinol as a treatment for anorexia associated with weight loss in patients with AIDS. *J Pain Symptom Manage.* 1995;10:89-97.
105. Nelson K, Walsh D, Deeter P, Sheehan F. A phase II study of delta-9-tetrahydrocannabinol for appetite stimulation in cancer-associated anorexia. *J Palliat Care.* 1994;10:14-18.
106. Strasser F, Luftner D, Possinger K, et al.; for the Cannabis-In-Cachexia-Study-Group. Comparison of orally administered cannabis extract and delta-9-tetrahydrocannabinol in treating patients with cancer-related anorexia-cachexia syndrome: a multicenter, phase III, randomized, double-blind, placebo-controlled clinical trial from the Cannabis-In-Cachexia-Study-Group. *J Clin Oncol.* 2006;24:3394-3400.
107. John M. Appetite stimulants. In: Hofbauer KG, Anker SD, Inui A, Jicholson JR, eds. *Pharmacotherapy of Cachexia.* Baco Raton: Taylor & Francis; 2006.
108. Pugh PJ, Jones TH, Channer KS. Acute haemodynamic effects of testosterone in men with chronic heart failure. *Eur Heart J.* 2003;24:909-915.
109. Cuerda C, Zugasti A, Bretón I, Camblor M, Miralles P, García P. Treatment with nandrolone decanoate and megestrol acetate in HIV-infected men. *Nutr Clin Pract.* 2005;20:93-97.
110. von Haehling S, Anker SD. Future prospects of anticytokine therapy in chronic heart failure. *Expert Opin Investig Drugs.* 2005;14:163-176.
111. Chung ES, Packer M, Lo KH, Fasanmade AA, Willerson JT; Anti-TNF Therapy Against Congestive Heart Failure Investigators. Randomized, double-blind, placebo-controlled, pilot trial of infliximab, a chimeric monoclonal antibody to tumor necrosis factor-alpha, in patients with moderate-to-severe heart failure: results of the anti-TNF Therapy Against Congestive Heart Failure (ATTACH) trial. *Circulation.* 2003;107:3133-3140.
112. Sampaio EP, Sarno EN, Galilly R, Cohn ZA, Kaplan G. Thalidomide selectively inhibits tumor necrosis factor production by stimulated human monocytes. *J Exp Med.* 1991;173: 699-703.
113. Calabrese L, Resztak K. Thalidomide revisited: pharmacology and clinical applications. *Expert Opin Investig Drugs.* 1998;7:2043-2060.
114. Zabel P, Schonharting MM, Schade UF, Schlaak M. Effects of pentoxifylline in endotoxinemia in human volunteers. *Prog Clin Biol Res.* 1991;367:207-213.
115. Sliwa K, Skudicky D, Candy G, Wisenbaugh T, Sareli P. Randomised investigation of effects of pentoxifylline on left-ventricular performance in idiopathic dilated cardiomyopathy. *Lancet.* 1998;351:1091-1093.
116. Sliwa K, Woodiwiss A, Kone VN, et al. Therapy of ischemic cardiomyopathy with the immunomodulating agent pentoxifylline: results of a randomized study. *Circulation.* 2004;109:750-755.
117. Skudicky D, Bergemann A, Sliwa K, Candy G, Sareli P. Beneficial effects of pentoxifylline in patients with idiopathic dilated cardiomyopathy treated with angiotensin-converting enzyme inhibitors and carvedilol: results of a randomized study. *Circulation.* 2001;103:1083-1088.
118. Bahrmann P, Hengst UM, Richartz BM, Figulla HR. Pentoxifylline in ischemic, hypertensive and idiopathic-dilated cardiomyopathy: effects on left-ventricular function, inflammatory cytokines and symptoms. *Eur J Heart Fail.* 2004;6:195-201.

Breathing Disturbances in Heart Failure

9

Resham Baruah and Darrel Francis

Chronic heart failure (CHF), a primary cardiac condition, manifests predominantly by the respiratory symptoms of breathlessness and fatigue, initially on exercise but with progression it occurs at lower and lower levels of activity and in severe cases is present at rest.

9.1
Pulmonary Abnormalities in Heart Failure

As the left ventricle fails, left ventricular end-diastolic pressure rises, causing left atrial and pulmonary venous and capillary pressures to rise.[1] The pulmonary vessels adapt to these chronically increased pressures with thickening of the media and intima.[2] Initially, despite increased pulmonary congestion, interstitial oedema is avoided as increased lymphatic clearage removes the excess fluid. Once the capacity for lymphatic clearage is exceeded, fluid begins to accumulate, first in the peribronchial and perivascular tissues as well as the interstitial spaces. Persistence of this fluid promotes fibroblast proliferation and fibrosis with remodeling of alveolar-capillary membrane.[3] Finally, if allowed to progress, alveolar oedema results.[4] This results in decreased lung compliance which is reflected by decreased vital capacity on spirometry, with increased work of breathing and hence increased metabolic demand.

Heart failure may be regarded as a pathological response to exercise, with initially pulmonary arterial pressure only elevated on exercise.[5] Simple spirometry in chronic heart failure patients reveals reduced vital capacity (VC), forced expiratory volume in 1 s (FEV$_1$), forced vital capacity (FVC) and total lung capacity (TLC) with relatively preserved forced expiratory vital capacity (FEVC); it is a restrictive pattern, which is considered to be secondary to interstitial and alveolar oedema and to a lesser extent compression from cardiomegaly, and the presence of pleural effusions.[6-8] Reduction in TLC reverses with reduction of the pulmonary capillary wedge pressure either by medical treatment[9] or lung transplantation[10] suggesting that the reduction in TLC is predominantly due to the fluid accumulation rather than the parenchymal and structural changes in the lungs. By

R. Baruah (✉)
National Heart and Lung Institute, Imperial College London, London, UK
e-mail: Resham.baruah@imperial.ac.uk

M.Y. Henein (ed.), *Heart Failure in Clinical Practice*,
DOI: 10.1007/978-1-84996-153-0_9, © Springer-Verlag London Limited 2010

contrast, in acute heart failure including acute exacerbations of chronic heart failure, patients often present with a predominantly obstructive picture which may be due to peri-bronchial vascular congestion producing increased airways resistance.[4] Gas transfer is reduced in CHF.[8] Patients have impaired transalveolar diffusion when measured using transcapillary carbon monoxide diffusion (DL_{CO}),[11] which is directly related to exercise tolerance[12] and the increased ventilatory response to exercise. This does not appear to be the effect of increased parenchymal fluid as it fails to improve with ultrafiltration[13] but does improve with angiotensin-converting enzyme inhibitors[14] and exercise training.[15]

Skeletal muscle, including the diaphragm and other respiratory muscles, demonstrate marked abnormalities in heart failure, which may contribute to the marked dyspnoea on exercise seen in heart failure. Abnormalities occur early in the disease progression and affect muscle structure, function, bulk and metabolic properties. Oxygen extraction from blood is also impaired, with a greater shift towards anaerobic metabolism and these are independent of reduced blood flow.[16] Indeed, in normal subjects with normal systolic func-tion, exercise appears to be ultimately limited by cardiac output; adding arm exercise when the subject is undergoing maximal leg exercise does not further increase the peak oxygen consumption (VO_2) on exercise testing. This compares with heart failure patients where the addition of further exercise, leads to a further increase in the peak oxygen consumption suggesting that cardiac output is not the limiting factor in these patients but rather the abil-ity of the muscle to extract oxygen.[17]

Not only do patients with heart failure complain of dyspnoea on exertion and increased fatiguability but there is also evidence of abnormal physiological reflex responses to exer-cise. Two major groups of ventilatory control reflexes have been found to be altered in heart failure patients compared to healthy controls: the ergoreflex and the chemoreflex.

9.2
Exercise Ventilatory Abnormalities in Heart Failure

Ergoreceptors are muscle receptors that are sensitive to metabolic products and act by increasing the ventilatory response on exercise and potentiating sympathetic mediated vas-constriction.[18, 19] There is an association between symptom severity, New York Heart Association (NYHA) functional class, muscle wasting[20] and ergoreflex overactivity.[21]

9.3
Exercise Testing

Cardiopulmonary exercise testing allows the real-time measurement of ventilatory param-eters such as respiratory rate, tidal volume, minute ventilation, inspired and expired frac-tions of O_2 and CO_2 as well oxygen uptake (VO_2) and carbon dioxide output (VCO_2). Peak exercise capacity has been defined as "the maximum ability of the cardiovascular system to deliver oxygen to exercising skeletal muscle and of the exercising muscle to extract oxygen from the blood".[22] Peak oxygen uptake (VO_2max) according to the Fick equation may be defined as follows:

$$VO_2 \, max = (SV \, max \times HR \, max) \times (CaO_2 - CvO_2),$$

where
SVmax is the maximum stroke volume (L/min)
HRmax is the maximum heart rate (bpm)
CaO_2 is the arterial oxygen content (kPa)
CvO_2 is the venous oxygen content (kPa)

In healthy subjects, the VO_2 appears to plateau close to peak exercise and this value of VO_2 is considered to be the VO_2max. Patients are not always able to achieve a plateau in VO_2 in which case the "peak oxygen uptake" (PVO_2) is used instead of VO_2max. In heart failure patients, PVO_2 has been demonstrated to be an extremely good predictor of outcome and has come to be an important parameter in assessing suitability for cardiac transplantation,[23,24] with a PVO_2 of less than 14 mL/kg/min and certainly less than 10 mL/kg/min suggestive that the risk: benefit ratio may be in favor of transplantation.[25,26]

The respiratory exchange ratio (RER), also known as the gas exchange ratio, is the ratio of carbon dioxide production to oxygen uptake (VCO_2/VO_2) and is measured on a breath-by-breath basis, at the mouth. Under steady state conditions this is equivalent to the respiratory quotient (RQ) which is the ratio at the tissue level of CO_2 production to O_2 consumption. The value of the RQ depends on the substrate for metabolism, with an RQ of 1 being utilization predominantly of carbohydrates (for example glucose):

$$C_6H_{12}O_6 + 6O_2 \rightarrow 6H_2O + 6CO_2$$

RQ is <1 when either fats or proteins are the major substrate being metabolized, because they have more carbon atoms per unit oxygen.

During exercise, ventilation and the carbon dioxide exhaled increase linearly, but in heart failure for a given production of carbon dioxide, the minute ventilation required is greater, or in other words the slope of this relationship (the VE/VCO_2 slope) is steeper.[27] This excessive ventilatory response or exercise hyperpnea, expressed as ventilation per unit of carbon dioxide produced or (VE/VCO_2) slope is a marker for poor prognosis in heart failure.[28,29] Moreover, the worse the exercise capacity, the more exaggerated is this respiratory response.[30]

Mathematically, the VE/VCO_2 ratio (which is similar in behavior to the slope) is determined by the following equation:

$$VE/VCO_2 = 863 \, mmHg \, / \, PaCO_2 \times (1 - VD \, / \, VT),$$

where
VE/VCO_2 is the ratio between ventilation and CO_2 production
863 mmHg is atmospheric pressure
$PaCO_2$ is the partial pressure of CO_2 in the arteries (mmHg)
VD is the deadspace (L)
VT is the tidal volume (L)

It is therefore clear that the parameters that can affect this relationship are the arterial CO_2, which is affected by metabolism and the balance between aerobic and anaerobic threshold on exercise, the dead-space ventilation, which would affect the plant gain, namely the change in CO_2 for a given change in ventilation and the chemoreflex, i.e., the change in ventilation that arises from a change in CO_2.

Respiratory muscle abnormalities have been noted including histological changes with increased type IIb muscular fibres expression,[31] early fatigue and early muscle deoxygenation.[32] An early switch to anaerobic respiration on exercise, with lactic acid production, has been postulated to drive down subsequent arterial CO_2, a finding common in heart failure; however, an increase in arterial lactate and hydrogen ions is correlated with a rise and not fall in arterial CO_2, and lactate levels in the recovery phase have not been found to correlate with the VE/VCO$_2$ slope.[33]

The relationship between carbon dioxide production (VCO$_2$) and ventilation (VE) is a linear one, and as arterial blood gases during exercise suggest that arterial carbon dioxide is at the lower end of the normal range, it is increased ventilation that drives the increased carbon dioxide production and not vice versa. Not only is the level of ventilation in heart failure patients greater than controls but the pattern of ventilation is abnormal at lower levels of exercise with heart failure patients displaying a higher respiratory rate but smaller tidal volume compared to controls.[34] As heart failure progresses, physiological dead space as a proportion of tidal volume increases.[6] Patients with a higher VE/VCO$_2$ slope have been demonstrated to have an increased VD/VT ratio and also lower arterial CO_2 during exercise.[35] This lower arterial CO2 therefore cannot be explained alone by inefficiency of gas exchange or an increased VD/VT ratio. There must a combination of this increased ratio and a primary increase in ventilatory drive. It has been proposed that this primary hyperventilation arises from activation of the ergoreflex. It seems that lactate levels within the muscle interstitum may differ considerably from the arterial lactate levels[32].

9.4
Chemoreceptors: The ventilatory Response to Changes in Arterial CO$_2$

Breathing free of conscious control, for example during sleep, is dependent on the activity of chemoreceptors. These receptors bring about a change in ventilation in response to a change in arterial carbon dioxide, oxygen or both. Chemoreceptors exist in the brainstem (central chemoreceptors) and at the aortic arch and carotid bodies collectively known as the peripheral chemoreceptors. Central chemoreceptors tend to respond primarily to local increases in the hydrogen ion concentration or arterial CO_2 whereas hypoxia acts as the predominant stimulus for the peripheral chemoreceptors; however, these responses are not absolute so that hypercapnia does lead to an increase in firing of the peripheral chemoreceptors. During sleep, particularly during rapid eye movement (REM) sleep, the responsiveness of the chemoreceptors to both hypoxia and hypercapnia and their ability to stimulate respiratory muscle afferents and increase ventilation are reduced.[36,37]

Animal work comparing the two anatomical groups of peripheral chemoreceptors suggests that there is a differential response to hypoxia between them; a fall in the arterial partial pressure of oxygen is followed by a greater increment in firing by the carotid chemoreceptors than by the chemoreceptors located at the aortic arch.[38] Moreover, the carotid body chemoreceptor stimulation by hypoxia drives an increase in respiratory rate and the depth of breathing whereas aortic body chemoreceptors produce a small increase in respiratory rate with very little effect on tidal volume.[39] Human studies, on patients who have had therapeutic bilateral carotid body resection appear to confirm that the carotid body chemoreceptors are responsible for the majority of the hypoxic response.[40–42]

The nucleus of the solitary tract in the dorsal medulla relays information both from the peripheral chemoreceptors and the pulmonary mechanoreceptors to other areas of the brainstem respiratory network. This network generates respiratory rhythm and controls the motor neurons that innervate respiratory muscles.[43]

Activation of either the hypoxic or hypercapnic responses not only produces a hyperventilation response but also sympathetic activation leading to an increase in blood pressure. The baroreflex then acts to inhibit the chemoreflex via negative feedback. Hyperventilation (following chemorecptor activation) leads to stretch of thoracic afferents. These act to inhibit chemoreflex mediated sympathetic activation particularly the peripheral chemoreceptors. Conversely when apnoea occurs and the thoracic afferents are not activated, and chemoreflex activation is potentiated with marked sympathetic activation. However, in studies of the carotid bodies of rabbits with pacing- induced heart failure despite an augmented ventilatory response, the sympathetic drive is augmented. The authors conclude that enhanced carotid body sensitivity as seen in heart failure has a considerable impact in the sympathetic over activation which is characteristic of and confers such great prognostic significance in heart failure.[38]

The increase in sympathetic outflow to vascular beds seen with chemoreflex activation probably acts, in health, to maintain arterial pressure despite the vasodilatory effects of hypoxia and hypercapnia.[44]

Patients with chronic heart failure consistently demonstrate an enhanced central chemoreflex with an exaggerated ventilatory response to hypercapnia although it has been more difficult to demonstrate exaggerated peripheral activity under normoxic conditions.[45]

9.5
Unstable Ventilatory Patterns/Sleep Apnoea in Heart Failure

Abnormal breathing patterns in patients with heart failure were first described by John Cheyne 1818 stating "it would entirely cease for a quarter of a minute then it would become perceptible though very low then by degrees it became heavy and quick and then it would gradually cease again: this revolution in the state of his breathing occupied about a minute during which there were about thirty acts of respiration".[46]

Around four decades later Dr William Stokes described "a symptom which appears to belong to a weakened state of heart, it consists in the occurrence of a series of inspirations, increasing to a maximum, and then declining in force and length, until a state of apparent apnoea is established..."

Today we recognize that sleep related breathing disorders are common in patients with heart failure.[47] Central sleep apnoea (CSA), which is prevalent in up to about 40% of heart failure patients is characterized by repetitive cessation of ventilation during sleep resulting from loss of central neural outflow or ventilatory drive. A central apnea is cessation in ventilation with no associated respiratory effort for greater than 10 s. Generally, five or more of such events per hour are considered abnormal. This frequency of apnoea may be accompanied by disrupted sleep and/or hypersomnolence during the day and is then considered to be CSA Syndrome. Cheyne–Stokes respiration, as first described by Cheyne and Stokes and characterized by a crescendo–decrescendo pattern of breathing with a central apnea or hypopnea at the nadir of ventilatory effort, is a form of periodic breathing. Periodic breathing (PB), which is characterized by cyclical rises and falls in ventilation but not necessarily with true periods of apnoea and both Cheyne–Stokes Respiration and PB, can occur in the daytime as well as during sleep.[48–50] Other types of CSA that do not become more prevalent in heart failure include altitude-induced PB, narcotic-induced central apnea, obesity hypoventilation syndrome (OHS) and idiopathic Cheyne–Stokes respiration.

Ventilatory oscillations are accompanied by oscillations in hemodynamic parameters such as blood pressure,[44] stroke volume[51] and even cerebral blood flow,[52] which may contribute to the increased mortality seen in patients with CSA and HF.

Patients with CSA in the context of heart failure may suffer from paroxysmal nocturnal dyspnoea and frequent nocturnal arousals and awakenings although reported daytime somnolence is not a prominent symptom. Despite this, objective assessment suggests that patients with CSA are sleepier compared to controls with lower daytime activity levels.[52] Data regarding the frequency of CSA and early morning headaches or symptomatically disturbed sleep are lacking.[53]

Cheyne–Stokes respiration and PB are associated with increased mortality both when present during sleep[54] and during the daytime.[45,55] In CSA, the ventilatory oscillations are accompanied by arousals from sleep and oscillations in blood pressure. While it has been postulated that the arousals provoke the recurrent elevations in blood pressure, studies in awake healthy volunteers who have voluntarily simulated PB demonstrate that peak blood pressure coincides with periods of hyperventilation, with troughs in blood pressure coincident with the apnoeic periods.[56] Studies of heart failure patients with both daytime and Cheyne–Stokes respiration during sleep recognized a similar pattern with respect to timing, with blood pressure falling during apnoeas and rising during the hyperpneas not only during wakefulness but also when both early and late arousals were present. The presence of late arousals further augmented the blood pressure oscillations but to a lesser degree than the ventilatory oscillations.[57]

9.6
Diagnosis of CSA

Current recommendations are that diagnosis and characterization of CSA requires full night polysomnography.[41] Detection of apnoeas is most successful with respiratory inductive plethysmography (RIP) or nasal pressure and less reliably with respiratory impedance devices such as bands, oro-nasal thermistors[58] or more recently novel techniques such as forehead venous pressure using photoplethysmography.[59] The differentiation of central hypopneas (rather than apneas) from hyponeas that are obstructive in nature, resulting from the partial upper airway obstruction, is more difficult. In both, respiratory effort continues but in obstructive events there will be thoraco-abdominal incoordination with evidence of airflow limitation nasally. However, the gold standard for differentiating the two underlying pathologies would be invasive tests such as intraoesophageal pressure measurements or diaphragmatic electromyograms.[53]

Overnight polysomnography in the sleep laboratory traditionally measures parameters such as an electroencephalogram (EEG), electromyography (EMG) and electroculography (EOG), which together allow the sleep stage to be identified, ventilation usually with a thermistor, video recording, oxygen saturations, body position and an ECG.

Overnight polysomnography allows parameters such as the apnoea–hypopnea index (AHI) to be derived. An event may be described as an apnoea if there is cessation of airflow accompanied by a fall in blood oxygen saturations and arousal, whereas if airflow is reduced then it may be classified as a hypopnea. As a result, many different laboratories have different thresholds for what they would define as either an apnoea or hypopnea, which clearly makes the interpretation of prevalence studies difficult. The AHI is the average number of apnoea and hypopnea per hour of sleep. Many of the diagnostic criteria in this field are historically on the basis of the initial work done on obstructive sleep apnoea (OSA) where a combination of sleepiness with an AHI>5 was diagnostic with mild disease being 5–15 events/h, moderate 15–30 events/h and severe being >30 events/h.[60] These OSA criteria have then been applied to CSA and indeed heart failure patients with an AHI >30 have been found to have a particularly poor outcome.[49] AHI might not be the ideal method of measuring severity in CSA, partly because of difficulties in deciding what truly equals an event and partly because the severity levels of the consequences of the event are not quantified, so a brief period of slight desaturation counts as one event as does a period of prolonged severe hypoxia. Moreover, patients who have longer cycle lengths cannot possibly achieve the same number of events as patients with shorter cycle lengths and therefore will score lower on AHI, even though such prolonged cycles are associated with slower circulation times typical of more advanced heart failure.[61]

9.7
Prevalence of CSA

CSA is more common in heart failure than in the general population. Prospective prevalence studies of heart failure patients with ejection fraction less than 45% suggest that there may be a prevalence of PB of up to 40%, and interestingly a relatively high proportion of the population (12%) demonstrate OSA.[62] Central and obstructive events coexist in many patients with heart failure[61,63] and may make it difficult to distinguish the two entities.[64] Indeed there may also be considerable overlap in the pathophysiology of CSA and OSA.[65]

9.8
Pathophysiology of Periodic Breathing

The pathophysiology of PB in heart failure is not fully understood. Cheyne's first description of abnormal respiration was in a patient with heart failure and likely low cardiac output and prolonged circulation time. He noted that in Cheyne–Stokes respiration there is a prolongation of the waxing and waning phase compared to the hyperventilation phase. It has since been demonstrated that the duration of the hyperpnoea phase is directly proportional to the circulation time and inversely proportional to cardiac output.[66] However, in animal studies, artificial prolongation of circulation time produces ventilatory instability only if prolonged to biological implausible lengths of 2–5 min.[67] Therefore, while prolonged circulation time contributes to PB in isolation, it is unlikely to cause it[63] and simple clinical observations such as this may explain some but not all of the underlying mechanisms predisposing to unstable ventilation. In fact, circulation delay appears to determine ventilatory cycle length with cycle length typically ranging from 2 to 2.5 times the circulatory delay.[68]

As a result, mathematical models based on negative feedback loop between arterial CO_2 allows individual risk factors is to be assessed independently. Critical to the pathogenesis of PB is an exaggerated ventilatory response to arterial carbon dioxide, i.e., increased chemosensitivity.[69,70] This enhanced response leads to an overshoot in ventilation which produces the characteristic oscillatory pattern seen in PB. The blood gas concentrations are dependent on the lung gas concentrations which also fluctuate with ventilation.[71]

Many mathematical models are developed from control theory which is an interdisciplinary branch of mathematics and engineering that can be used to describe dynamic systems. Control gain in ventilation corresponds with the chemoreflex gain, namely the change in ventilation that results from a change in end-tidal CO_2. The chemoreflex response curve describes this relationship over a range of end-tidal CO_2.

The resultant physical effect of the change in ventilation on end-tidal CO_2 is the exhalation or plant gain. Assuming that end-tidal CO_2 exhaled is proportional to CO_2 produced by metabolism, it can be seen that end-tidal CO_2 is linked to ventilation by a hyperbolic curve.

As a result of these two relationships, at any one point there can only be one possible combination of ventilation and end-tidal CO_2 – the potential steady state. Graphically, this point is the intercept between the metabolism curve and the chemoreflex response curve.

When a small perturbation is added, for example when CO_2 is added to the system, where the system responds by returning to the potential steady state, the system is considered stable. Hence, following a deviation, the ventilatory oscillations spontaneously decay as the system returns to the steady state and the loop gain is less than 1. Where a small deviation triggers larger deviations away from the steady state, the system is unstable. In this case, the system oscillates around a central point, the steady state in potential form. The loop gain[72] is therefore greater than 1.

Six principal physiological variables have been identified using mathematical modeling as being important in making unstable ventilation more likely. These are a steep chemoreflex slope, long lag to chemoreflex response, low ventilation, low cardiac output, high alveolar-atmospheric CO_2 difference and small lung volume. All these factors decrease ventilatory stability by exaggerating either the ventilatory response to CO_2 (chemoreflex) or the CO_2 response to ventilation (plant gain). Any such exaggeration, increases overall loop gain and it is likely that such overshoot in response leads to the cyclical oscillations seen in PB. Of all these factors, chemoreflex enhancement and prolonged lag to ventilatory response may be the most important factors in heart failure patients.[63]

When chemoreflex gain is increased, the gradient of the chemoreflex curve is higher and the intercept between the metabolic hyperbola and the chemoreflex curve is higher. As a result mean alveolar ventilation must be higher and mean end-tidal CO_2 lower, as is seen clinically in patients with PB. Therefore, heart failure patients with high mean ventilation should be suspected of disguising a high chemoreflex gain.[63]

It has long been recognized that patients with PB have low mean arterial CO_2 levels compared with heart failure patients with stable breathing. Moreover, a period of hyper-ventilation appears to trigger PB and it has been hypothesized that ventilation becomes unstable when arterial CO_2 falls below an apnoeic threshold which is pathologically elevated in patients prone to unstable ventilation.[73–75] However, mathematical modeling suggests that increased mean alveolar ventilation and decreased arterial CO_2 also both favor stability.

In clinical practice, it is impossible to tease out the individual effects of chemoreflex gain, apnoea threshold and potential steady state end-tidal CO_2. Therefore, a novel mathematical model that allows the chemoreflex curve to bend so that it can pass through any designated apnoeic threshold but retain the required gradient at the potential steady state was developed.[67] In isolation, when apnoeic threshold was varied, but chemoreflex gain and steady state fractional end-tidal CO_2 were kept constant at values at the edge of stability, apnoeic threshold had no overall effect on system stability. This compared with chemoreflex gain, where even very small changes in chemoreflex gain resulted in large changes in system stability. Interestingly, using this model to vary potential steady state CO_2, but keeping apnoeic threshold and chemoreflex gain constant, revealed that higher rather than lower CO_2 levels favor instability. This was a counter-intuitive finding particularly given that low arterial CO_2 is a powerful predictor of CSA in heart failure patients.[70] It is believed that this is because in clinical practice very small changes in CO_2 can conceal extremely large changes in chemoreflex gain. This can be seen from the following equation:

$$S = \frac{\overline{VCO_2}}{\overline{C}\left(\overline{C} - C_{apn}\right)}$$

where
S is the chemoreflex gain (L/min/mmHg)
$\overline{VCO_2}$ is the steady-state CO_2 production (kPa)
$\overline{C}$ is the steady-state alveolar CO_2 fraction
C_{apn} is the apnoea threshold expressed as a fraction of CO_2

Therefore any change in $\overline{C}$ is squared and can therefore produce a much bigger change in S.

This fails to explain why when supplemental CO_2 is delivered, unstable breathing is often stabilized. Flux of carbon dioxide into and out of the lungs is dependent on metabolism, ventilation and the solubility of carbon dioxide in the blood. Normally the inspired CO_2 in air is negligible and CO_2 diffuses freely from the blood to the alveolar space down its concentration gradient from where it is expelled during expiration. When supplemental CO_2 is inhaled less CO_2 moves from the blood to alveoli and therefore less is cleared. Therefore, the effective plant gain is reduced as the effective CO_2 elimination from the body for a given ventilation rate is reduced and the overall gain of the system is reduced. This can be seen from the following equation:

$$\overline{VA} = \frac{\overline{VCO_2}}{FETCO_2 - FICO_2},$$

where

$\overline{VA}$ is the mean alveolar ventilation (L/min)

$\overline{VCO_2}$ is the carbon dioxide output (kPa)

$FETCO_2$ is the fraction of end-tidal CO_2

$FICO_2$ is the fraction of inspired CO_2

This equation also explains why a higher mean ventilation favors stability. For example, if the alveolar ventilation goes from 4 to 5 L/min, with an initial end-tidal CO_2 of 4.5 kPa and a constant metabolic production of CO_2, then the resultant absolute decrease in end-tidal CO_2 is 0.9 kPa (from 4.5 to 3.6 kPa). If the alveolar ventilation goes from 9 to 10 L/min with an initial end-tidal CO_2 of 4.5 kPa, then the absolute decrease in end-tidal CO_2 is 0.45 kPa (from 4.5 to 4.05 kPa). Therefore, the resultant absolute change in end-tidal CO_2 concentration for a given change in alveolar ventilation is lower, the higher the mean alveolar ventilation. In other words, the higher the mean alveolar ventilation, the lower the plant gain.

9.9
CSA and Mortality

Heart failure patients with Cheyne–Stokes respiration and a high AHI have been observed to have an increased mortality compared to patients with a similar degree of heart failure but stable ventilation overnight.[49,76] However, these patients also have worse left ventricular impairment (as measured by ejection fraction), suggesting that Cheyne–Stokes respiration maybe a measure of heart failure severity rather than an independent risk factor for mortality. Daytime Cheyne–Stokes respiration also appears to confer an adverse prognosis in heart failure patients; indeed, approximately 16% of patients who demonstrate abnormalities during the day have a worse outcome than those who demonstrated nocturnal Cheyne–Stokes respiration alone.[77]

Despite robust evidence that beta-blockers and drugs that block the rennin-angiotensin system reduce mortality in heart failure, there is a lack of evidence that these drugs have significantly affected the prevalence of sleep disordered breathing in heart failure.[78,79] This may in part reflect differing population characteristics and also differing diagnostic criteria for Cheyne–Stokes respiration. If prevalence has not changed at all despite improved management of heart failure, then it may be that unstable ventilation is not simply a marker of heart failure severity. Recent data suggest that mortality is increased in patients where the etiology of the heart failure is ischemic but not in those where the underlying pathology is nonischemic.[80]

9.10
Treatment of CSA

One way of establishing causality with respect to Cheyne–Stokes respiration and increased mortality, would be if treatments that specifically target and treat unstable ventilation could reduce mortality. Unfortunately, most treatments also have an effect on cardiac output as well as ventilation.

Certainly following heart transplantation, CSA is abolished in most patients[81] and there have been reports of left ventricular assist devices also abolishing CSA.[82] Therefore, increasing cardiac output in itself appears to reduce the prevalence of CSA. There has been conflicting evidence regarding whether atrial overdrive pacing reduces the prevalence of sleep apnoea syndrome; whilst initial studies were positive, follow-up studies failed to replicate these results.[83, 84] One explanation would be that atrial overdrive pacing eradicates sleep apnoea syndrome only when it successfully increases cardiac output considerably. Cardiac resynchronization therapy (CRT) improves cardiac efficiency, increasing cardiac output without increasing metabolic demand. It has been demonstrated to improve mortality in heart failure.[85] CRT has also been demonstrated to reduce the prevalence of CSA and also leads to an improvement in sleep quality as well as the VE/VCO$_2$ slope.[86]

Drug therapies have also been used in CSA: there have been some reports that beta-blockers reduce the prevalence of CSA[87–89] presumably by reducing the sympathetic potentiation of the chemoreflex. Theophylline has been tried and has been demonstrated to reduce the AHI and desaturations but failed to reduce the number of arousals.[90] Theophylline acts as a competitive antagonist of adenosine and therefore acts as a respiratory stimulant, and it may thereby increase mean ventilation and hence stabilize breathing. Acetazolamide, another respiratory stimulant has been used to similar effect.[91]

On the basis of the observation that arterial CO$_2$ levels are low in patients with CSA and the observation that CSA is triggered when arterial CO$_2$ falls below the apnoeic threshold, CO$_2$ has been administered to patients. This also abolishes the CSA but does not reduce the number of arousals. This may be because CO$_2$, in high doses, may act directly to potentiate the sympathetic nervous system.[92] The addition of dead space, which also increases inspired CO$_2$, has been demonstrated to reduce the AHI, the number of desaturations and the number of arousals during sleep but with no improvement in hemodynamic parameters.[93] These methods act by increasing mean ventilation and hence metabolic demand, which heart failure patients may already be struggling to meet.[94]

Continuous positive airways pressure (CPAP) has been extensively investigated in CSA. While it has been shown to reduce the AHI, improve ejection fraction by reducing transmural pressure and decrease sympathetic activity, a large multicentre randomized trial failed to demonstrate any mortality benefit.[95] This was probably because of a large proportion of the participants failing to comply with CPAP and as a result the study being underpowered. Indeed, a post-hoc analysis of the trial suggests that in those patients who were compliant and in whom the AHI was successfully suppressed by CPAP, mortality may have been reduced.[96] It may be that some of the benefit of CPAP in CSA is by increasing lung volume, which stabilizes breathing.

9.11
Periodic Breathing During Exercise

Up to 19% of heart failure patients referred for cardiopulmonary testing demonstrate PB on exercise, known as exercise oscillatory ventilation (EOV) where it is associated with more severe disease and a poorer prognosis.[97–99] Patients with EOV have lower end-tidal CO_2 at rest, which decreases further on exercise illustrating the hyperventilation that occurs in heart failure.[100] There is a pathophysiological interdependence between EOV and the cyclical ventilatory disorders seen during sleep.[101]

9.12
Conclusion

The predominant symptom of the syndrome of heart failure is breathlessness, which suggests that abnormality of the myocardium affects cardiorespiratory interaction. Indeed there are key abnormalities in heart failure patients' response to exercise, their other muscles, metabolism and reflex control of breathing. Indeed, despite often having abnormalities in their static lung function, it appears that much of the breathlessness that they suffer on exertion is due to structural and metabolic changes in skeletal muscle, the so- called muscle hypothesis. The exaggerated ventilatory response to exercise can in part be explained by increased dead space ventilation and hyperventilation, which maybe driven by ergoreceptors and to a much lesser extent by chemoreceptors. CSA is a common condition affecting heart failure patients which appears to be associated with an adverse prognosis. While a great deal of progress has been made in elucidating the mechanisms underlying the condition, a good deal remains unknown or fiercely contested. Until its role in heart failure is better understood, it is unlikely that we will develop therapies which can successfully completely eradicate CSA and its consequences.

References

1. Gazetopoulos N, Davies H, Oliver C, Deuchar D. Ventilation and haemodynamics in heart disease. *Br Heart J*. 1966;28:1-15.
2. Smith RC, Burchell HB, Edwards JE. Pathology of the pulmonary vascular tree IV. Structural changes in the pulmonary vessels in chronic left ventricular failure. *Circulation*. 1954;10: 801-808.

3. Guazzi M. Alveolar-capillary membrane dysfunction in heart failure: evidence of a pathophysiologic role. *Chest.* 2003;124:1090-1102.
4. Chua TP, Coats AJ. The lungs in chronic heart failure. *Eur Heart J.* 1995;16(7):882-887.
5. Sullivan MJ, Higginbotham MB, Cobb FR. Increased exercise ventilation in patients with chronic heart failure: intact ventilatory control despite hemodynamic and pulmonary abnormalities. *Circulation.* 1988;77:552-559.
6. Wasserman K, Zhang YY, Gitt A, et al. Lung function and exercise gas exchange in chronic heart failure. *Circulation.* 1997;96:2221-2227.
7. Collins JV, Clark TJH, Brown DJ. Airway function in healthy subjects and patients with left heart disease. *Clin Sci Mol Med.* 1975;49:217-228.
8. Wright RS, Levine MS, Bellamy PE, Simmons MS, Batra P, Stevenson LW. Ventilatory and diffusion abnormalities in potential heart transplant recipients. *Chest.* 1990;98:816-820.
9. Faggiano P, Lombardi C, Sorgato A, Ghizzoni G, Spedini C, Rusconi C. Pulmonary function tests in patients with congestive heart failure: effects of medical therapy. *Cardiology.* 1993; 83:30-35.
10. Hosenpud JD, Stibolt TA, Atwal K, Shelley D. Abnormal pulmonary function specifically related to congestive heart failure: comparison of patients before and after cardiac transplantation. *Am J Med.* 1990;88:493-496.
11. Puri S, Baker BL, Oakley CM, Hughes JM, Cleland JG. Increased alveolar/capillary membrane resistance to gas transfer in patients with chronic heart failure. *Br Heart J.* 1994;72:140-144.
12. Puri S, Baker BL, Dutka DP, Oakley CM, Hughes JMB, Cleland JGF. Reduced alveolar–capillary membrane diffusing capacity in chronic heart failure : its pathophysiological relevance and relationship to exercise performance. *Circulation.* 1995;91:2769-2774.
13. Agostoni PG, Guazzi M, Bussotti M, Grazi M, Palermo P, Marenzi G. Lack of improvement of lung diffusing capacity following fluid withdrawal by ultrafiltration in chronic heart failure. *J Am Coll Cardiol.* 2000;36:1600-1604.
14. Guazzi M, Marenzi G, Alimento M, Contini M, Agostoni P. Improvement of alveolar–capillary membrane diffusing capacity with enalapril in chronic heart failure and counteracting effect of aspirin. *Circulation.* 1997;95:1930-1936.
15. Guazzi M, Reina G, Tumminello G, Guazzi MD. Improvement of alveolar-capillary membrane diffusing capacity with exercise training in chronic heart failure. *J Appl Physiol.* 2004; 97:1866-1873.
16. Massie BM, Conway M, Rajagopalan B, et al. Skeletal muscle metabolism during exercise under ischemic conditions in congestive heart failure. Evidence for abnormalities unrelated to blood flow. *Circulation.* 1988;78(2):320-326.
17. Jondeau G, Katz SD, Zohman L, et al. Active skeletal muscle mass and cardiopulmonary reserve. Failure to attain peak aerobic capacity during maximal bicycle exercise in patients with severe congestive heart failure. *Circulation.* 1992;86(5):1351-1356.
18. Clark AL. Origin of symptoms in chronic heart failure. *Heart.* 2006;92(1):12-16.
19. Tumminello G, Guazzi M, Lancellotti P, Piérard LA. Exercise ventilation inefficiency in heart failure: pathophysiological and clinical significance. *Eur Heart J.* 2007;28(6): 673-678.
20. Anker SD, Ponikowski P, Varney S, et al. Wasting as independent risk factor for mortality in chronic heart failure. *Lancet.* 1997;349:1050-1053.
21. Ponikowski PP, Chua TP, Francis DP, Capucci A, Coats AJ, Piepoli MF. Muscle ergoreceptor overactivity reflects deterioration in clinical status and cardiorespiratory reflex control in chronic heart failure. *Circulation.* 2001;104:2324-2330.
22. Dennis C. Rehabilitation of patients with coronary artery disease. In: Braunwald E, ed. *Heart Disease, A Textbook Of Cardiovascular Medicine.* 4th ed. Philadelphia: Saunders; 1992: 1382.
23. Szlachcic J, Massie BM, Kramer BL, Topic N, Tubau J. Correlates and prognostic implication of exercise capacity in chronic congestive heart failure. *Am J Cardiol.* 1985;55(8):1037-1042.

24. Likoff MJ, Chandler SL, Kay HR. Clinical determinants of mortality in chronic congestive heart failure secondary to idiopathic dilated or to ischemic cardiomyopathy. *Am J Cardiol.* 1987;59(6):634-638.
25. Mancini DM, Eisen H, Kussmaul W, Mull R, Edmunds LH Jr, Wilson JR. Value of peak exercise oxygen consumption for optimal timing of cardiac transplantation in ambulatory patients with heart failure. *Circulation.* 1991;83(3):778-786.
26. Hunt SA, Abraham WT, Chin MH, et al.; American College of Cardiology Foundation; American Heart Association. 2009 Focused update incorporated into the ACC/AHA 2005 Guidelines for the Diagnosis and Management of Heart Failure in Adults A Report of the American College of Cardiology Foundation/American Heart Association Task Force on Practice Guidelines Developed in Collaboration With the International Society for Heart and Lung Transplantation. *J Am Coll Cardiol.* 2009;53(15):e1-e90.
27. Buller NP, Poole-Wilson PA. Mechanism of the increased ventilatory response to exercise in patients with chronic heart failure. *Br Heart J.* 1990;63(5):281-283.
28. Chua TP, Ponikowski P, Harrington D, et al. Clinical correlates and prognostic significance of the ventilatory response to exercise in chronic heart failure. *J Am Coll Cardiol.* 1997; 29:1585-1590.
29. Ponikowski P, Francis DP, Piepoli MF, et al. Enhanced ventilatory response to exercise in patients with chronic heart failure and preserved exercise tolerance : marker of abnormal cardiorespiratory reflex control and predictor of poor prognosis. *Circulation.* 103:967-972.
30. Davies SW, Emery TM, Watling MI, Wannamethee G, Lipkin DP. A critical threshold of exercise capacity in the ventilatory response to exercise in heart failure. *Br Heart J.* 1991; 65(4):179-183.
31. Lipkin DP, Jones DA, Round JM, Poolen-Wilson PA. Abnormalities of skeletal muscle in patients with chronic heart failure. *Int J Cardiol.* 1988;18:187-195.
32. Mancini DM, Henson D, LaManca J, Levine S. Evidence of reduced respiratory muscle endurance in patients with heart failure. *J Am Coll Cardiol.* 1994;24(4):972-981.
33. Wensel R, Francis DP, Georgiadou P, et al. Exercise hyperventilation in chronic heart failure is not caused by systemic lactic acidosis. *Eur J Heart Fail.* 2005;7:1105-1111.
34. Clark AL, Volterrani M, Swan JW, Coats AJ. The increased ventilatory response to exercise in chronic heart failure: relation to pulmonary pathology. *Heart.* 1997;77(2):138-146.
35. Wensel R, Georgiadou P, Francis DP, et al. Differential contribution of dead space ventilation and low arterial pCO2 to exercise hyperpnea in patients with chronic heart failure secondary to ischemic or idiopathic dilated cardiomyopathy. *Am J Cardiol.* 2004;93(3): 318-323.
36. Wiegand L, Zwillich CW, White DP. Sleep and the ventilatory response to resistive loading in normal men. *J Appl Physiol.* 1988;64:1186-1195.
37. White DP, Douglas NJ, Pickett CK, et al. Hypoxic ventilatory response during sleep in normal premenopausal women. *Am Rev Respir Dis.* 1982;126:530-533.
38. Lahiri S, Nishino A, Mulligan E, Nishino T. Comparison of aortic and carotid chemoreceptor response to hypercapnia and hypoxia. *J Appl Physiol.* 1981;51:55-61.
39. Hopp FA, Seagard JL, Bajic J, Zuperku EJ. Respiratory responses to aortic and carotid chemoreceptor activation in the dog. *J Appl Physiol.* 1991;70:2359-2550.
40. Lugliani R, Whipp BJ, Seard C, Wasserman K. Effect of bilateral carotid body resection on ventilatory control at rest and during exercise in man. *N Engl J Med.* 1971;285:1105-1111.
41. Swanson GD, Whipp BJ, Kaufman RD, Aqleh KA, Winter B, Belville JW. Effect of hypercapnia on hypoxic ventilatory drive in normal and carotid body-resected man. *J Appl Physiol.* 1978;45:971-977.
42. Honda Y, Watanabe S, Hashizume I, et al. Hypoxic chemosensitivity in asthmatic patients two decades after carotid body resection. *J Appl Phsyiol.* 1979;46:632-638.
43. Feldman JL, Mitchell GS, Nattie EE. Breathing: rhythmicity, plasticity, chemosensitivity. *Annu Rev Neuro Sci.* 26:239-266.
44. Schultz HD, Li YL. Carotid body function in heart failure. *Respir Physiol Neurobiol.* 2007; 157(1):171-185.

45. Chua T, Clark AL, Amadi AA, Coats AJ. Relation between chemosensitivity and the ventilatory response to exercise in chronic heart failure. *J Am Coll Cardiol.* 1996;27:650-657.
46. Ito A, Lorenz R. The definition of Cheyne-Stokes rhythms. *Acta Neurochirurgica.* 1978; 43(1):61-76.
47. Somers VK, White DP, Amin R, et al.; American Heart Association Council for High Blood Pressure Research Professional Education Committee, Council on Clinical Cardiology; American Heart Association Stroke Council; American Heart Association Council on Cardiovascular Nursing; American College of Cardiology Foundation. Sleep apnea and cardiovascular disease: an American Heart Association/American College Of Cardiology Foundation Scientific Statement from the American Heart Association Council for High Blood Pressure Research Professional Education Committee, Council on Clinical Cardiology, Stroke Council, and Council On Cardiovascular Nursing. In collaboration with the National Heart, Lung, and Blood Institute National Center on Sleep Disorders Research (National Institutes of Health). *Circulation.* 2008;118(10):1080-1111.
48. Feld H, Priest S. A cyclic breathing pattern in patients with poor left ventricular function and compensated heart failure: a mild form of Cheyne-Stokes respiration? *J Am Coll Cardiol.* 1993;21:971-974.
49. Mortara A, Sleight P, Pinna GD, et al. Abnormal awake respiratory patterns are common in chronic heart failure and may prevent evaluation of autonomic tone by measures of heart rate variability. *Circulation.* 1997;96:246-252.
50. Ponikowski P, Anker SD, Chua TP, Francis D, et al. Oscillatory breathing patterns during wakefulness in patients with chronic heart failure: clinical implications and role of augmented peripheral chemosensitivity. *Circulation.* 1999;100(24):2418-2424.
51. Maze SS, Kotler MN, Parry WR. Doppler evaluation of changing cardiac dynamics during Cheyne-Stokes respiration. *Chest.* 1989;95:525-529.
52. Franklin KA, Sandstrom E, Johansson G, Balfors EM. Hemodynamics, cerebral circulation, and oxygen saturation in Cheyne-Stokes respiration. *J Appl Physiol.* 1997;83:1184-1191.
53. Hastings PC, Vazir A, O'Driscoll DM, Morrell MJ, Simonds AK. Symptom burden of sleep-disordered breathing in mild-to-moderate congestive heart failure patients. *Eur Respir J.* 2006;27(4):748-755.
54. Lanfranchi PA, Bragiroli A, Bosimini E, et al. Prognostic value of nocturnal Cheyne-Stokes respiration in chronic heart failure. *Circulation.* 1999;99:1435-1440.
55. Andreas S, Hagenah G, Moller C, et al. Cheyne-Stokes respiration and prognosis in congestive heart failure. *Am J Cardiol.* 1996;78:1260-1264.
56. Lorenzi-Filho G, Dajani HR, Leung RS, Floras JS, Bradley TD. Entrainment of blood pressure and heart rate oscillations by periodic breathing. *Am J Respir Crit Care Med.* 1999;159(4 Pt 1):1147-1154.
57. Trinder J, Merson R, Rosenberg JI, Fitzgerald F, Kleiman J, Douglas Bradley T. Pathophysiological interactions of ventilation, arousals, and blood pressure oscillations during cheyne-stokes respiration in patients with heart failure. Am J Respir Crit Care Med. 2000;162(3 pt 1):808-813.
58. Yumino D, Bradley TD. Central sleep apnea and Cheyne-Stokes respiration. *Proc Am Thorac Soc.* 2008;5(2):226-236.
59. Popovic D, King C, Guerrero M, Levendowski DJ, Henninger D, Westbrook PR. Validation of forehead venous pressure as a measure of respiratory effort for the diagnosis of sleep apnea. *J Clin Monit Comput.* 2009;23(1):1-10.
60. Sleep-related breathing disorders in adults: recommendations for syndrome definition and measurement techniques in clinical research. The report of an American academy of sleep medicine task force. *Sleep* 1999;22(5):667-689.
61. Thomas RJ, Terzano MG, Parrino L, Weiss JW. Obstructive sleep-disordered breathing with a dominant cyclic alternating pattern–a recognizable polysomnographic variant with practical clinical implications. *Sleep.* 2004;27(2):229-234.
62. Javaheri S. Sleep disorders in systolic heart failure: a prospective study of 100 male patients: the final report. *Int J Cardiol.* 2006;106:21-28.

63. Sleep-related breathing disorders in adults: recommendations for syndrome definition and measurement techniques in clinical research. The Report of an American Academy of Sleep Medicine Task Force. *Sleep.* 1999;22:667-689.

64. MacDonald M, Fang J, Fittman SD, et al. The current prevalence of sleep disordered breathing in congestive heart failure patients treated with beta-blockers. *J Clin Sleep Med.* 2008;4: 38-42.

65. Eckert DJ, Malhotra A, Jordan AS. Mechanisms of apnea. *Prog Cardiovasc Dis.* 2009;51(4): 313-323.

66. Hall MJ, Xie A, Rutherford R, Ando S, Floras JS, Bradley TD. Cycle length of periodic breathing in patients with and without heart failure. *Am J Respir Crit Care Med.* 1996;154: 376-381.

67. Guyton AG, Crowell JW, Moore JW. Basic oscillating mechanisms of Cheyne-Stokes breathing. *Am J Physiol.* 1956;187:395-401.

68. Francis DP, Willson K, Davies LC, Coats AJ, Piepoli M. Quantitative general theory for periodic breathing in chronic heart failure and its clinical implications. *Circulation.* 2000;102(18): 2214-2221.

69. Douglas C, Haldane J. The causes of periodic or Cheyne-Stokes breathing. *J Physiol.* 1909;38: 401-419.

70. Cherniack NS, von Euler EC, Homma I, Kao FF. Experimentally induced Cheyne-Stokes breathing. *RespirPhysiol.* 1979;37:185-200.

71. Bradley TD, Phillipson EA. Central sleep apnea. In: Phillipson EA, Bradley TD, eds. *Clinics in Chest Medicine.* Philadelphia: WB Saunders; 1992:493-506.

72. Manisty CH, Willson K, Wensel R, et al. Development of respiratory control instability in heart failure: a novel approach to dissect the pathophysiological mechanisms. *J Physiol.* 2006;577(Pt 1):387-401.

73. Skatrud JB, Dempsey JA. Relative effectiveness of acetazolamide versus medroxyprogesterone acetate in correction of chronic carbon dioxide retention. *Am Rev Respir Dis.* 1983; 127(4):405-412.

74. Modarreszadeh M, Bruce EN, Hamilton H, Hudgel DW. Ventilatory stability to CO_2 disturbances in wakefulness and quiet sleep. *J Appl Physiol.* 1995;79(4):1071-1081.

75. Javaheri S, Corbett WS. Association of low PaCO2 with central sleep apnea and ventricular arrhythmias in ambulatory patients with stable heart failure. *Ann Intern Med.* 1998;128(3):204-207.

76. Hanly PJ, Zuberi-Khokhar NS. Increased mortality associated with Cheyne-Stokes respiration in patients with congestive heart failure. *Am J Respir Crit Care Med.* 1996;153(1):272-276.

77. Brack T, Thüer I, Clarenbach CF, et al. Daytime Cheyne-Stokes respiration in ambulatory patients with severe congestive heart failure is associated with increased mortality. *Chest.* 2007;132(5):1463-1471.

78. Hagenah G, Beil D. Prevalence of Cheyne-Stokes respiration in modern treated congestive heart failure. *Sleep Breath.* 2009;13(2):181-185.

79. Yumino D, Wang H, Floras JS, et al. Bradley TD Prevalence and physiological predictors of sleep apnea in patients with heart failure and systolic dysfunction. *J Card Fail.* 2009;15(4):279-285.

80. Yumino D, Wang H, Floras JS, et al. Relationship between sleep apnoea and mortality in patients with ischaemic heart failure. *Heart.* 2009;95(10):819-824.

81. Mansfield DR, Solin P, Roebuck T, et al. The effect of successful heart transplant treatment of heart failure on central sleep apnea. *Chest.* 2003;124:1675-1681.

82. Vazir A, Hastings PC, Morrell MJ, et al. Resolution of central sleep apnoea following implantation of a left ventricular assist device. *Int J Cardiol.* 2008 Aug 25.

83. Garrigue S, Bordier P, Jais P, et al. Benefit of atrial pacing in sleep apnea syndrome. *N Engl J Med.* 2002;346:404-412.

84. Pépin JL, Defaye P, Garrigue S, Poezevara Y, Lévy P. Overdrive atrial pacing does not improve obstructive sleep apnoea syndrome. *Eur Respir J.* 2005;25(2):343-347.

85. Cleland JG, Daubert JC, Erdmann E, et al.; Cardiac Resynchronization-Heart Failure (CARE-HF) Study Investigators. The effect of cardiac resynchronization on morbidity and mortality in heart failure. *N Engl J Med*. 2005;352(15):1539-1549.
86. Sinha AM, Skobel EC, Breithardt OA, et al. Cardiac resynchronization therapy improves central sleep apnea and Cheyne-Stokes respiration in patients with chronic heart failure. *J Am Coll Cardiol*. 2004;44(1):68-71.
87. Köhnlein T, Welte T. Does beta-blocker treatment influence central sleep apnoea? *Respir Med*. 2007;101(4):850-853.
88. Tamura A, Kawano Y, Naono S, Kotoku M, Kadota J. Relationship between beta-blocker treatment and the severity of central sleep apnea in chronic heart failure. *Chest*. 2007;131(1): 130-135.
89. Tamura A, Kawano Y, Kadota J. Carvedilol reduces the severity of central sleep apnea in chronic heart failure. *Circ J*. 2009;73(2):295-298.
90. Javaheri S, Parker TJ, Wexler L, Liming JD, Lindower P, Roselle GA. Effect of theophylline on sleep-disordered breathing in heart failure. *N Engl J Med*. 1996;335(8):562-567.
91. Javaheri, S. Acetazolamide improves central sleep apnea in heart failure. A double blind prospective trial. *Am J Respir Crit Care Med*. 2006;173:234-237.
92. Szollosi I, Jones M, Morrell MJ, Helfet K, Coats AJ, Simonds AK. Effect of CO2 inhalation on central sleep apnea and arousals from sleep. *Respiration*. 2004;71(5):493-498.
93. Khayat RN, Xie A, Patel AK, Kaminski A, Skatrud JB. Cardiorespiratory effects of added dead space in patients with heart failure and central sleep apnea. *Chest*. 2003;123(5): 1551-1560.
94. Naughton MT, Lorenzi-Filho G. Sleep in heart failure. *Prog Cardiovasc Dis*. 2009;51(4): 339-349.
95. Bradley TD, Logan AG, Kimoff RJ, et al. Continuous positive airway pressure for central sleep apnea and heart failure. *N Engl J Med*. 2005;353:2025-2033.
96. Arzt M, Floras JS, LoganAG, et al. Suppression of central sleep apnea by continuous positive airway pressure and transplant-free survival in heart failure. A post hoc analysis of the Canadian Continuous Positive Airway Pressure for Patients With Central Sleep Apnea and Heart Failure Trial (CANPAP). *Circulation*. 2007;115:3173-3180.
97. Ribeiro JP, Knutzen A, Rocco MB, Hartley LH, Colucci WS. Periodic breathing during exercise in severe heart failure: reversal with milrinone or cardiac transplantation. *Chest*. 1987; 92:555-556.
98. Corrà U, Giordano A, Bosimini E, et al. Oscillatory ventilation during exercise in patients with chronic heart failure: clinical correlates and prognostic implications. *Chest*. 2002;121: 1572-1580.
99. Leite JJ, Mansur AJ, de Freitas HF, et al. Periodic breathing during incremental exercise predicts mortality in patients with chronic heart failure evaluated for cardiac transplantation. *J Am Coll Cardiol*. 2003;41:2175-2181.
100. Olson LJ, Arruda-Olson AM, Somers VK, Scott CG, Johnson BD. Exercise oscillatory ventilation: instability of breathing control associated with advanced heart failure. *Chest*. 2008; 133(2):474-481.
101. Corra U, Pistono M, Mezzani A, et al. Sleep and exertional periodic breathing in chronic heart failure: prognostic importance and interdependence. *Circulation*. 2006;113:44-50.

Stress Echocardiography

10

Eugenio Picano

Heart failure is a progressive, lethal syndrome characterized by accelerating deterioration.[1] Its estimated prevalence in the United States is around 2.0%, with an increased prevalence of 6–10% in patients >65 years old.[2] The prognosis of heart failure is uniformly poor if the underlying problem cannot be rectified; half of all patients carrying a diagnosis of heart failure will die within 4 years, and in patients with severe heart failure more than 50% will die within 1 year.[2] The actual rate of deterioration is highly variable and depends on the nature and causes of the overload, the age of the patient, and many other factors (Fig. 10.1).

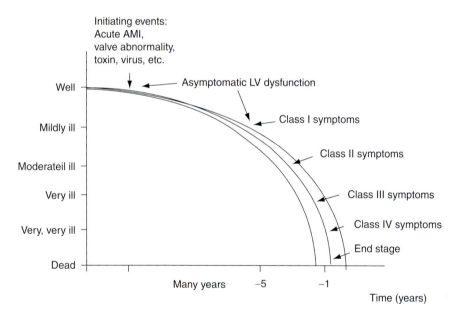

Fig. 10.1 The natural history of cardiomyopathy (modified from Katz[3])

E. Picano
CNR, Institute of Clinical Physiology, Pisa, Italy
e-mail: picano@ifc.cnr.it

M.Y. Henein (ed.), *Heart Failure in Clinical Practice*,
DOI: 10.1007/978-1-84996-153-0_10, © Springer-Verlag London Limited 2010

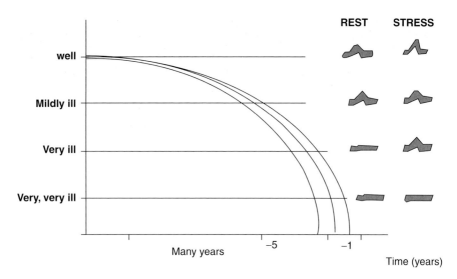

Fig. 10.2 The role of stress echo in prognostic titration of cardiomyopathy. At an early stage, baseline function is normal but inotropic reserve is depressed. At an advanced stage, the baseline function is depressed but there is inotropic reserve. At a very advanced stage, the resting function is depressed and the inotropic response is abolished

Following a period of asymptomatic left ventricular dysfunction that can last more than a decade, survival after the onset of significant symptoms averages about 5 years.[3] Stress echo has a role in the initial and advanced stages (Fig. 10.2). In formulating the 2001 document, also endorsed in the 2005 document, ACC/AHA guidelines developed a new approach to the classification of heart failure, identifying four stages: stage A (at high risk, but without structural heart disease, e.g., hypertension); stage B (structural heart disease but without signs and symptoms of heart failure, e.g., previous myocardial infarction or asymptomatic valvular heart disease); stage C (structural heart disease with current or prior symptoms of heart failure) and stage D (refractory heart failure requiring specialized interventions). According to this staging approach, which is conceptually similar to that achieved by staging in other diseases such as cancer, patients would be expected to either not advance at all or to advance from one stage to the next, unless progression of the disease was slowed or stopped by treatment. The recent realization that therapies aimed at symptomatic heart failure may improve outcomes in patients with asymptomatic left ventricular dysfunction has increased the importance of recognizing and treating patients with the asymptomatic stage A and B condition – possibly even more frequent than overt heart failure. In the early stage, in patients with normal left ventricular function a reduced inotropic reserve can unmask initial damage. In advanced stages, stress echo complements resting echo, identifying a heterogenous prognostic profile that underlies a similar resting echocardiographic pattern (Table 10.1).

Table 10.1 Stress echo response and the four stages of dilated cardiomyopathy

Disease class (ACC/AHA)	Stage of disease	Resting global function (EF)	Longitudinal function	Stress function	Coronary flow reserve
A	Absent	Normal	Normal	Normal	Normal
B	Initial	Normal	Abnormal	Blunted hyperkinesia	$\downarrow \rightarrow$
C	Overt	Abnormal	Very abnormal	Functional recovery	$\downarrow$
D	Advanced	Abnormal	Very abnormal	No functional recovery	$\downarrow\downarrow$

10.1
Incipient or Latent Cardiomyopathy

Some patients are exposed to potentially cardiotoxic conditions, such as chemotherapy in cancer or iron overload in thalassemia. The clinical natural history of these conditions is characterized by a very short interval between the onset of cardiac symptoms and end-stage cardiac failure. The detection of preclinical cardiac involvement can be important in order to start a more aggressive therapy. There are two possible, and not mutually exclusive, approaches for the early detection of incipient myocardial damage when ejection fraction is still normal. The first possibility is to assess longitudinal function, impaired at an earlier stage of disease than Ejection Fraction, which may remain normal due to super-normal compensatory radial function. The selective early impairment of longitudinal global function can be easily measured with M-mode mitral annulus plane systolic excursion or with myocardial velocity imaging, as decreased systolic S wave velocity of basal (septal and/or lateral) segments with tissue Doppler and/or strain rate imaging. The early reduction in longitudinal function, with normal ejection fraction, has been described in several conditions, from systemic sclerosis[4] to diabetic[5] or hypertensive[6] cardiomyopathy.

The second approach is to assess the segmental and global contractile reserve during inotropic challenge. The rationale of applying stress echo in these conditions is that structural impairments of the myocardial wall can be subtle enough so as not to impair resting systolic function, but severe enough to blunt or even exhaust the contractile response to the inotropic stimulation. At low doses (≤ 10 mcg/kg/min), dobutamine selectively stimulates beta-1 myocardial receptors, determining a mild, sustained inotropic stimulation with little if any effect on either systemic hemodynamic parameters or loading conditions. With these low dobutamine doses, the infero-basal wall shows a blunted increase in % systolic thickening, or in peak systolic velocity on myocardial velocity imaging, which helps detect early damage. The blunted regional cardiac contractile reserve, (Fig. 10.2.), has also proved useful in detecting subtle forms of cardiac involvement in several diseases, such as doxorubicin chemotherapy,[7] thalassemia,[8] diabetic,[9] or hypertrophic cardiomyopathy.[10] In

Table 10.2 Prognosis in dilated cardiomyopathy: from bad to worse

	M-mode	2D	Color	CW	Pulsed TDI	Chest
TAPSE	√					
LV end-systolic volume		√				
Mitral insufficiency			√			
PASP increase				√		
E/e′ (restrictive)					√	
ULC						√

all these conditions, the reduction in myocardial contractile reserve – best observed with dobutamine stress – is also accompanied by impaired coronary flow reserve, best detected today by vasodilator stress combined with pulsed Doppler of mid-distal left anterior descending coronary artery.[11] The reduction of coronary flow reserve at a very early clinical stage, when symptoms are absent or minimal and left ventricular ejection fraction is normal at baseline,[12] has been described in several clinical conditions such as systemic sclerosis,[13] and diabetic[14] or hypertensive[15] heart disease. Contractile reserve focuses on the myocytes, whereas coronary flow reserve assessed the coronary microcirculation. Both impaired contractile reserve and decreased coronary flow reserve are therefore very early, and possibly diagnostically relevant, markers of initial cardiomyopathy, at a stage when any form of intervention (lifestyle or drugs) is more likely to be efficacious (Table 10.2).

10.2
Dilated Cardiomyopathy

Dilated cardiomyopathy is a condition that predominantly affects ventricular systolic function. Nevertheless, indices of global systolic dysfunction as measured at rest are inadequate for depicting the severity of the disease and are poorly correlated with symptoms, exercise capacity, and prognosis.[16] In contrast, the assessment of contractile reserve by pharmacological challenge, rather than baseline indices, is an important means of quantifying the degree of cardiac impairment and refining prognostic prediction.[17] In general, all of the twelve available studies on several hundreds of patients have shown a beneficial effect of a preserved inotropic response on prognosis, although disparate methodology, selection criteria (including both idiopathic and ischemic dilated cardiomyopathy) and prognostic endpoint were utilized.[18-30] The contractile reserve can be identified through wall motion index improvement (greater than 0.20) or with a reduction of end-systolic volume during stress. A specific application has been proposed in patients with long-lasting atrial fibrillation and dilated cardiomyopathy. Atrial fibrillation can cause a reversible form of dilated cardiomyopathy, with restoration of normal left ventricular function after cardioversion to sinus rhythm. The distinction between idiopathic dilated cardiomyopathy and tachycardiomyopathy is important because restoration of sinus rhythm leads to a significant improvement in left ventricular function only in the latter case.[19]

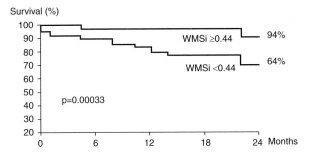

Fig. 10.3 Kaplan–Meier survival curves in patients with dilated cardiomyopathy separated on the basis of preserved (Δ WMSI >0.44) or impaired (Δ WMSI <0.44) left ventricular contractile reserve during dobutamine stress (modified from Pratali et al[24])

The dobutamine infusion protocol is similar to the one followed in patients with ischemic heart disease, but without atropine administration. In patients with dilated cardiomyopathy and heart failure, a lack of increase in left ventricular function is associated with higher mortality (Fig. 10.3). However, limiting minor side effects occur in about 10–20% of these patients, who have a depressed ejection fraction and are more vulnerable to arrhythmic side effect of the drug. In patients with contraindications to or submaximal, nondiagnostic dobutamine stress echo, alternative tests may offer comparable information. Dipyridamole may elicit a prognostically meaningful increase in function, comparable to the one provided with the more arrhythmogenic dobutamine.[31] With dipyridamole, the prognostic information is further expanded by the assessment of coronary flow reserve on the left anterior descending artery (Fig. 10.4) and, when possible, the posterior descending right coronary artery. The prognosis is worse in patients with CFR on LAD <2,[32] and worst when the coronary flow reserve is depressed in both coronaries.[33] The prognostic information derived from stress echo can be added on the top of the versatility of data provided by resting transthoracic echocardiography. A reduced tricuspid annulus plane systolic excursion and increased pulmonary artery systolic pressure may further worsen the prognostic

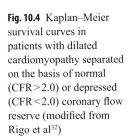

Fig. 10.4 Kaplan–Meier survival curves in patients with dilated cardiomyopathy separated on the basis of normal (CFR > 2.0) or depressed (CFR < 2.0) coronary flow reserve (modified from Rigo et al[32])

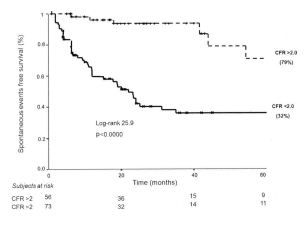

outlook (Table 10.2), dominated by the "deadly quartet": (1) dilated (end-systolic volume >90 mL/m²) left ventricle; (2) severe mitral insufficiency; (3) diastolic restrictive pattern (or E/e′ value >15); (4) increased extravascular lung water detectable as Ultrasound Lung Comets on chest sonography.[34,35]

10.3
Differentiation Between Ischemic and Nonischemic Dilated Cardiomyopathy

The detection of coronary artery disease in a patient with global left ventricular dysfuction and dilatation has important therapeutic and prognostic implications. The diagnosis of ischemic cardiomyopathy may either be straightforward or impossible on a noninvasive basis. At one end of the clinical spectrum, the ischemic etiology is obvious when an unequivocal history of ischemic heart disease and infarction can be collected. As a rule, several episodes of myocardial necrosis have progressively reduced pump function; after repeated infarctions, marked global dysfunction ensues; anginal symptoms are reduced and progressively replaced by dyspnea. At the other end of the clinical spectrum, ischemic cardiomyopathy can be completely superimposable on an idiopathic form with signs and symptoms of congestive heart failure. Dyspnea can be an angina equivalent, and on the other hand angina may be present in idiopathic and absent in ischemic cardiomyopathy. Several noninvasive clues to this differentiation have been proposed (Table 10.3). Ischemic patients more frequently show akinetic segments and a more elliptical shape at resting echocardiography, a smaller and less compromised right ventricle, and larger stress-induced defects during perfusion imaging, with scintigraphy or echocardiography. Encouraging results have also been reported with dobutamine stress echocardiography. Of particular value is the "biphasic" response in at least two segments and/or the extensive "ischemic" response.[36-38] However, all stress-imaging clues concerning the distinction between ischemic and idiopathic cardiomyopathy cannot always be considered clinically significant, although they have been reported to be statistically significant in some studies. Cardiomyopathy is one of the most frequent sources of "false-positive" ischemic response and no wall motion abnormalities can be evoked in an ischemic cardiomyopathy when

Table 10.3 Differential diagnosis of dilated cardiomyopathy

	Ischemic	Nonischemic
History of infarction	Yes/no	No
Resting echo: regional abnormality	Yes/no	No/yes
Stress echo: inducible abnormalities	Yes/no	No/yes
CMR	Subendocardial transmural scar	Patchy, subepicardial fibrosis
MSCT	Severe CAD	Normal

fibrosis is extensive. CMR can be more helpful, identifying a subendocardial-transmural regional pattern in ischemia as opposed to a patchy, diffuse scar pattern in nonischemic dilated cardiomyopathy. Coronary angiography (or its noninvasive counterpart of MSCT) is quite often the only way to firmly establish the differential diagnosis between ischemic and idiopathic cardiomyopathy. In these patients, the role of stress echo is mainly focused on the prognostic stratification dictating the therapy. In ischemic cardiomyopathy, only the presence of significant (≥4 left ventricular segments) contractile reserve warrants a prognostically beneficial revascularization.[39]

10.4
Stress Echo and CRT

Cardiac resynchronization therapy (CRT) is a promising technique in patients with end-stage heart failure. Current selection criteria include New York Heart Association class III or IV heart failure, left ventricular ejection fraction ≤35%, and wide QRS complex (>120 ms). The majority of patients selected according to these criteria respond well to CRT, but 30% (by echocardiographic criteria) do not respond. The most frequently used clinical marker is the improvement of ≥1 grade in NYHA class; the most frequently used echocardiographic marker is an antiremodeling effect defined as a reduction ≥15% in left ventricular end-systolic volume.[40] In the majority of patients there is full agreement between clinical and echocardiographic response, but 25% of patients show discordant results, more often with clinical but not echocardiographic response. The large number of nonresponders for a costly, risky and demanding therapy such as CRT led researchers to look for better selection criteria. In the failing heart, cardiac dyssynchrony is present on three levels: (1) atrio-ventricular; (2) interventricular (right vs. left ventricle); (3) intraventricular (within the left ventricle). Echocardiography can assess intra- and interventricular dyssynchrony. The assessment of interventricular dyssynchrony is simple, standardized, reproducible but basically useless[40]; the assessment of intraventricular dyssynchrony is complex, deregulated with dozens of different methods proposed in the last 10 years, suffers from higher variability[41] and is equally worthless.[42] M-mode echocardiography is the simplest technique, and a short axis view is used to measure the so-called septal-to-posterior wall motion delay, the interval between the systolic excursion of the antero-septum and of the infero-lateral wall.[41] Unfortunately, with this method only two segments (out of 17!) are sampled and the parameter cannot be assessed in 50% of patients, when the septum is akynetic, especially in ischemic cardiomyopathy. Tissue Doppler imaging (TDI) is probably the most popular technique for assessing LV dyssynchrony (Figs. 10.5 and 10.6). It measures peak systolic velocities in different regions of the myocardium and the time-intervals between electrical activity (the QRS complex) and the mechanical activity (segmental peak systolic velocity). The 2-, 4- or 11-segment approach has been used (the apical segments are unreadable with this technique). Tissue synchronization imaging is more visually oriented. It automatically calculates the peak systolic velocities from TDI and displays them as a color map, for direct visualization of the early activated segments (displayed in green) and late activated segments (displayed in red). With strain imaging – and more specifically with strain

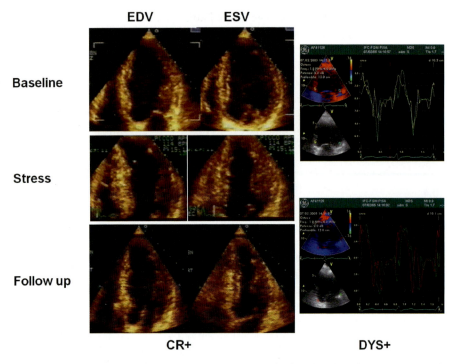

Fig. 10.5 An example of CRT responder. Echocardiographic four-chamber view at rest, at peak stress and at follow-up of a patients with contractile reserve (CR+) (*left*) and tissue Doppler criteria of intraventricular dyssynchrony (Rest DYS+) (*right*) (modified from Ciampi et al[44])

rate imaging measures of the rate of myocardial deformation – the extent of left ventricular dyssynchrony is assessed by measuring time to peak systolic strain. With RT3D echocardiography, a series of plots is obtained representing the change in volume for each segment throughout the cycle. However, in the presence of left ventricular dyssynchrony, minimum volume will be reached for each segment at different times, and the extent of this dispersion reflects the left ventricular dyssynchrony.[40,41] Responders have a higher systolic dyssynchrony than nonresponders (Fig. 10.7).

At present, TDI is probably the most popular technique for assessing LV dyssynchrony,[40,41] but not the most useful, since all proposed parameters tested in the multicenter PROSPECT trial failed, and did not add anything to clinical and ECG stratification.[42]

Recently, disappointment with the mechanical dyssynchrony approach led several investigators to integrate the "electrical" approach with a more functional one. In fact, it is probably unrealistic to expect a response to CRT if there is not enough muscle to be resynchronized. In other words, it is unlikely that home comfort will benefit from a brand-new electric system if there are no walls and no ceiling left. Indeed, this "functional" approach appears to be much more gratifying in selecting candidates for CRT. In patients with depressed ejection fraction, lack of a substantial ($\geq$5 segments) viability response to

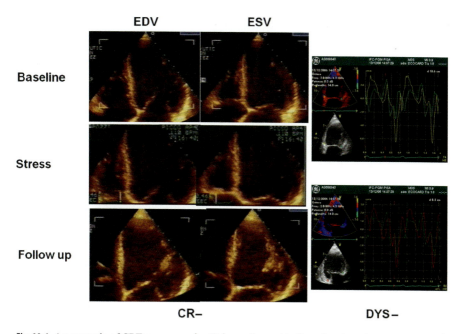

EDV   ESV

Baseline

Stress

Follow up

CR−   DYS−

Fig. 10.6 An example of CRT nonresponder. Echocardiographic four-chamber view at rest, at peak stress and at follow-up of a patient without contractile reserve (CR−) (*left*) without tissue Doppler criteria of intraventricular dyssynchrony (Rest DYS−) (*right*) (modified from Ciampi et al[44])

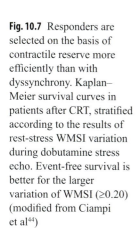

Fig. 10.7 Responders are selected on the basis of contractile reserve more efficiently than with dyssynchrony. Kaplan–Meier survival curves in patients after CRT, stratified according to the results of rest-stress WMSI variation during dobutamine stress echo. Event-free survival is better for the larger variation of WMSI (≥0.20) (modified from Ciampi et al[44])

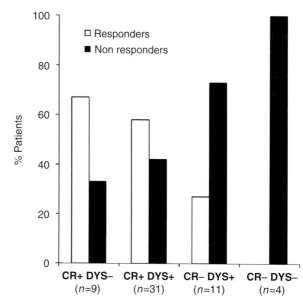

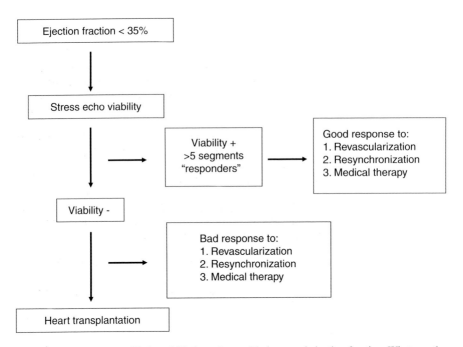

Fig. 10.8 The importance of being viable in patients with depressed ejection fraction. Whatever the underlying disease, response to therapy is dependent upon underlying mortality. The type of therapy obviously depends on the underlying etiology: coronary revascularization in coronary artery disease, aortic valve replacement in low-flow, low-gradient aortic stenosis, cardiac resynchronization therapy in nonischemic cardiomyopathy (modified from Ciampi et al[44])

dobutamine stress echo is invariably associated with a lack of response to CRT (Fig. 10.8).[43,44] This is the same pattern that has been described in ischemia cardiomyopathy patients undergoing revascularization[39] or cardiomyopathy patients on beta-blockers or other medical therapy[45] or low-flow, low-gradient aortic stenosis patients undergoing aortic valve replacement.[46] The beneficial effect of medical, mechanical or electrical therapy in heart failure patients requires the presence of a critical mass of target tissue: "No muscle, no party!"[47] Also, this shift in diagnostic forms from electrical synchronicity to functional reserve dramatically simplifies the screening of the CRT candidate; stress echo is simpler, much faster and more reproducible than CRT criteria. Echocardiographic evaluation of dyssynchrony may add something to the risk stratification, but only in patients with viability. This approach can be made even simpler and more quantitative in CRT, when the single most important stress echo parameter is variation in end-systolic volume, which today can be estimated even more accurately with RT3D. This stress-echo-driven approach to selection of CRT-responders is now mature and ready for large-scale validation.

Acknowledgement   Reproduced from Picano E, Stress echocardiography, Fifth edition, Springer, Berlin, 2009.

References

1. Swedberg K, Cleland J, Dargie H, et al.; Task Force for the Diagnosis and Treatment of Chronic Heart Failure of the European Society of Cardiology. Guidelines for the diagnosis and treatment of chronic heart failure: executive summary (update 2005): The Task Force for the Diagnosis and Treatment of Chronic Heart Failure of the European Society of Cardiology. *Eur Heart J.* 2005;26:1115-40

2. Hunt SA, Abraham WT, Chin MH, et al.; American College of Cardiology; American Heart Association Task Force on Practice Guidelines; American College of Chest Physicians; International Society for Heart and Lung Transplantation; Heart Rhythm Society. ACC/AHA 2005 guideline update for the diagnosis and management of chronic heart failure in the adult: a report of the American College of Cardiology/American Heart Association Task Force on Practice Guidelines (Writing Committee to Update the 2001 Guidelines for the Evaluation and Management of Heart Failure): developed in collaboration with the American College of Chest Physicians and the International Society for Heart and Lung Transplantation: endorsed by the Heart Rhythm Society. *Circulation.* 2005;112:e154-235.

3. Katz AM. *Heart Failure. Pathophysiology, Molecular Biology and Clinical Management.* Philadelphia: Lippincott Williams and Wilkins; 2001.

4. Henein MY, Cailes J, O'Sullivan C, et al. Abnormal ventricular long-axis function in systemic sclerosis. *Chest.* 1995;108:1533-1540.

5. Fang ZY, Najos-Valencia O, Leano R, et al. Patients with early diabetic heart disease demonstrate a normal myocardial response to dobutamine. *J Am Coll Cardiol.* 2003;42:446-453.

6. Kobayashi T, Tamano K, Takahashi M, et al. Myocardial systolic function of the left ventricle along the long axis in patients with essential hypertension: a study by pulsed tissue Doppler imaging. *J Cardiol.* 2003;41:175-182.

7. Klewer SE, Goldberg SJ, Donnerstein RL, et al. Dobutamine stress echocardiography: a sensitive indicator of diminished myocardial function in asymptomatic doxorubicin-treated long-term survivors of childhood cancer. *J Am Coll Cardiol.* 1992;19:394-401.

8. Mariotti E, Agostini A, Angelucci E, et al. Reduced left ventricular contractile reserve identified by low dose dobutamine echocardiography as an early marker of cardiac involvement in asymptomatic patients with thalassemia major. *Echocardiography.* 1996;13:463-472.

9. Ha JW, Lee HC, Kang ES, et al. Abnormal left ventricular longitudinal functional reserve in patients with diabetes mellitus: implication for detecting subclinical myocardial dysfunction using exercise tissue Doppler echocardiography. *Heart.* 2007;93:1571-1576.

10. Kawano S, Ilda K, Fujeda K, et al. Response to isoproterenol as a prognostic indicator of evolution from hypertrophic cardiomyopathy to a phase resembling dilated cardiomyopathy. *J Am Coll Cardiol.* 1995;25:687-692.

11. Picano E. Diabetic cardiomyopathy. The importance of being earliest. *J Am Coll Cardiol.* 2003;42:454-457.

12. Neglia D, Parodi O, Gallopin M, et al. Myocardial blood flow response to pacing tachycardia and to dipyridamole infusion in patients with dilated cardiomyopathy without overt heart failure. A quantitative assessment by positron emission tomography. *Circulation.* 1995;92:796-804.

13. Montisci R, Vacca A, Garau P, et al. Detection of early impairment of coronary flow reserve in patients with systemic sclerosis. *Ann Rheum Dis.* 2003;62:890-893.

14. Galderisi M, Capaldo B, Sidiropulos M, et al. Determinants of reduction of coronary flow reserve in patients with type 2 diabetes mellitus or arterial hypertension without angiographically determined epicardial coronary stenosis. *Am J Hypertens.* 2007;20:1283-1290.

15. Bartel T, Yang Y, Müller S, et al. Noninvasive assessment of microvascular function in arterial hypertension by transthoracic Doppler harmonic echocardiography. *J Am Coll Cardiol.* 2002; 39:2012-2018.

16. Agricola E, Oppizzi M, Pisani M, et al. Stress echocardiography in heart failure. *Cardiovasc Ultrasound*. 2004;2:11.
17. Neskovic AN, Otasevic P. Stress-echocardiography in idiopathic dilated cardiomyopathy: instructions for use. *Cardiovasc Ultrasound*. 2005;3:3.
18. Nagaoka H, Isobe N, Kubota S, et al. Myocardial contractile reserve as prognostic determinant in patients with idiopathic dilated cardiomyopathy without overt heart failure. *Chest*. 1997;111:344-350.
19. Paelinck B, Vermeersch P, Stockman D, et al. Usefulness of low-dose dobutamine stress echocardiography in predicting recovery of poor left ventricular function in atrial fibrillation dilated cardiomyopathy. *Am J Cardiol*. 1999;83:1668-1671.
20. Naqvi TZ, Goel RK, Forrester JS, et al. Myocardial contractile reserve on dobutamine echocardiography predicts late spontaneous improvement in cardiac function in patients with recent onset idiopathic dilated cardiomyopathy. *J Am Coll Cardiol*. 1999;34:1537-1544.
21. Kitaoka H, Takata J, Yabe T, et al. Dobutamine stress echocardiography can predict the improvement of left ventricular systolic function in dilated cardiomyopathy. *Heart*. 1999; 81:523-527.
22. Scrutinio D, Napoli V, Passantino A, et al. Low-dose dobutamine responsiveness in idiopathic dilated cardiomyopathy: relation to exercise capacity and clinical outcome. *Eur Heart J*. 2000;21:927-934.
23. Paraskevaidis IA, Adamopoulos S, Kremastinos DT. Dobutamine echocardiographic study in patients with nonischemic dilated cardiomyopathy and prognostically borderline values of peak exercise oxygen consumption: 18-month follow-up study. *J Am Coll Cardiol*. 2001; 37:1685-1691.
24. Pratali L, Picano E, Otasevic P, et al. Prognostic significance of dobutamine echocardiography test in idiopathic dilated cardiomyopathy. *Am J Cardiol*. 2001;88:1374-1378.
25. Pinamonti B, Perkan A, Di Lenarda A, et al. Dobutamine echocardiography in idiopathic dilated cardiomyopathy: clinical and prognostic implications. *Eur J Heart Fail*. 2002;4: 49-61.
26. Drozdz J, Krzeminska-Pakula M, Plewka M, et al. Prognostic value of low-dose dobutamine echocardiography in patients with idiopathic dilated cardiomyopathy. *Chest*. 2002;121: 1216-1222.
27. Otasevic P, Popovic ZB, Vasiljevic JD, et al. Head-to-head comparison of indices of left ventricular contractile reserve assessed by high-dose dobutamine stress echocardiography in idiopathic dilated cardiomyopathy: five-year follow up. *Heart*. 2006;92:1253-1258.
28. Williams MJ, Odabashian J, Lauer MS, et al. Prognostic value of dobutamine echocardiography in patients with left ventricular dysfunction. *J Am Coll Cardiol*. 1996;27:132-139.
29. Marron A, Schneeweiss A. Prognostic value of noninvasively obtained left ventricular contractile reserve in patients with severe heart failure. *J Am Coll Cardiol*. 1997;29:422-428.
30. Pratali L, Otasevic P, Rigo F, et al. The additive prognostic value of restrictive pattern and dipyridamole-induced contractile reserve in idiopathic dilated cardiomyopathy. *Eur J Heart Fail*. 2005;7:844-851.
31. Pratali L, Otasevic P, Neskovic A, et al. DIP Prognostic value of pharmacologic stress echocardiography in patients with idiopathic dilated cardiomyopathy: a prospective, head-to-head comparison between dipyridamole and dobutamine test. *J Card Fail*. 2007;13:836-842.
32. Rigo F, Gherardi S, Galderisi M, et al. The prognostic impact of coronary flow-reserve assessed by Doppler echocardiography in non-ischaemic dilated cardiomyopathy. *Eur Heart J*. 2006;27:1319-1323.
33. Rigo F, Richieri M, Pasanisi E, et al. Usefulness of coronary flow reserve over regional wall motion when added to dual-imaging dipyridamole echocardiography. *Am J Cardiol*. 2003; 91:269-273.

34. Pinamonti B, Zecchin M, Di Lenarda A, et al. Persistence of restrictive left ventricular filling pattern in dilated cardiomyopathy: an ominous prognostic sign. *J Am Coll Cardiol.* 1997; 29:604-612.

35. Frassi F, Gargani L, Tesorio P, et al. Prognostic value of extravascular lung water assessed with ultrasound lung comets by chest sonography in patients with dyspnea and/or chest pain. *J Card Fail.* 2007;13:830-835.

36. Sharp SM, Sawada SG, Segar DS, et al. Dobutamine stress echocardiography: detection of coronary artery disease in patients with dilated cardiomyopathy. *J Am Coll Cardiol.* 1994; 24:934-939.

37. Vigna C, Russo A, De Rito V, et al. Regional wall motion analysis by dobutamine stress echocardiography to distinguish between ischemic and non-ischemic dilated cardiomyopathy. *Am Heart J.* 1996;131:537-543.

38. Cohen A, Chauvel C, Benhalima B, et al. Is dobutamine stress echocardiography useful for noninvasive differentiation of ischemic from idiopathic dilated cardiomyopathy? *Angiology.* 1997;48:783-793.

39. Allman KC, Shaw LJ, Hachamovitch R, et al. Myocardial viability testing and impact of revascularization on prognosis in patients with coronary artery disease and left ventricular dysfunction: a meta-analysis. *J Am Coll Cardiol.* 2002;39:1151-1158.

40. Galderisi M, Cattaneo F, Mondillo S. Doppler echocardiography and myocardial dyssynchrony: a practical update of old and new ultrasound technologies. *Cardiovasc Ultrasound.* 2007;5:28.

41. Gorcsan J III, Abraham T, Agler DA, et al.; American Society of Echocardiography Dyssynchrony Writing Group. Echocardiography for cardiac resynchronization therapy: recommendations for performance and reporting--a report from the American Society of Echocardiography Dyssynchrony Writing Group endorsed by the Heart Rhythm Society. *J Am Soc Echocardiogr.* 2008;21:191-213.

42. Chung ES, Leon AR, Tavazzi L, et al. Results of the predictors of response to CRT (PROSPECT) trial. *Circulation.* 2008;2008(117):2608-2616.

43. Da Costa A, Thévenin J, Roche F, et al. Prospective validation of stress echocardiography as an identifier of cardiac resynchronization therapy responders. *Heart Rhythm.* 2006;3:406-413.

44. Ciampi Q, Pratali L, Citro R, et al (2009) Identification of responders to CRT by stress echo: no contractile reserve, no party. *Eur J Heart Failure.* 2009;11:489-496.

45. Jourdain P, Funck F, Fulla Y, et al. Myocardial contractile reserve under low doses of dobutamine and improvement of left ventricular ejection fraction with treatment by carvedilol. *Eur J Heart Fail.* 2002;4:269-276.

46. Schwammenthal E, Vered Z, Moshkowitz Y, et al. Dobutamine echocardiography in patients with aortic stenosis and left ventricular dysfunction: predicting outcome as a function of management strategy. *Chest.* 2001;119:1766-1777.

47. Ciampi Q, Villari B. Role of echocardiography in diagnosis and risk stratification in heart failure with left ventricular systolic dysfunction. *Cardiovasc Ultrasound.* 2007;5:34.

Echocardiography in Heart Failure

11

Per Lindqvist, Stellan Mörner, and Michael Y. Henein

It is generally accepted that Doppler echocardiography is the mainstay investigation for the diagnosis and management of patients with heart failure. Its noninvasive nature makes it patient friendly as well as a unique tool for repeat studies during various stages of the disease process. It provides detailed information, with high temporal resolution, on cardiac structure and function, which guide clinicians to the optimum management plan. Even if resting information fails to explain the patient's symptoms, stress echo findings usually provide accurate explanation and guide toward direct management. We hereby discuss the use of echocardiography in heart failure in detail.

11.1
Resting Echocardiography

Global ventricular function: Being the first requested investigation for a heart failure patient, Doppler echocardiography aims at providing information on cardiac structure and function. It is unique in accurately assessing valve anatomy and function. Having excluded significant valve disease as a cause for the patient's symptoms, detailed assessment of ventricular structure and function is undertaken. Ventricular dimensions are measured, and systolic function is evaluated using various techniques as well as atrial size and function. Systolic left ventricular function is usually presented as ejection fraction, normally >50%. The commonest heart failure presentation is that of ischemic heart disease and dilated cardiomyopathy when the left ventricle is enlarged and its systolic function is impaired with an ejection fraction <45%. Left ventricular cavity, in some patients with heart failure, may be normal in size, with well preserved end-diastolic volume but increased end-systolic volume (end-systolic dimension >40 mm). This results in a similar degree of systolic function impairment as that seen in dilated cavity. Most patients with dilated left ventricle exhibit some degree of mitral regurgitation, which is usually described as functional, since the leaflets appear normal and not prolapsing. However, critical study of the mitral valve apparatus in

P. Lindqvist (✉)
Heart Centre, Public Health and Clinical Medicine, Umeå University Hospital, Umeå, Sweden
e-mail: Per.lindqvist@medicin.umu.se

M.Y. Henein (ed.), *Heart Failure in Clinical Practice*,
DOI: 10.1007/978-1-84996-153-0_11, © Springer-Verlag London Limited 2010

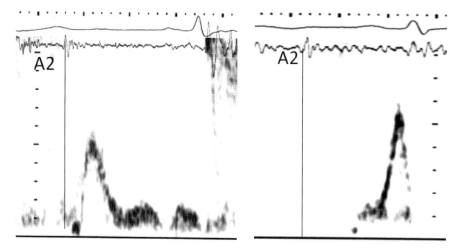

Fig. 11.1 Pulsed wave Doppler of LV filling from two patients with heart failure, one with restrictive filling (*left*) and the other with predominant late diastolic filling (*right*)

these patients may reveal leaflet tethering and annular dilatation as a cause for the imperfect coaptation and valve regurgitation. Untreated patients usually present with dilated left atrium, which has been shown to predict clinical outcome in those with heart failure.[1]

It has been recognized that up to 50% of patients with heart failure have preserved ejection fraction[2] and most of them show evidence of diastolic dysfunction.[3,4] Therefore, Left ventricular diastolic function, assessed by filling pattern, has become an integral part of the overall cardiac performance, and hence is considered of great importance, particularly in heart failure patients. The commonest presentation is the "predominant late diastolic filling pattern" that is consistent with some degree of slow relaxation or ventricular incoordination.[5] A less common picture is the "restrictive filling pattern" (Fig. 11.1), which is characterized by dominant "E" wave with short deceleration time, short isovolumic relaxation time, and a small "A" wave with a respective flow reversal component, of a longer duration, in the pulmonary veins.[6] All patients with restrictive filling pattern have some degree of mitral regurgitation, even if it is mild.[7] Restrictive filling pattern is consistent with a high left atrial pressure, which is known to reflect unstable cardiac physiology and the potential development of atrial arrhythmia.[8] An isovolumic relaxation time of zero is consistent with left atrial pressure of 30 mmHg. Successful treatment of such patients with vasodilators often reverses the filling pattern into the more stable and less serious "incoordination pattern."[9] Once successfully achieved, cardiac function shows clear evidence for improved left ventricular subendocardial function, regression of left atrial size, and reduction or disappearance of mitral regurgitation. The least common filling pattern is that of the "isolated A wave" (Fig. 11.2) in which there is virtually complete suppression of early diastolic LV filling component due to severe cavity asynchrony.[10] Patients with long standing raised left atrial pressure often present with signs of pulmonary hypertension. This is easily reflected on the retrograde pressure drop across the tricuspid valve, with values exceeding 40 mmHg, particularly in patients with insignificant tricuspid regurgitation. If

Fig. 11.2 LV lateral wall and septal long axis M-mode recordings showing severe degree of asynchrony, suppressing early diastolic LV filling (*left*)

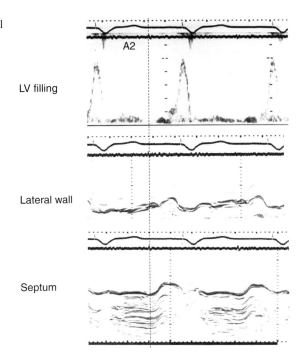

LV filling

Lateral wall

Septum

ignored such patients may develop right ventricular dilatation and worsening severity of pulmonary hypertension. The right ventricle, with its thin walls, might eventually fail to support such degree of afterload and hence dilate further at the level of tricuspid annulus, giving rise to significant tricuspid regurgitation with systolic flow reversal in the SVC, IVC, and hepatic veins. This can easily be confirmed by color Doppler and pulsed wave Doppler recording with proper timing landmarks.

Left ventricular segmental function: Left ventricular segmental function is of great importance in suggesting the possible underlying etiology as well as means of management. In patients with dilated left ventricle, segmental wall motion abnormalities, and/or scarring are often seen, suggesting coronary artery disease as the most probable underlying cause. Even in the absence of epicardial coronary artery disease, wall motion abnormalities may be detected in up to 50% of heart failure cases.[11] In patients with known coronary artery disease and cavity dysfunction, end-diastolic segmental thickness is a useful marker for myocardial viability. A value ≥6 mm is a good sign for viable myocardium that warrants revascularisation.[12] Thickened ventricular walls are commonly seen with increased afterload, for example systemic hypertension or aortic stenosis. In the absence of both, the diagnosis of hypertrophic cardiomyopathy is made, whether symmetrical or asymmetrical.[13] If the hypertrophy is confined to the apex, it may represent the isolated apical form of hypertrophic cardiomyopathy, but if the apex appears extensively trabeculated a diagnosis of myocardial non compaction disease is envisaged.[14] Finally, thickened left ventricular walls that poorly thicken in systole, particularly in the absence of evidence for raised after load are very suggestive of infiltrative myocardial disease the commonest example in the elderly is amyloid left ventricular disease

Fig. 11.3 M-mode recording of LV minor axis from a patient with amyloid heart disease showing thick walls, which fail to thicken in systole

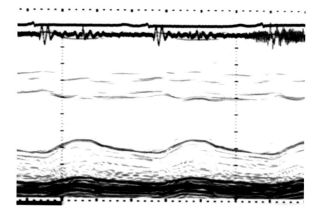

(Fig. 11.3). In those patients, the left ventricle is normal in size, but systolic function is very poor, myocardial echo intensity is raised, and cavity filling is of the restrictive pattern.[15] A similar picture can be seen in the right side of the heart. Amyloid pathology may also invade other cardiac structures, for example, valves and interatrial septum. The very poor thickening fraction itself in amyloid disease has been shown to predict significantly limited survival.[16] Finally, the atria are not usually enlarged in cardiac amyloidosis because of its myocardial infiltration; hence, most patients remain in sinus rhythm, in contrast to other forms of restrictive cardiomyopathy.[17] Idiopathic restrictive cardiomyopathy is the commonest presentation in which the left ventricle is normal in size and systolic function but the left atrium is large in the absence of obvious mitral valve disease. In addition to being much commoner, idiopathic restrictive cardiomyopathy is a benign condition and carries good survival.

Synchronous ventricular function: Mild degree of segmental left ventricular asynchrony normally exists, particularly between its long and short axes.[18] This has been shown to have an important role in maintaining left ventricular pressure development during ejection. Even between the two ventricles, time differences have been shown with the right ventricle completing its tension development before the left ventricle.[19] The commonest cause of pathological asynchrony is coronary artery disease, which usually responds, even partially, to successful revascularization, whether interventional or surgical.[20-22] Another cause of pathological asynchrony is chronic afterload, for example aortic stenosis and peripheral vascular stenosis.[23] This too responds to removal of afterload, although residual disturbances may remain. Irreversible asynchrony may feature in severe left ventricular disease despite full medical therapy. Although this has been shown to be related to intracavitary conduction disease, it may also occur in patients with normal QRS duration.[24] Left ventricular asynchrony manifested in the form of significant time delay between segments >100 ms, which results in inefficient cavity performance and reduced stroke volume.[25] Various echo techniques; M-mode, myocardial tissue velocities, strain and strain rate or speckle tracking can be used to demonstrate segmental asynchrony, with varying sensitivities (Fig. 11.4).[26-29] A simplified way of assessing global cavity asynchrony is by measuring total isovolumic time, which represents the wasted time in the cardiac cycle when the ventricle is neither filling nor ejecting.[26] The longer the isovolumic time, the more asynchronous is the left ventricle and the worse compromised are filling and ejection times.

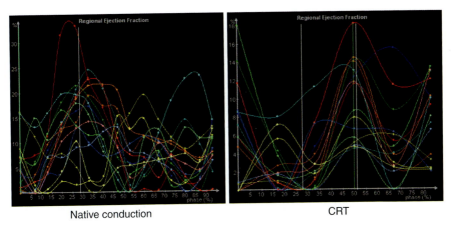

Fig. 11.4 Three-dimensional echocardiographic recordings from a patient with asynchronous LV (*left*) during native conduction, which has become less asynchronous with CRT (*right*)

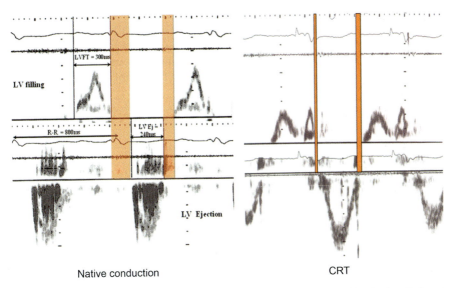

Fig. 11.5 A composite of LV filling and ejection from a patient with heart failure before (*left*) and with (*right*) CRT showing a fall of total isovolumic time from 23 to 11 s/min with treatment as shown by the *orange blocks*

This method has shown great applicability in identifying patients who should benefit from cardiac resynchronization therapy for symptomatic improvement.[30] A total isovolumic time of >15 s/min has been proposed as a cut off value for such treatment (Fig. 11.5). It should be mentioned that patients with restrictive filling pattern, despite full medical therapy, are unlikely to benefit from cardiac resynchronization therapy since their main limiting physiology is pressure rise irrespective of the degree of asynchrony.[31]

11.2
Echocardiography in Resistant Fluid Retention

The commonest cause of fluid retention in heart failure is concomitant right-sided failure with its consequences. In these patients various degrees of right ventricular dysfunction and tricuspid regurgitation are seen, even if the primary cause is left ventricular dysfunction. Conventional treatment with diuretics, vasodilators, and fluid restriction usually settle cardiac function for a while. Patients with systemic congestion who do not respond to such treatment represent a clinical challenge. The differential diagnosis is either left and/or right ventricular restrictive myocardial disease or pericardial constrictive disease. Although the two conditions have similar clinical presentation, their management is completely different. Restrictive myocardial disease is characterized by raised right ventricular end-diastolic pressure, early diastolic "Y" descent on the JVP associated with respective right atrial filling component. These features could easily be demonstrated by Doppler blood velocities of the SVC, IVC, or hepatic veins.[32] Pericardial constriction, in contrast, is characterized by deep "X" descent in the JVP and systolic right atrial filling component. In addition, the ventricles are usually normal in size. While restrictive right ventricular myocardial disease is treated only medically, pericardial constriction may need surgical intervention i.e., pericardiectomy, in order to control symptoms. Rapid increase in cardiac size, mainly ventricles, within a limited pericardial space may present in a similar picture to that of pericardial constriction, which subsides as ventricular size regress with medical treatment.

11.3
Stress Echocardiography

Stress echocardiography is an essential investigation for patients with exertional symptoms, in whom cardiac cause is sought of. The unique advantage of stress Doppler echocardiography, by either physiological or pharmacological means, is its ability to assess cardiac function at the time of symptom development with high reproducibility.

Ischemic cardiomyopathy: In these patients, the clinical question is always related to the presence of viable myocardium that should benefit from revascularization. A segmental biphasic response during dobutamine stress, i.e., increased segmental activity at low dose and reduced activity at high dose, is consistent with the diagnosis of viable myocardium.[33] The same principle applies to long axis measurements, with segments increasing their amplitude and velocities at low dobutamine dosage, which fall with high dosage.

Conduction disease: The second question is evidence for ischemia in patients with conduction disease, for example left bundle branch block. No other noninvasive technique has been shown sensitive enough to answer this question, but echocardiography, because of their well known limitations. Even LV wall motion analysis does not add any clinical value in such patients.[34] Stress ventricular long axis function is unique in this respect, an increase in segmental amplitude associated with a fall in QRS duration rules out coronary artery disease as a possible cause for heart failure. This has significant implications in managing patients with dilated cardiomyopathy of unknown etiology.[35]

Exertional breathlessness: The third common question is the cause of breathlessness in patients with dilated or hypertrophied left ventricle. A stress-induced development of restrictive filling pattern suggests a very stiff left ventricle that causes significant rise in left atrial pressure, which needs aggressive pressure offloading therapy, for example vasodilators.[9] Such patients, if not managed appropriately, carry unsatisfactory prognosis, and hence ICD implantation may be recommended for prognostic reasons. Those who develop global or segmental asynchrony may need revascularization but in the absence of coronary artery disease (Fig. 11.6), cardiac resynchronization therapy should be envisaged as the best management option. When dealing with the ischemic cardiomyopathy scenario, breathlessness might be caused by stress-induced significant mitral regurgitation, probably secondary to ischemic myocardial dysfunction, although this rarely happens.[36] When these patients are planned for surgical revascularization, they should be recommended for additional mitral valve ring insertion. Finally, basal septal hypertrophy, commonly seen in long

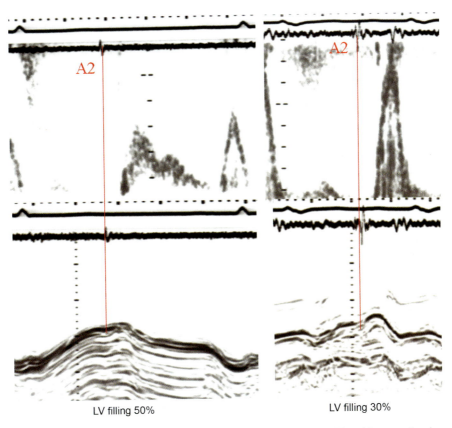

LV filling 50%   LV filling 30%

Fig. 11.6 LV filling and long axis recordings from a patient with exertional breathlessness showing stress-related asynchrony and abbreviation of filling time from 50 to 30% R–R interval

standing elderly hypertensives, could be the cause of exertional breathlessness, in patients presenting with heart failure symptoms and normal left ventricular ejection fraction.[37] In those patients, the increase in heart rate results in left ventricular outflow tract obstruction caused by systolic anterior movement of the mitral valve (SAM) (Fig. 11.7), in a similar

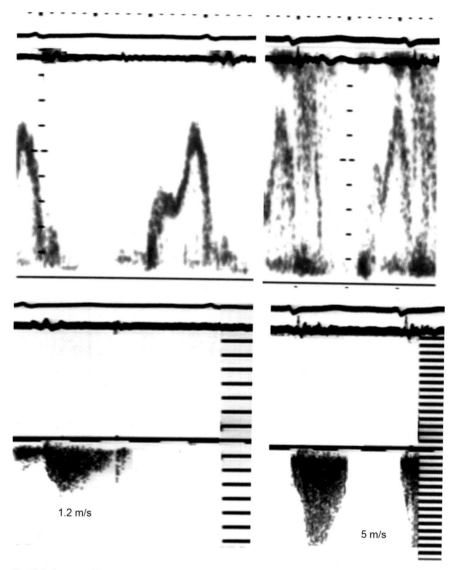

1.2 m/s

5 m/s

Fig. 11.7 A composite of LV filling and outflow tract velocities from a patient with exertional breathlessness, who was found to have basal septal hypertrophy on resting echocardiographic study. The patient developed significant signs of LV outflow tract obstruction, increased velocities from 1.5 to 5 m/s (consistent with pressure drop of 100 mmHg with dobutamine stress). At that stage the blood pressure dropped by 20 mmHg, and there was also a clear evidence for systolic anterior movement of the mitral valve

fashion to that occurring in hypertrophic cardiomyopathy. LV outflow tract obstruction causes acute drop in systolic blood pressure and development of mitral regurgitation. While the former may cause the patient's systemic symptoms, the latter results in acute rise of left atrial pressure and pulmonary venous pressure, and hence breathlessness. This condition is fairly common and needs heart rate control with beta blockers or verapamil.[38] In the absence of obvious cause of breathlessness, patients might have subclinical primary pulmonary hypertension, manifested only with slightly raised pulmonary vascular resistance at rest.[39,40] Stress echo for detailed assessment of pulmonary artery pressure and vascular resistance should be sought in these patients.[41,42] Aggressive treatment of such patients with vasodilators and specific pulmonary hypertension agents (sildenafil or Bosentan) may slow or delay the disease process.[43]

References

1. Rossi A, Cicoira M, Florea VG, et al. Chronic heart failure with preserved left ventricular ejection fraction: diagnostic and prognostic value of left atrial size. *Int J Cardiol.* 2006; 110(3):386-392.
2. Vasan RS, Larson MG, Benjamin EJ, Evans JC, Reiss CK, Levy D. Congestive heart failure in subjects with normal versus reduced left ventricular ejection fraction: prevalence and mortality in a population-based cohort. *J Am Coll Cardiol.* 1999;33(7):1948-1955.
3. Owan TE, Hodge DO, Herges RM, Jacobsen SJ, Roger VL, Redfield MM. Trends in prevalence and outcome of heart failure with preserved ejection fraction. *N Engl J Med.* 2006; 355(3):251-259.
4. Bhatia RS, Tu JV, Lee DS, et al. Outcome of heart failure with preserved ejection fraction in a population-based study. *N Engl J Med.* 2006;355(3):260-269.
5. Zile MR, Brutsaert DL. New concepts in diastolic dysfunction and diastolic heart failure: Part I: diagnosis, prognosis, and measurements of diastolic function. *Circulation.* 2002;105(11): 1387-1393.
6. Nagueh SF, Appleton CP, Gillebert TC, et al. Recommendations for the evaluation of left ventricular diastolic function by echocardiography. *Eur J Echocardiogr.* 2009;10(2):165-193.
7. Beinart R, Boyko V, Schwammenthal E, et al. Long-term prognostic significance of left atrial volume in acute myocardial infarction. *J Am Coll Cardiol.* 2004;44(2):327-334.
8. Tsang TS, Gersh BJ, Appleton CP, et al. Left ventricular diastolic dysfunction as a predictor of the first diagnosed nonvalvular atrial fibrillation in 840 elderly men and women. *J Am Coll Cardiol.* 2002;40(9):1636-1644.
9. Henein MY, Amadi A, O'Sullivan C, Coats A, Gibson DG. ACE inhibitors unmask incoordinate diastolic wall motion in restrictive left ventricular disease. *Heart.* 1996;76(4):326-331.
10. Henein MY, Gibson DG. Suppression of left ventricular early diastolic filling by long axis asynchrony. *Br Heart J.* 1995;73(2):151-157.
11. Medina R, Panidis IP, Morganroth J, Kotler MN, Mintz GS. The value of echocardiographic regional wall motion abnormalities in detecting coronary artery disease in patients with or without a dilated left ventricle. *Am Heart J.* 1985;109(4):799-803.
12. La Canna G, Rahimtoola SH, Visioli O, et al. Sensitivity, specificity, and predictive accuracies of non-invasive tests, singly and in combination, for diagnosis of hibernating myocardium. *Eur Heart J.* 2000;21(16):1358-1367.
13. Elliott P, McKenna WJ. Hypertrophic cardiomyopathy. *Lancet.* 2004;363(9424):1881-1891.

14. Spirito P, Autore C. Apical hypertrophic cardiomyopathy or left ventricular non-compaction? A difficult differential diagnosis. *Eur Heart J.* 2007;28(16):1923-1924.

15. Falk RH. Diagnosis and management of the cardiac amyloidoses. *Circulation.* 2005;112(13): 2047-2060.

16. Cueto-Garcia L, Reeder GS, Kyle RA, et al. Echocardiographic findings in systemic amyloidosis: spectrum of cardiac involvement and relation to survival. *J Am Coll Cardiol.* 1985; 6(4):737-743.

17. Perugini E, Rapezzi C, Reggiani LB, Poole-Wilson P, Branzi A, Henein MY. Comparison of ventricular long-axis function in patients with cardiac amyloidosis versus idiopathic restrictive cardiomyopathy. *Am J Cardiol.* 2005;95(1):146-149.

18. Lindqvist P, Borgstrom E, Gustafsson U, Morner S, Henein MY. Asynchronous normal regional left ventricular function assessed by speckle tracking echocardiography: appearances can be deceptive. *Int J Cardiol.* 2009;134(2):195-200.

19. Dell'Italia LJ. The right ventricle: anatomy, physiology, and clinical importance. *Curr Probl Cardiol.* 1991;16(10):653-720.

20. Henein MY, Priestley K, Davarashvili T, Buller N, Gibson DG. Early changes in left ventricular subendocardial function after successful coronary angioplasty. *Br Heart J.* 1993;69(6):501-506.

21. Duncan A, Francis D, Gibson D, Pepper J, Henein M. Electromechanical left ventricular resynchronisation by coronary artery bypass surgery. *Eur J Cardiothorac Surg.* 2004;26(4):711-719.

22. Bajraktari G, Duncan A, Pepper J, Henein M. Prolonged total isovolumic time predicts cardiac events following coronary artery bypass surgery. *Eur J Echocardiogr.* 2008;9:779-783.

23. Henein MY, Das SK, O'Sullivan C, Kakkar VV, Gillbe CE, Gibson DG. Effect of acute alterations in afterload on left ventricular function in patients with combined coronary artery and peripheral vascular disease. *Heart.* 1996;75(2):151-158.

24. Yu CM, Lin H, Zhang Q, Sanderson JE. High prevalence of left ventricular systolic and diastolic asynchrony in patients with congestive heart failure and normal QRS duration. *Heart.* 2003;89(1):54-60.

25. Penicka M, Bartunek J, De Bruyne B, et al. Improvement of left ventricular function after cardiac resynchronization therapy is predicted by tissue Doppler imaging echocardiography. *Circulation.* 2004;109(8):978-983.

26. Duncan AM, Lim E, Clague J, Gibson DG, Henein MY. Comparison of segmental and global markers of dyssynchrony in predicting clinical response to cardiac resynchronization. *Eur Heart J.* 2006;27(20):2426-2432.

27. Bleeker GB, Mollema SA, Holman ER, et al. Left ventricular resynchronization is mandatory for response to cardiac resynchronization therapy. analysis in patients with echocardiographic evidence of left ventricular dyssynchrony at baseline. *Circulation.* 2007;116:1440-1448.

28. Bertola B, Rondano E, Sulis M, et al. Cardiac dyssynchrony quantitated by time-to-peak or temporal uniformity of strain at longitudinal, circumferential and radial level: implications for resynchronization therapy. *J Am Soc Echocardiogr.* 2009;22:665-671.

29. Nesser HJ, Winter S. Speckle tracking in the evaluation of left ventricular dyssynchrony. *Echocardiography.* 2009;26(3):324-336.

30. Duncan AM, Lim E, Gibson DG, Henein MY. Effect of dobutamine stress on left ventricular filling in ischemic dilated cardiomyopathy: pathophysiology and prognostic implications. *J Am Coll Cardiol.* 2005;46(3):488-496.

31. Salukhe TV, Francis DP, Clague JR, Sutton R, Poole-Wilson P, Henein MY. Chronic heart failure patients with restrictive LV filling pattern have significantly less benefit from cardiac resynchronization therapy than patients with late LV filling pattern. *Int J Cardiol.* 2005;100(1):5-12.

32. Henein MY, Rakhit RD, Sheppard MN, Gibson DG. Restrictive pericarditis. *Heart.* 1999;82(3):389-392.

33. Marwick TH. Measurement of strain and strain rate by echocardiography: ready for prime time? *J Am Coll Cardiol.* 2006;47(7):1313-1327.

34. Duncan AM, Francis DP, Gibson DG, Henein MY. Limitation of exercise tolerance in chronic heart failure: distinct effects of left bundle-branch block and coronary artery disease. *J Am Coll Cardiol*. 2004;43(9):1524-1531.

35. Duncan AM, Francis DP, Gibson DG, Henein MY. Differentiation of ischemic from nonischemic cardiomyopathy during dobutamine stress by left ventricular long-axis function: additional effect of left bundle-branch block. *Circulation*. 2003;108(10):1214-1220.

36. Shiran A, Merdler A, Ismir E, et al. Intraoperative transesophageal echocardiography using a quantitative dynamic loading test for the evaluation of ischemic mitral regurgitation. *J Am Soc Echocardiogr*. 2007;20(6):690-697.

37. Henein MY, O'Sullivan C, Sutton GC, Gibson DG, Coats AJ. Stress-induced left ventricular outflow tract obstruction: a potential cause of dyspnea in the elderly. *J Am Coll Cardiol*. 1997;30(5):1301-1307.

38. Al-Nasser F, Duncan A, Sharma R, et al. Beta-blocker therapy for dynamic left-ventricular outflow tract obstruction. *Int J Cardiol*. 2002;86(2–3):199-205.

39. Grunig E, Weissmann S, Ehlken N, et al. Stress Doppler echocardiography in relatives of patients with idiopathic and familial pulmonary arterial hypertension: results of a multicenter European analysis of pulmonary artery pressure response to exercise and hypoxia. *Circulation*. 2009;119(13):1747-1757.

40. Huez S, Roufosse F, Vachiery JL, et al. Isolated right ventricular dysfunction in systemic sclerosis: latent pulmonary hypertension? *Eur Respir J*. 2007;30(5):928-936.

41. Dabestani A, Mahan G, Gardin JM, et al. Evaluation of pulmonary artery pressure and resistance by pulsed Doppler echocardiography. *Am J Cardiol*. 1987;59(6):662-668.

42. Bossone E, Rubenfire M, Bach DS, Ricciardi M, Armstrong WF. Range of tricuspid regurgitation velocity at rest and during exercise in normal adult men: implications for the diagnosis of pulmonary hypertension. *J Am Coll Cardiol*. 1999;33(6):1662-1666.

43. Galie N, Rubin L, Hoeper M, et al. Treatment of patients with mildly symptomatic pulmonary arterial hypertension with bosentan (EARLY study): a double-blind, randomised controlled trial. *Lancet*. 2008;371(9630):2093-2100.

Cardiac Radionuclide Imaging in the Assessment of Patients with Heart Failure

12

James Stirrup and Constantinos Anagnostopoulos

In patients with heart failure, the identification and treatment of reversible causes of left ventricular (LV) dysfunction are paramount. Establishment of underlying ischemic heart disease as a cause of LV dysfunction is therefore crucial, as its treatment may improve symptoms, ventricular function, and, importantly, long-term outcome. Radionuclide imaging techniques, using either single-photon (SPECT) or positron emitting (PET) radiotracers, are helpful for management decisions in this setting because of their ability to assess accurately not only the level of LV dysfunction but also the ischemic burden and extent and magnitude of myocardial viability. The term "myocardial viability" is often used in a broad and sometimes confusing context as an interchangeable term for myocardium that recovers function after revascularization. In reality, viability relates simply to the presence of living myocardium, without reference to the state of perfusion, metabolism, or function. In this way, infarcted tissue is considered nonviable and any noninfarcted myocardium will be viable. Beyond this simple classification, there exist other states where myocardium may be viable but dysfunctional. These are referred to as "stunning" and "hibernation" (described elsewhere in this book), and it is the identification of these areas that will determine management strategy in a patient with LV dysfunction. Cardiac radionuclide imaging has been used extensively in this setting and contributed significantly to our understanding of the underlying pathophysiology. Each technique makes use of different physiological processes to image myocardial viability (Table 12.1) and can delineate irreversibly scarred from dysfunctional but viable myocardium with varying sensitivity and specificity (see below). Myocardial perfusion, cell membrane integrity, mitochondrial function, and glucose utilization may all be assessed, and their presence or absence relates to the severity of ultrastructural damage at the myocyte level.

Part of the above chapter is based on the review article "Radionuclide Imaging in Ischaemic Heart Failure" published in the British Medical Bulletin.

J. Stirrup (✉)
Department of Nuclear Medicine, Royal Brompton Hospital,
London, UK
e-mail: J.Stirrup@rbht.nhs.uk

Table 12.1 Radionuclide techniques for imaging myocardial viability and hibernation

Technique	Physiological process	Agent	Localisation of agent	Basis of interpretation
ECG-gated SPECT	Perfusion and wall motion assessment	Thallium-201 ^{99m}Tc-MIBI ^{99m}Tc-Tetrofosmin	Flow dependent uptake by cardio-myocytes	Ischemia and/or disproportionate wall motion abnormality
PET	Glucose metabolism	^{18}F-FDG	Uptake by glucose using cardio-myocytes	Mismatched metabolism to perfusion
	Myocardial Perfusion	^{13}NH3/^{15}O-H$_2$O		

12.1
Positron Emission Tomography

PET has been considered for many years to be the "gold-standard" for assessment of myo-cardial viability using metabolic tracers. The high energy photons released from the anni-hilation of positrons confer a spatial resolution superior to SPECT. Furthermore, high count statistics in combination with attenuation correction allow quantitative analysis of regional myocardial blood flow and metabolism. When assessments of myocardial perfu-sion and glucose metabolism are combined, the normal, stunned, hibernating, and infarcted myocardium can be distinguished.

The advantage of PET is the ability to label naturally occurring elements in the body such as carbon, oxygen, and nitrogen (Table 12.2). For assessment of myocardial perfu-sion, oxygen-15 water, nitrogen-13 ammonia, and rubidium-82 chloride can be used. Currently available tracers for the assessment of myocardial metabolism are the glucose analog flourine-18 fluorodeoxyglucose and carbon-11 acetate. Nitrogen-13 ammonia/fluorine-18 fluorodeoxyglucose (NH$_3$/FDG) PET or rubidium-82/FDG are the most common combinations for detection of myocardial hibernation in clinical practice. Dysfunctional myocardial segments with higher FDG uptake compared with that of NH$_3$ or rubidium-82 (mismatch between metabolism and perfusion) represent hibernating myocardium. It should be emphasized that resting flow in hibernating myocardial seg-ments may not be decreased to the extent that would account for the degree of cardiac dysfunction[1] and in most cases, there is impairment of coronary flow reserve,[2] with reduction of resting blood flow seen in only the most advanced cases. Hibernation may therefore represent a spectrum from chronic repetitive stunning,[3] normal, or near normal resting blood flow and impaired flow reserve to truly reduced resting blood flow. Accordingly, hibernating myocardium can be defined as viable but dysfunctional myo-cardium that is susceptible to myocardial ischemia. The sensitivity and specificity of FDG-PET for segmental recovery of hibernating myocardium after revascularization are 89 and 57%, respectively, with positive and negative predictive values of 73 and 90%, respectively.[4]

Table 12.2 Common radiopharmaceuticals for PET imaging

Radionuclide	Physical half life	Radiopharmaceutical	Application
^{82}Rb	76 s	Rubidium chloride	Blood flow, membrane integrity
^{15}O	120 s	Water	Blood flow, perfusable tissue index
^{13}N	10 min	Ammonia	Blood flow
^{18}F	110 min	Deoxyglucose (FDG)	Glucose metabolism

The major disadvantages of PET are its limited availability and cost. For example, although oxygen-15 water has a myocardial extraction fraction of virtually 100% and is hence an excellent tracer of myocardial perfusion, it must be manufactured using an on-site cyclotron because of its very short half-life. Nitrogen-13 NH$_3$ is also difficult to access unless there is an on-site cyclotron. In clinical practice, therefore, rubidium-82 is the most widely used PET radiotracer for assessment of myocardial perfusion as it is generator rather than cyclotron produced. A rubidium generator lasts for 1 month and is relatively expensive (approximately €30,000). To overcome the limitations related to PET perfusion tracers, some centers have adopted a hybrid (SPECT/PET) approach combining FDG-PET with a SPECT perfusion tracer such as thallium-201 or technetium-99m. Although conceptually this is an interesting combination,[5] there are technical issues regarding the comparison of PET and SPECT images.

12.2
Single Photon Emission Computed Tomography Tracers

SPECT is a well-established and widely available technique. Thallium-201 is a tracer of both perfusion and myocardial viability due to the reliance of tracer uptake on both myocardial blood flow and sarcolemmal integrity. It has therefore been used widely for identifying myocardial hibernation. A common threshold for defining clinically significant viability is ≥50% of maximal myocardial uptake, although the best threshold may be higher. As thallium redistribution may be slow or incomplete in regions of reduced perfusion, the usual stress/redistribution protocol can underestimate myocardial viability and additional steps may be required. These include late redistribution imaging at 8–72 h after stress injection, reinjection of tracer at rest after redistribution imaging, and a resting injection on a separate day with both early and delayed imaging.

Technetium-99m sestamibi and tetrofosmin have also been used for the detection of viable and hibernating myocardium. In theory, these tracers may underestimate viability in areas with reduced resting perfusion, because they do not redistribute and therefore cannot allow independent distinction of perfusion and viability. Some studies have therefore found thallium MPS to be a more sensitive test for the assessment of viability.[6] However, the use of sublingual nitrates improves resting perfusion and thus the detection of myocardial viability using technetium tracers. Whichever tracer is used, SPECT assessments generally have higher sensitivity but poorer specificity when compared with dobutamine stress echocardiography for the detection of myocardial viability. The higher sensitivity of SPECT is likely to be due to the reliance of tracer uptake on myocyte membrane integrity, which may be preserved even after loss of myocyte contractile reserve. The use of a ≥50% threshold of maximal myocardial uptake to identify viability may contribute to the poorer specificity. A myocardial segment with 60% of the maximal myocardial uptake will be classified as viable, even though the reduction may be due to partial thickness myocardial damage, which will not recover after revascularization.

The higher energy photons released from technetium-99m tracers results in better image quality, which may in itself improve the detection of viability. However, the greatest advantage is the ability to perform ECG gating and thus assess ventricular function. Since detection of hibernation requires knowledge of viability, perfusion, and function, ECG-gated SPECT can provide information on regional ventricular wall motion and thickening without the need for extra radiation or separate imaging equipment. Comparative studies between magnetic resonance imaging and gated SPECT have shown good correlation for myocardial wall motion and wall thickening where myocardial tracer uptake is present.[7] However, in areas of transmural myocardial infarction, tracer uptake may be reduced or negligible. Although less accurate, global function may still be estimated reasonably because gating software is able to detect endo- and epicardial contours even when counts are as low as 5% of normal. The addition of ECG gating to standard MPS results in improved specificity for the detection of hibernating myocardium without compromising sensitivity.[7] Pooled data analysis from studies using thallium-201 and technetium-99m reveals that the sensitivity and specificity of SPECT MPS for segmental recovery of hibernating myocardium after revascularization are 89 and 68%, respectively, with positive and negative predictive values of 73 and 84%, respectively.[4]

In the absence of hibernation, MPS may still identify inducible ischemia, the treatment of which may lead to symptomatic improvement. Conversely, if myocardial perfusion is normal or near normal in patients with left ventricular dysfunction, the likelihood of significant coronary disease is low. While the negative predictive value of MPS for the exclusion of CAD in patients with heart failure is close to 100%, its positive predictive value is only 40–50%. This is because significant myocardial fibrosis[8] and impaired coronary flow reserve during hyperemic stress[9,10] may all occur in the absence of epicardial coronary obstruction with resultant abnormalities that can mimic significant CAD on MPS. Usually, patients with underlying CAD as a cause for LV dysfunction have more extensive and severe defects, which lie within a typical coronary distribution; those with nonischemic LV dysfunction tend to have smaller, milder defects, which do not correspond to any particular coronary territory.[11] However, even in nonischemic LV dysfunction, larger and more extensive inducible abnormalities are associated with increased mortality.[12]

12.3
Assessment of Cardiac Neuronal Function

Although the myocardium represents the focus of most investigations in heart failure, there is growing evidence that other aspects of cardiac physiology may be of relevance. In particular, assessment of myocardial sympathetic innervation using the noradrenaline analog iodine-123 metaiodobenzylguanidine (MIBG) has become a subject of substantial research interest. As sympathetic nerves supplying the heart are more sensitive to ischemia than myocardium,[13] periods of ischemia insufficient to cause myocardial necrosis may nonetheless lead to sympathetic nerve death in the territory of the compromised coronary artery and thus heterogeneity of global myocardial sympathetic distribution. Myocardium that is viable but sympathetically denervated has a greater propensity for arrythmogenesis.[14] Assessment of regional myocardial sympathetic supply using MIBG may therefore help in the selection of patients for implantable cardiac defibrillators. A more global approach is to assess the total myocardial sympathetic supply through planar MIBG imaging. Total MIBG uptake within the heart may be compared with a reference area, usually the mediastinum, to calculate the heart-mediastinum ratio (HMR). This is a measure of the integrity of the cardiac sympathetic nervous system and a low HMR indicates poor uptake of MIBG and diminished total cardiac sympathetic coverage. Images acquired soon after injection of MIBG may be compared with those acquired several hours later, with the ratio of the respective HMRs representing the washout rate of MIBG and thus the function of the sympathetic nerves of the heart. A high washout rate indicates elevated spillover of NA from presynaptic nerve terminals and thus elevated sympathetic nerve activity. Elevated sympathetic tone in heart failure has been suggested by the measurement of plasma[15] and coronary sinus[16] noradrenaline levels, heart rate variability[17] and muscle sympathetic nerve activity.[18] Low HMR and high washout rates correlate with a poorer prognosis in heart failure.[19] These parameters may be useful in predicting response to cardiac resynchronization therapy and thus allow stratification of patients to either conservative or interventional management strategies. Cardiac sympathetic and parasympathetic receptors may also be assessed by positron-emission labeled tracers. These include the catecholamine analog [11C] hydroxyephedrine and tracers for the measurement of β-adrenoceptor and muscarinic receptors. Like the studies performed with MIBG, PET imaging of myocardial neural function and innervation has been shown to have strong prognostic value in patients with heart failure. Cost and availability remain important limitations hampering the widespread use of these PET tracers in clinical practice.[20]

12.4
Myocardial Fatty Acid Metabolism

Fatty acids serve as the primary source of energy for the myocardium. During periods of ischemia, however, stores are quickly exhausted and myocardial metabolism switches to glucose. This switch may persist for several hours, even after restoration of normal myocardial perfusion. Myocardial metabolism may be imaged through the use of radio-labeled fatty acid analogs, of which the most widely studied is iodine-123 beta-methyl-iodophenylpentadecanoic acid (BMIPP). This tracer is taken up by metabolically active myocardium but not by infarcted tissue or myocytes that have switched to glucose as their primary energy source. BMIPP imaging therefore offers the opportunity to detect myocardial ischemia even after it has resolved, a phenomenon referred to as "ischemic memory." In those with chronic CAD, myocardial segments demonstrating inducible ischemia may have larger resting BMIPP defects compared with resting thallium-201 images, suggesting that the metabolic abnormality may be more severe than would be expected from the defect in perfusion.[21] Uptake within areas of infarcted myocardium is similar for both BMIPP and thallium-201. In patients with chronic CAD and depressed LV function, the presence and extent of discordant BMIPP uptake compared with both thallium-201[22] and technetium-99m-labeled agents[23] is a good predictor of functional recovery after revascularization.

12.5
Other Applications of Radionuclide Imaging in Heart Failure

Assessment of apoptosis is possible through the use of ^{99m}Tc annexin-5.[24] This radiotracer has been used to identify early rejection in heart transplant recipients[25] as well as in patients with progressive worsening of symptoms in the setting of dilated cardiomyopathy and may be useful in the identification of patients with accelerated myocardial cell loss.[24] Other biological targets for molecular imaging in chronic dysfunctional myocardium may be extracellular matrix activation, collagen deposition, or inflammation. Imaging of matrix metalloproteinase (MMP) activity may come to play an important role in defining the process of left ventricular remodeling after myocardial infarction.[26] At the experimental level, an emerging application of PET involves the use of reporter genes and labeled reporter probes for noninvasive imaging of transgene expression. This technique is based on a vector-mediated transfer of genes, which translate into protein products such as enzymes or receptors that may then be targeted by radiotracers. Accumulation of tracer thus indirectly reflects gene expression in target tissue. Several experimental studies have reported proof of this principle for cardiac imaging.[27,28] Stem cell transplantation is another approach that holds potential promise for treatment of ischemic heart disease. In clinical studies, changes in myocardial perfusion, viability, and perfusion are assessed with SPECT and PET imaging thus allowing evaluation of response to treatment.[20] Finally, multimodality imaging in the form of PET/CT or SPECT/CT may be of special value in chronic left ventricular dysfunction by incorporating morphological data that complement the physiological or biological information obtained by PET or SPECT imaging alone. The precise role of multimodality imaging in this setting is currently under investigation.

12.6
Radionuclide Ventriculography

Radionuclide ventriculography (RNV) is widely used in the setting of heart failure setting. Red blood cells are labeled with technetium-99m pertechnate and reinjected into the patient. Once these have equilibrated within the blood pool, the left ventricle is imaged in static planar anterior, left anterior oblique and lateral projections. Counts within the left ventricular blood pool are directly proportional to blood pool volume and, through the use of ECG-gating, left ventricular volumes can be calculated at different phases of the cardiac cycle. Comparison of end-systolic and end-diastolic phases allows calculation of left ventricular ejection fraction. This is a highly accurate and reproducible technique[29] and thus changes in ventricular dimensions and function on RNV may be used to gauge LV remodeling after heart failure therapy. RNV is also able to evaluate left and right ventricular phase, a variable that represents the timing of ventricular contraction. Phase analysis allows quantification of the temporal sequence of systolic ventricular wall motion and is displayed as a color-coded histogram in which the y-axis usually represents the number of pixels and x-axis the phase angle. The latter corresponds to the relative sequence and pattern of ventricular contraction of each pixel within the left ventricular blood pool. The mean phase angle is used to evaluate regional synchrony. The difference between mean phase angles of the right and left ventricles can be used to determine interventricular synchrony. The standard deviation of the phase angle indicates the spread of different phase angles within a ventricle and is thus a marker of intraventricular synchrony. Such assessment can be useful in predicting both response to cardiac resynchronization therapy[30] and likelihood of cardiac death[31] in heart failure patients.

12.7
Conclusion

Cardiac radionuclide imaging has a wide variety of applications in heart failure. As for the investigation of CAD, experience with these techniques can be measured over decades and evidence supports their integration into diagnostic strategies for the investigation of heart failure. PET and SPECT techniques are widely validated for both the diagnosis of obstructive CAD as a cause for LV dysfunction and the identification of hibernating myocardium requiring revascularization on prognostic grounds. For this reason, the use of these techniques is heavily embedded in US and European guidelines for the management of patients with heart failure. Beyond myocardial perfusion, radionuclide techniques can be used to assess left and right ventricular function, myocardial innervation and metabolism, and response to heart failure therapy. Cardiac radionuclide imaging therefore comprises a broad suite of techniques that have high clinical utility in patients with heart failure.

References

1. Camici PG, Wijns W, Borgers M, et al. Pathophysiological mechanisms of chronic reversible left ventricular dysfunction due to coronary artery disease (hibernating myocardium). *Circulation*. 1997;96(9):3205-3214.
2. Pagano D, Fath-Ordoubadi F, Beatt KJ, Townend JN, Bonser RS, Camici PG. Effects of coronary revascularisation on myocardial blood flow and coronary vasodilator reserve in hibernating myocardium. *Heart*. 2001;85(2):208-212.
3. Vanoverschelde JL, Wijns W, Depre C, et al. Mechanisms of chronic regional postischemic dysfunction in humans. New insights from the study of noninfarcted collateral-dependent myocardium. *Circulation*. 1993;87(5):1513-1523.

4. Camici PG, Prasad SK, Rimoldi OE. Stunning, hibernation, and assessment of myocardial viability. *Circulation.* 2008;117(1):103-114.
5. Slart RH, Bax JJ, De Boer J, et al. Comparison of 99mTc-sestamibi/18FDG DISA SPECT with PET for the detection of viability in patients with coronary artery disease and left ventricular dysfunction. *Eur J Nucl Med Mol Imaging.* 2005;32(8):972-979.
6. Gunning MG, Anagnostopoulos C, Knight CJ, et al. Comparison of 201Tl, 99mTc-tetrofosmin, and dobutamine magnetic resonance imaging for identifying hibernating myocardium. *Circulation.* 1998;98(18):1869-1874.
7. Gunning MG, Anagnostopoulos C, Davies G, Forbat SM, Ell PJ, Underwood SR. Gated technetium-99m-tetrofosmin SPECT and cine MRI to assess left ventricular contraction. *J Nucl Med.* 1997;38(3):438-442.
8. Hudson RE. Pathology of cardiomyopathy. *Cardiovasc Clin.* 1972;4(1):3-59.
9. Cannon RO III, Cunnion RE, Parrillo JE, et al. Dynamic limitation of coronary vasodilator reserve in patients with dilated cardiomyopathy and chest pain. *J Am Coll Cardiol.* 1987;10(6):1190-1200.
10. Pasternac A, Noble J, Streulens Y, Elie R, Henschke C, Bourassa MG. Pathophysiology of chest pain in patients with cardiomyopathies and normal coronary arteries. *Circulation.* 1982;65(4):778-789.
11. Danias PG, Ahlberg AW, Clark BA III, et al. Combined assessment of myocardial perfusion and left ventricular function with exercise technetium-99m sestamibi gated single-photon emission computed tomography can differentiate between ischemic and nonischemic dilated cardiomyopathy. *Am J Cardiol.* 1998;82(10):1253-1258.
12. Doi YL, Chikamori T, Tukata J, et al. Prognostic value of thallium-201 perfusion defects in idiopathic dilated cardiomyopathy. *Am J Cardiol.* 1991;67(2):188-193.
13. Zipes DP. Influence of myocardial ischemia and infarction on autonomic innervation of heart. *Circulation.* 1990;82(4):1095-1105.
14. Kammerling JJ, Green FJ, Watanabe AM, et al. Denervation supersensitivity of refractoriness in noninfarcted areas apical to transmural myocardial infarction. *Circulation.* 1987;76(2):383-393.
15. Cohn JN, Levine TB, Olivari MT, et al. Plasma norepinephrine as a guide to prognosis in patients with chronic congestive heart failure. *N Engl J Med.* 1984;311(13):819-823.
16. Matsui T, Tsutamoto T, Kinoshita M. Relationship between cardiac 123I-metaiodobenzylguanidine imaging and the transcardiac gradient of neurohumoral factors in patients with dilated cardiomyopathy. *Jpn Circ J.* 2001;65(12):1041-1046.
17. Ajiki K, Murakawa Y, Yanagisawa-Miwa A, et al. Autonomic nervous system activity in idiopathic dilated cardiomyopathy and in hypertrophic cardiomyopathy. *Am J Cardiol.* 1993;71(15):1316-1320.
18. Ferguson DW, Berg WJ, Sanders JS. Clinical and hemodynamic correlates of sympathetic nerve activity in normal humans and patients with heart failure: evidence from direct microneurographic recordings. *J Am Coll Cardiol.* 1990;16(5):1125-1134.
19. Yamada T, Shimonagata T, Fukunami M, et al. Comparison of the prognostic value of cardiac iodine-123 metaiodobenzylguanidine imaging and heart rate variability in patients with chronic heart failure: a prospective study. *J Am Coll Cardiol.* 2003;41(2):231-238.
20. Knuuti J, Bengel FM. Positron emission tomography and molecular imaging. *Heart.* 2008;94(3):360-367.
21. Taki J, Nakajima K, Matsunari I, Bunko H, Takada S, Tonami N. Impairment of regional fatty acid uptake in relation to wall motion and thallium-201 uptake in ischaemic but viable myocardium: assessment with iodine-123-labelled beta-methyl-branched fatty acid. *Eur J Nucl Med.* 1995;22(12):1385-1392.
22. Taki J, Nakajima K, Matsunari I, et al. Assessment of improvement of myocardial fatty acid uptake and function after revascularization using iodine-123-BMIPP. *J Nucl Med.* 1997;38(10):1503-1510.

23. Hambye AS, Dobbeleir AA, Vervaet AM, Van den Heuvel PA, Franken PR. BMIPP imaging to improve the value of sestamibi scintigraphy for predicting functional outcome in severe chronic ischemic left ventricular dysfunction. *J Nucl Med.* 1999;40(9):1468-1476.

24. Boersma HH, Kietselaer BL, Stolk LM, et al. Past, present, and future of annexin A5: from protein discovery to clinical applications. *J Nucl Med.* 2005;46(12):2035-2050.

25. Narula J, Acio ER, Narula N, et al. Annexin-V imaging for noninvasive detection of cardiac allograft rejection. *Nat Med.* 2001;7(12):1347-1352.

26. Su H, Spinale FG, Dobrucki LW, et al. Noninvasive targeted imaging of matrix metalloproteinase activation in a murine model of postinfarction remodeling. *Circulation.* 2005;112(20): 3157-3167.

27. Bengel FM, Anton M, Avril N, et al. Uptake of radiolabeled 2′-fluoro-2′-deoxy-5-iodo-1-beta-D-arabinofuranosyluracil in cardiac cells after adenoviral transfer of the herpesvirus thymidine kinase gene: the cellular basis for cardiac gene imaging. *Circulation.* 2000;102(9):948-950.

28. Lan X, Yin X, Wang R, Liu Y, Zhang Y. Comparative study of cellular kinetics of reporter probe [(131)I]FIAU in neonatal cardiac myocytes after transfer of HSV1-tk reporter gene with two vectors. *Nucl Med Biol.* 2009;36(2):207-213.

29. Wackers FJ, Berger HJ, Johnstone DE, et al. Multiple gated cardiac blood pool imaging for left ventricular ejection fraction: validation of the technique and assessment of variability. *Am J Cardiol.* 1979;43(6):1159-1166.

30. Somsen GA, Verberne HJ, Burri H, Ratib O, Righetti A. Ventricular mechanical dyssynchrony and resynchronization therapy in heart failure: a new indication for Fourier analysis of gated blood-pool radionuclide ventriculography. *Nucl Med Commun.* 2006;27(2):105-112.

31. Fauchier L, Marie O, Casset-Senon D, Babuty D, Cosnay P, Fauchier JP. Interventricular and intraventricular dyssynchrony in idiopathic dilated cardiomyopathy: a prognostic study with fourier phase analysis of radionuclide angioscintigraphy. *J Am Coll Cardiol.* 2002;40(11): 2022-2030.

Cardiovascular Magnetic Resonance in Heart Failure

13

Bengt Johansson

13.1
Introduction

Cardiovascular magnetic resonance (CMR) is an increasingly used imaging tool in cardiology. Initially, technical resources and access to trained staff were limited to a few centers. As scanners become more available and thanks to widespread training of cardiologists and technicians, CMR can now be performed in most cardiology centers. Without exposing the patient to ionizing radiation, a comprehensive cardiac study can be performed in 30–45 min, depending on clinical problem and scanner capabilities. A typical cardiac exam consists of anatomical images for gross anatomy and cine images for the evaluation of ventricular function. Depending on the clinical problem, a number of additional techniques can be added. Using chelated gadolinium contrast agents, first pass myocardial perfusion can be analyzed during pharmacological stress for the diagnosis of coronary artery disease. After injection of contrast in a peripheral vein, high resolution angiography can be performed. Phase contrast velocity maps (which despite the terminology it does not include contrast agents) can also be used to analyze intrathoracic vascular blood flow and flow velocity.

A central question in the evaluation of a patient with recent diagnosis of heart failure is the underlying cause and whether it is treatable. The most common first line diagnostic modality is conventionally echocardiography. CMR is, however, always an alternative to echocardiography, particularly in patients with technically limited image acquisition. CMR is also complimentary to echocardiography in providing data on myocardial viability (Fig. 13.1), myocardial perfusion, tissue composition and flow variables. A more detailed discussion of the application of CMR in the diagnosis and management of heart failure follows below.

B. Johansson
Heart Centre, Umeå University Hospital, Umeå, Sweden
e-mail: Bengt.johansson@medicin.umu.se

M.Y. Henein (ed.), *Heart Failure in Clinical Practice*,
DOI: 10.1007/978-1-84996-153-0_13, © Springer-Verlag London Limited 2010

Fig. 13.1 Short-axis inversion recovery image showing the left ventricle at the papillary muscle level. There is late gadolinium enhancement in the anteroseptal wall which is seen as bright signal (*arrows*). The central area of the infarct is transmural whereas the lateral part only affects the subendocardium. Viable myocardium appears as black

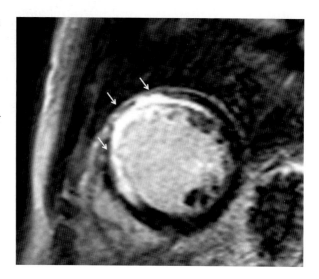

13.2
Ventricular Function

Because of its high accuracy and reproducibility, CMR is currently considered the "gold standard" for evaluation of right and left ventricular volumes, ejection fraction and myocardial mass. CMR has also been carefully validated against other imaging modalities and ex vivo (autopsy) hearts. Compared with echocardiography, studies are much less operator dependent. With adequately trained staff and use of standardized protocols, the inter- and intra-investigator variability is usually very low. Acquisition of data for calculation of ventricular volumes is quick and the analysis is performed within minutes. Normal age, sex and body surface area (BSA) adjusted reference values have been documented, for both the left[1] and right[2] ventricles. An adult's heart is usually covered by approximately ten sequential short-axis cine images along its long-axis. For cine images, the sequence used is steady state free precession (SSFP) which provides high spatial resolution and high myocardium-blood-pool contrast. In clinical practice, the time resolution is approximately 50 ms which is less than echocardiography but better than computerized tomography (CT). The SSFP sequence is ECG-gated and thus sensitive for arrhythmia, similar to many other imaging modalities. Arrhythmia rejection algorithms however, do exist and if there still are problems, real time imaging may be an alternative. As the entire heart is included in the analysis, there is no need for using geometrical models as is the case in 2D-echocardiography. This is of importance when ventricular morphology is altered e.g., after myocardial infarction, in cardiomyopathy and in congenital heart disease. In diastole, a time-volume curve can be obtained and the diastolic transmitral valve flow can be measured. With improved imaging speed and time resolution, CMR may become more important in evaluating diastolic ventricular function. Regional systolic ventricular function can currently be assessed visually but quantitative tools such as strain and velocity encoding has recently been developed for accurate assessment. Cardiac output in the systemic and pulmonary circulation is calculated either from volumetric calculated stroke volumes or from phase velocity map stroke volumes and heart rate. More technical details on the use of CMR in assessment of ventricular function can be obtained from Epstein[3] and Keenan and Pennell.[4]

13.3
Viability and Coronary Arteries

Regional left ventricular wall motion abnormalities can be visually detected by cine CMR as with echocardiography but is usually of limited etiological diagnostic value. After 10–15 min of gadolinium injection, the contrast accumulates in the extracellular space of myocardial scars, thus allowing clear identification of focal areas of fibrosis (late Gadolinium enhancement, LGE) as is the case with myocardial infarcts (Fig. 13.1) and other cardiac pathologies. This information is of particular importance when evaluating patients for revascularization. A myocardial scar which occupies more than 50% of the transmural thickness has low probability to recover its contractile function after revascularization compared to a scar of LGE <25% of the thickness.[5] A viability study can then be combined with a perfusion scan or CMR during dobutamine stress. Furthermore, the coronary arteries can be investigated non-invasively with high resolution and without contrast but valuable results are currently limited to the left main stem disease and for the detection of proximal large branch disease. At present, the main indication for CMR coronary imaging is for the diagnosis of anomalous coronary arteries and coronary artery aneurysms.

13.4
Perfusion

During the first-pass of gadolinium contrast through the myocardium with adenosine stress, areas of hypoperfusion appear darker than the surrounding normally perfused myocardium. This is helpful when the clinical significance of a coronary artery stenosis is in doubt. The CMR study can also reveal coronary artery disease as the underlying cause of ventricular dysfunction prior to angiography. The two main indications for CMR perfusion is presently the evaluation of microvascular obstruction after myocardial infarction and the detection of ischemia in suspected coronary disease.[6]

13.5
Dilated Cardiomyopathy

Dilated cardiomyopathy (DCM) is characterized by uni- or biventricular dilatation, impaired systolic function (Fig. 13.2) and normal coronary lumens on angiography. A LGE scan usually shows viable myocardium without scars. In approximately 30% of such

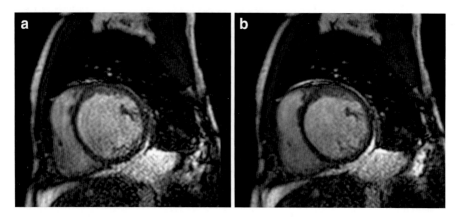

Fig. 13.2 Short axis steady state free presession cine images in diastole (**a**) and systole (**b**). There is marked dilatation of the left ventricle, 350 mL in diastole and 290 mL in systole with ejection fraction 17%

patients, mid-myocardial hyper-enhancement, typically in the interventricular septum, is seen. This localization is in contrast to the characteristic subendocardial hyper-enhancement of ischemic pathology. The latter has been shown to be present in approximately 10% of patients with DCM,[7] hence indicating a potential coronary recanalization or other forms of ischemic etiology. As far as prognosis in DCM is concerned, mid-wall fibrosis carries the worse prognosis in terms of all-cause mortality, sudden death, serious arrhythmia and frequency of hospitalization.[8] Finally, the greater extent of LGE has been shown to carry poor prognosis in ischemic cardiomyopathy.[9]

13.6
Cardiac Resynchronization Therapy

Critical selection of patients for cardiac resynchronization therapy (CRT) is very important. Besides clinical and ECG-criteria, evaluation of mechanical dyssynchrony has been tried by various echocardiographic techniques including tissue Doppler imaging. The latter, in particular, has been shown to have limited reproducibility. In contrast, CMR has high reproducibility and has the ability to evaluate strain and velocity in addition to visualization of myocardial scars. These features make CMR a strong candidate for future patient selection for CRT. Only few published studies on the use of CMR in the field of CRT currently exist. Early results showed that scar burden shown by "late enhancement," scar transmurality and posterolateral scar localization, are all negative predictors for successful CRT.[10-12] Finally, CMR can reliably map cardiac venous anatomy which may help in planning of left ventricular lead positioning.

13.7
Hypertrophic Cardiomyopathy

In hypertrophic cardiomyopathy (HCM), CMR clearly shows the anatomy and calculate ventricular volumes, systolic function and mass (Fig. 13.3). Intracavitary flow jets indicating subvalvular obstruction can be detected in cine images and quantified with phase contrast velocity maps. LGE studies may detect ventricular fibrosis, a finding that may have prognostic value and in the future help in risk-stratifying.[13]

13.8
Valvular Heart Disease

Valvular heart disease is a potentially treatable cause for ventricular dysfunction and heart failure. Echocardiography is usually the first line imaging modality in such patients, but CMR can always provide similar and complimentary information. With phase velocity maps, the regurgitant fraction and absolute regurgitant volume can be calculated in aortic (Fig. 13.4) and pulmonary regurgitation. These volume based measurements can be more reliable than those obtained from echocardiography since they provide a linear rather than categorical description of valvular regurgitation. CMR is the method of choice to assess and quantify pulmonary regurgitation. Aortic stenosis is evaluated using the continuity[14] or simplified continuity equations.[15] By combining phase velocity maps and ventricular volume data, mitral regurgitation can be assessed, (Fig. 13.5)[16] and more so the site of regurgitation can be accurately determined.[17]

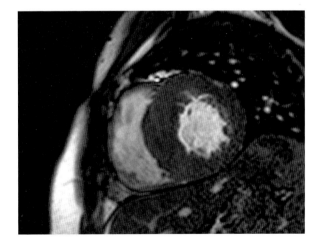

Fig. 13.3 Short axis steady state free presession cine image in diastole showing marked thickening of the interventricular septum in a patient with hypertrophic cardiomyopathy

Fig. 13.4 Oblique steady state free presession cine image of the left ventricular outflow in diastole with a jet of aortic regurgitation (*arrow*). In this study, phase velocity velocity maps showed regurgitant fraction 38%. The left ventricle was dilated to 234 mL in diastole

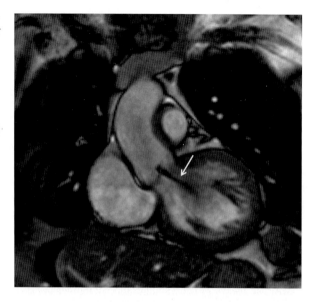

Fig. 13.5 Four chamber steady state free presession cine image in systole showing dilated left ventricle and left atrium and a jet of mitral regurgitation (*arrow*). The left ventricle was dilated in diastole, 350 mL, with preserved ejection fraction which must be interpreted in the context of significant mitral regurgitation. The regurgitant fraction was approximately 50%

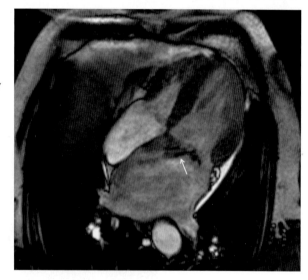

13.9
Sarcoidosis

Sarcoidosis is a systemic granulomatous disease that can affect any organ. Cardiac involvement has been reported in up to 50% of fatal sarcoidosis and sudden cardiac death may be the first symptom. Almost 25% of patients with cardiac sarcoidosis die from progressive heart failure. LGE can detect cardiac involvement with high sensitivity. Lesions are often located subepicardially at the basal left ventricle regions.[18] Localized thinning of the ventricular wall and regional motion abnormalities have also been described. A structured combined assessment with CMR and FDG-PET has proved more sensitive for cardiac sarcoidosis compared with the previously established clinical criteria.[19]

13.10
Amyloidosis

In cardiac amyloidosis, the amyloid material is deposited in the myocardial interstitium and the ventricular walls become thick and stiff, leading to diastolic dysfunction and restrictive physiology. The myocardial mass is often increased (Fig. 13.6). Typical LGE distribution is in the form of global subendocardial enhancement, which corresponds to the histological distribution of amyloid, coupled with abnormal gadolinium myocardial and blood-pool kinetics.[20] The risk of mortality in cardiac amyloidosis has been shown to be related to gadolinium kinetics which in turn reflects the total cardiac amyloid burden.[21] When scanning a patient with known or suspected cardiac amyloidosis it is difficult to set the scanning parameter inversion time (TI) to adequately "null" the signal from the myocardium, which in fact is a clue to accurate diagnosis in previously undiagnosed cases.

13.11
Myocarditis

Mild regional or global left ventricular dysfunction is common, however not diagnostic, in the acute phase of myocarditis. Indications for CMR in suspected myocarditis are relevant symptoms and evidence for ongoing or recent myocardial injury and suspected

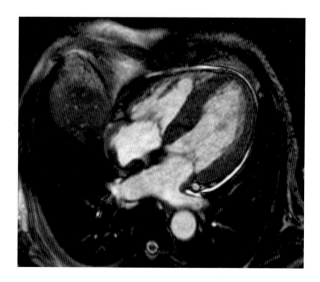

Fig. 13.6 Four chamber steady state free presession cine image in diastole showing left ventricular hypertrophy with increased mass in a patient with systemic amyloidosis. There is also thickening of the atrial septum

Fig. 13.7 Four chamber
inversion recovery
sequence showing late
gadolinium enhancement
in the basal, lateral left
ventricular wall. There are
also small foci in the
interventricular septum and
in the apex. This patient
presented with chest pain,
ECG indicating ischemia,
positive troponin and recent
suspected viral infection.
The coronary arteries were
normal. Note that the lesion
in the basal, lateral wall is
mainly epicardial

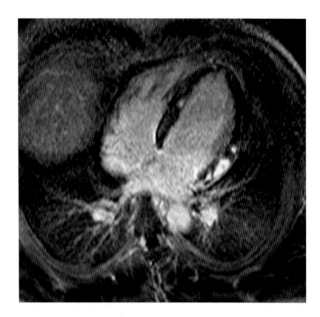

viral aetiology.[22] Suggested CMR criteria for myocarditis are edema visualized by
T2-weighted images, signs of hyperemia and capillary leakage (early gadolinium enhancement) and signs of necrosis and fibrosis shown by LGE.[22] Myocardial involvement in
myocarditis is typically at the epicardial level as opposed to ischemic injury and does not
follow patterns of coronary artery territory distribution (Fig. 13.7). Finally, in a recent
study CMR signs of myocarditis were reported in 30% of patients presenting with chest
pain, elevated troponin and normal coronary arteries.[23]

13.12
Peripatum Cardiomyopathy

Peripartum cardiomyopathy occurs in 1:15,000 of pregnancies in the US and complete
recovery occurs in about 50–60% of patients. A considerable proportion of those patients
may thus remain with various degrees of ventricular dysfunction. CMR data is scarce but
there are two case reports where one patient with no left ventricular LGE recovered while
the other, with left ventricular LGE, persisted with left ventricular dysfunction.[24] Despite
the lack of a definitive role for CMR in peripartum cardiomyopathy, it may in the future be
a potential technique for providing prognostic information.

13.13
Pulmonary Arterial Hypertension

Pulmonary hypertension (PAH) causes right ventricular pressure overload with right ventricular hypertrophy and eventually ventricular dysfunction and death in severe cases. CMR has advantages over echocardiography in assessing the right ventricle due to the ability of imaging complex geometrical structures. Typical findings are right ventricular hypertrophy and flattening of the interventricular septum or bulging towards the left side, in systole. In PAH right ventricular function is related to prognosis. Increased right ventricular volumes and small stroke volumes diagnosed with CMR are predictors of mortality and treatment failure.[25] Furthermore, small left ventricular end diastolic volume was related to a worse prognosis[25] which is explained by the poor transpulmonary flow due to right ventricular-left ventricular interaction with compromised left ventricular filling.[26] In a small study, CMR estimation of pulmonary arterial distensibility reflected the response to pulmonary vasodilators.[27] Proximal pulmonary artery distensibility itself carries prognostic value and stiff vessels are related to worse outcome.[28] Finally, CMR seems to be a promising imaging modality for noninvasive follow-up in PAH.[29]

13.14
Congenital Heart Disease

Despite the significant improvement of survival in the congenital heart disease population, for many reasons, various degrees of ventricular dysfunction are common. Patients may have undergone one or more cardiac operation on cardiopulmonary by-pass, there may be residual lesions, a varying preoperative period with central cyanosis, previous ventricular incisions with scarring and finally conditions specific to the congenital lesion. An example of the latter is congenitally corrected transposition of the great arteries where the systemic ventricle has right ventricular morphology. When planning a CMR scan in a patient with congenital heart disease, it is very helpful to have complete surgical history before planning imaging. Scanning and reporting should ideally be limited to individuals with vast experience and knowledge in congenital heart disease. Patients with complex anomalies should be studied in, or in collaboration with, a center with expertise in congenital heart disease.

In the symptomatic patient, or in routine out-patient follow-up, CMR is an excellent imaging tool with ability to evaluate cardiac structures such as conduits, baffles, tunnels, valves and shunts. Ventricular dysfunction may, as mentioned, be expected in many patients. Individuals with transposition of the great arteries with a previous atrial switch operation (Mustard or Senning operation) have systemic right ventricles which often develope systolic dysfunction over time. In patients with a previous Fontan or total cavo-pulmonary correction (TCPC) procedure, ventricular morphology and function may deviate significantly

Fig. 13.8 Four chamber steady state free presession cine image in diastole showing dilated right ventricle and right atrium. There is a large secundum atrial septal defect (*arrow*) The Qp/Qs was 2:1

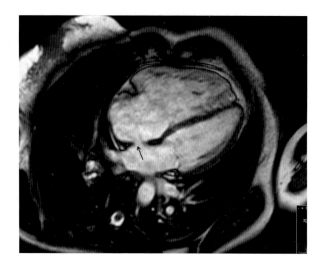

from what is seen in the biventricular heart. CMR is ideal for assessing ventricular volumes in these patients often have unusual ventricular geometry. After repair of tetralogy of Fallot, phase contrast velocity maps are sensitive in quantifying severity of pulmonary regurgitation complimented with cines for right ventricular volumes and systolic function. Echocardiography can identify clinically significant regurgitation but cannot quantify the regurgitant flow.

New diagnosis of congenital heart disease is relatively uncommon in adults. An incidental finding on echocardiography of right ventricular dilatation usually leads to a series of further investigations (Fig. 13.8). Depending on clinical history and other findings, most likely differential diagnoses are left-right shunts at the atrial level or arrythmogenic right ventricular cardiomyopathy (ARVC). Primum or secundum atrial septal defects are usually detected with transthoracic echocardiography whereas sinus venosus defects and anomalous pulmonary venous drainage may be more difficult to visualize by echocardiography. In such situations CMR is usually diagnostic. Phase contrast velocity maps in the pulmonary artery and the aorta quantifies the shunt ratio (Qp/Qs). Furthermore, the right ventricular volumes can be estimated, thus a comprehensive evaluation of shunt anatomy, size and consequences is achieved.

13.15
Contraindications/Limitations of CMR

CMR is still considered contraindicated in patients with pacemakers and implantable defibrillators but in the future CMR-safe devices will hopefully be developed. Other implantable electronic devices such as cochlear implants also limit the use of CMR. However, CMR has been performed safely in patients with pacemakers and implantable defibrillators[30] but this requires individual and qualified risk–benefit analysis and access to electrophysiological expertise during the scan. Among other problems, the pacemaker may be inhibited during the scan which is life threatening in pacemaker dependent patients. In fact, most MRI related deaths are related to pacemakers. Moreover, the rapidly changing magnetic field may trigger anti-tachycardia treatments in implantable defibrillators and such algorithms must be turned off prior to scanning to prevent inappropriate shocks. Retained pacemaker electrodes also contraindicate the use of CMR. Intracranial vascular clips must be checked for being safe before scanning. If there is suspicion of an intraocular metallic foreign body, this has to be excluded with a plain X-ray prior to scanning. All metallic heart valve prostheses, intracoronary stents and other interventional devices such as ASD/PFO occluders and coils are usually safe but may cause image artifacts. If in any doubt, expertise must be consulted before allowing the patient into the scanner. Claustrophobia is sometimes a problem in adults but may be overcome with reassurance and use of mild sedation. Metallic piercing has to be removed. Sometimes patients with heart failure may be unable or uncomfortable to stay in the supine position and all efforts must be undertaken to reduce the scanning time. Likewise, breath-holding (up to 15–20s) may be problematic and sometimes real-time scanning is an alternative. Furthermore, atrial fibrillation is common in heart failure and may pose a problem, but scanning can often be performed, in adequately rate-controlled patients, although at the cost of some blurring of the cine images. In other cases arrhythmia rejection algorithms or real time scanning may be the solution. Finally, gadolinium containing contrast agents used in viability, perfusion and angiographic studies has been associated with nephrogenic systemic sclerosis (NSF) which is a serious complication with high mortality. Fortunately, NSF is very rare and also now largely preventable as it has only been reported in individuals with very poor renal function. Thus, renal function must be known before administration of gadolinium.[31,32]

The author is supported by the Swedish heart and lung foundation.

References

1. Maceira AM, Prasad SK, Khan M, Pennell DJ. Normalized left ventricular systolic and diastolic function by steady state free precession cardiovascular magnetic resonance. *J Cardiovasc Magn Reson.* 2006; 8(3):417-426.
2. Maceira AM, Prasad SK, Khan M, Pennell DJ. Reference right ventricular systolic and diastolic function normalized to age, gender and body surface area from steady-state free precession cardiovascular magnetic resonance. *Eur Heart J.* 2006;27(23):2879-2888.
3. Epstein FH. MRI of left ventricular function. *J Nucl Cardiol.* 2007;14(5):729-744.
4. Keenan NG, Pennell DJ. CMR of ventricular function. *Echocardiography.* 2007;24(2):185-193.
5. Kim RJ, Wu E, Rafael A, et al. The use of contrast-enhanced magnetic resonance imaging to identify reversible myocardial dysfunction. *N Engl J Med.* 2000;343(20):1445-1453.
6. Gerber BL, Raman SV, Nayak K, et al. Myocardial first-pass perfusion cardiovascular magnetic resonance: history, theory, and current state of the art. *J Cardiovasc Magn Reson.* 2008;10(1):18.
7. McCrohon JA, Moon JC, Prasad SK, et al. Differentiation of heart failure related to dilated cardiomyopathy and coronary artery disease using gadolinium-enhanced cardiovascular magnetic resonance. *Circulation.* 2003;108(1):54-59.

8. Assomull RG, Prasad SK, Lyne J, et al. Cardiovascular magnetic resonance, fibrosis, and prognosis in dilated cardiomyopathy. *J Am Coll Cardiol.* 2006;48(10):1977-1985.

9. Kwon DH, Halley CM, Carrigan TP, et al. Extent of left ventricular scar predicts outcomes in ischemic cardiomyopathy patients with significantly reduced systolic function: a delayed hyperenhancement cardiac magnetic resonance study. *JACC Cardiovasc Imaging.* 2009; 2(1):34-44.

10. Bleeker GB, Kaandorp TA, Lamb HJ, et al. Effect of posterolateral scar tissue on clinical and echocardiographic improvement after cardiac resynchronization therapy. *Circulation.* 2006;113(7):969-976.

11. Chalil S, Foley PW, Muyhaldeen SA, et al. Late gadolinium enhancement-cardiovascular magnetic resonance as a predictor of response to cardiac resynchronization therapy in patients with ischaemic cardiomyopathy. *Europace.* 2007;9(11):1031-1037.

12. White JA, Yee R, Yuan X, et al. Delayed enhancement magnetic resonance imaging predicts response to cardiac resynchronization therapy in patients with intraventricular dyssynchrony. *J Am Coll Cardiol.* 2006;48(10):1953-1960.

13. O'Hanlon R, Assomull RG, Prasad SK. Use of cardiovascular magnetic resonance for diagnosis and management in hypertrophic cardiomyopathy. *Curr Cardiol Rep.* 2007;9(1):51-56.

14. Caruthers SD, Lin SJ, Brown P, et al. Practical value of cardiac magnetic resonance imaging for clinical quantification of aortic valve stenosis: comparison with echocardiography. *Circulation.* 2003;108(18):2236-2243.

15. Yap SC, van Geuns RJ, Meijboom FJ, et al. A simplified continuity equation approach to the quantification of stenotic bicuspid aortic valves using velocity-encoded cardiovascular magnetic resonance. *J Cardiovasc Magn Reson.* 2007;9(6):899-906.

16. Hellgren L, Landelius J, Stridsberg M, et al. Severe mitral regurgitation-relations between magnetic resonance imaging, echocardiography and natriuretic peptides. *Scand Cardiovasc J.* 2008;42(1):48-55.

17. Chan KM, Wage R, Symmonds K, et al. Towards comprehensive assessment of mitral regurgitation using cardiovascular magnetic resonance. *J Cardiovasc Magn Reson.* 2008;10(1):61.

18. Ichinose A, Otani H, Oikawa M, et al. MRI of cardiac sarcoidosis: basal and subepicardial localization of myocardial lesions and their effect on left ventricular function. *AJR Am J Roentgenol.* 2008;191(3):862-869.

19. Sharma S. Cardiac imaging in myocardial sarcoidosis and other cardiomyopathies. *Curr Opin Pulm Med.* 2009;15(5):507-512.

20. Maceira AM, Joshi J, Prasad SK, et al. Cardiovascular magnetic resonance in cardiac amyloidosis. *Circulation.* 2005;111(2):186-193.

21. Maceira AM, Prasad SK, Hawkins PN, Roughton M, Pennell DJ. Cardiovascular magnetic resonance and prognosis in cardiac amyloidosis. *J Cardiovasc Magn Reson.* 2008;10(1):54.

22. Friedrich MG, Sechtem U, Schulz-Menger J, et al. Cardiovascular magnetic resonance in myocarditis: A JACC White Paper. *J Am Coll Cardiol.* 2009;53(17):1475-1487.

23. Assomull RG, Lyne JC, Keenan N, et al. The role of cardiovascular magnetic resonance in patients presenting with chest pain, raised troponin, and unobstructed coronary arteries. *Eur Heart J.* 2007;28(10):1242-1249.

24. Marmursztejn J, Vignaux O, Goffinet F, et al. Delayed-enhanced cardiac magnetic resonance imaging features in peripartum cardiomyopathy. *Int J Cardiol.* 2009;137(3):e63-e64.

25. van Wolferen SA, Marcus JT, Boonstra A, et al. Prognostic value of right ventricular mass, volume, and function in idiopathic pulmonary arterial hypertension. *Eur Heart J.* 2007; 28(10):1250-1257.

26. Gan CT, Lankhaar JW, Marcus JT, et al. Impaired left ventricular filling due to right-to-left ventricular interaction in patients with pulmonary arterial hypertension. *Am J Physiol Heart Circ Physiol.* 2006;290(4):H1528-H1533.

27. Jardim C, Rochitte CE, Humbert M, et al. Pulmonary artery distensibility in pulmonary arterial hypertension: an MRI pilot study. *Eur Respir J.* 2007;29(3):476-481.
28. Gan CT, Lankhaar JW, Westerhof N, et al. Noninvasively assessed pulmonary artery stiffness predicts mortality in pulmonary arterial hypertension. *Chest.* 2007;132(6):1906-1912.
29. McLure LE, Peacock AJ. Cardiac magnetic resonance imaging for the assessment of the heart and pulmonary circulation in pulmonary hypertension. *Eur Respir J.* 2009;33(6):1454-1466.
30. Nazarian S, Roguin A, Zviman MM, et al. Clinical utility and safety of a protocol for noncardiac and cardiac magnetic resonance imaging of patients with permanent pacemakers and implantable-cardioverter defibrillators at 1.5 tesla. *Circulation.* 2006;114(12):1277-1284.
31. Canavese C, Mereu MC, Aime S, et al. Gadolinium-associated nephrogenic systemic fibrosis: the need for nephrologists' awareness. *J Nephrol.* 2008;21(3):324-336.
32. Graziani G, Montanelli A, Brambilla S, Balzarini L. Nephrogenic systemic fibrosis an unsolved riddle. *J Nephrol.* 2009;22(2):203-207.

Principles of Treatment and Pharmacotherapy

14

Lip-Bun Tan, Ashish Y. Patwala, and Michael Y. Henein

Within the medical career covering the past 3–4 decades, heart failure (HF) management has been transformed from that of resignation and mainly palliative treatments to options of proactive prophylactic pharmacological, device and interventional treatments. The prognosis and quality of life of HF patients have also significantly improved over the same period, although they are generally still far below that of normal healthy subjects. A most gratifying of triumphs is that of observing occasionally reversals of severe failure towards normality in cardiac function. However, we are far from being able to ensure such a process in every patient, perhaps until cardiac or myocardial replacement therapy can in practice be as standard a procedure as valve or pacemaker replacement therapies.

Departing from the conventional textbook approaches of listing beneficial medical therapies that have already been comprehensively compiled in various compendiums, formularies, pharmacological and medical textbooks, journal reviews and websites, this chapter aims to empower the clinician reader so that more rational treatment regimens can be instituted for greater benefits of HF patients. Memorizing drug names, doses, pharmacological properties and which clinical trials form the basis for evidence of their benefits are basic knowledge which every medical student is trained to acquire and retain, but the wisdom of how the agents interact with individual heterogeneous patients with different sets of pathophysiological processes at play, the timing of which drug to introduce first and which later, how to assess the responses both adverse and beneficial, taking into account compliance issues, of when and how to detect iatrogenic harms and withdraw treatments appropriately, and optimizing the combination of drugs and their doses to maximize actual benefits to individual patients, require more than just memory banks and robotic adherence to guidelines. It is the aim of this chapter to provide an outline of some principles and considerations which will enhance clinical care of unfortunate HF patients, but we would also apologize in advance that due to limitations in space and time, it has been impossible to be exhaustive in this coverage.

L.-B. Tan (✉)
Leeds General Infirmary, Leeds, LS1 3EX, UK
e-mail: lbtan99@hotmail.com

M.Y. Henein (ed.), *Heart Failure in Clinical Practice*,
DOI: 10.1007/978-1-84996-153-0_14, © Springer-Verlag London Limited 2010

14.1
Principles of Modern Heart Failure Treatment

Clinicians and patients have been dealt with a number of conflicting agenda in HF therapy by various authorities, which can be quite confusing and some not necessarily in the best interests of individual patients. Some of these agenda have been imposed under the guise of "evidence-based medicine" with rather selective bias in the choice of admissible evidences. The agenda of medical therapy has sometimes been hijacked from the patients and clinicians to subserve other objectives, such as healthcare economics or "payment by results" policies imposed by various health care organizations. For example, a general practitioner group looking after a disproportionate number of elderly HF patients would have their income deducted for failing to exceed arbitrarily set percentages of patients receiving beta-blockers or ACE inhibitors for HF through a Quality and Outcomes Framework. It is therefore important to revisit the basic principles of clinical HF therapy.

14.1.1
Objectives of Heart Failure Therapy

A number of categories of therapeutic objectives exist in actual practice, and these may include the following:-

1. Improvements in the culprit organ dysfunction and the underlying cause(s) responsible for the dysfunction.
2. Identifiable clinical improvements (e.g., improved symptoms, exercise capacity, prognosis).
3. Improvements in surrogate measures (e.g., ventricular remodeling, ejection fraction, plasma BNP, 6-minute walk tests, aggregate prognostic scores).
4. Improving the income/cost ratios of the institutions and/or clinicians responsible for managing the patients.

Since the root cause of HF lies primarily in the malfunction of the organ, the cardiac pump, in line with science-based Western medical practice, a primary objective must therefore be objective 1, to improve organ function and prevent its future deterioration. If true improvement in organ dysfunction (not surrogate measures) can be achieved, it will then lead to clinical improvements (objective 2) and justifiably lead to objectives 3 and 4. However, when there is no further scope to improve organ function, improving symptoms and patient well-being and postponing demise may be achieved through judicious use of palliative therapies.

A fundamental issue that needs to be established is who has the final say on the objectives of treatment, whether it should be the individual patient, family or carers, clinicians, guideline-publishing committees, institutional managers, medical insurance companies or funding authorities or the government? Since our societal values are founded on the basic moral and legal principle of "best interests of the patient," if compos mentis, the patient must be the final arbiter on this issue, within the constraints of available resources. Based on this premise, the clinical objectives (#2 above) of HF therapy would consist of the following:-

(a) To improve quality of life.
  1. To relieve symptoms.
  2. To improve exercise intolerance.
  3. To reduce hospitalization rates.
(b) To improve quantity of life (longevity).

It is therefore essential to discuss with the patients in detail, at the first opportunity and at subsequent consultations, to ascertain the wishes of each individual HF patient such as whether improving quality of life is of greater importance than prolonging survival or vice versa. Most published Guidelines tend to emphasize treatments which prolong survival more than those that improve symptoms or qualities of life. Once the patients' preferences have been ascertained, then it is possible for the caring clinicians to determine which HF drugs need to be continued or withdrawn. The principles underlying this depend on which drugs are mainly for:-

(a) Prophylactic therapy to improve HF prognosis.
(b) Symptom relief $\pm$ improvement in functional capacity.

14.1.2
Mortality Reduction or Prolonging Longevity

Because of the simplicity and unambiguity in determining life or death of patients, it is much easier to obtain definitive outcome data by quantifying the number of deaths within a period of study follow-up, as opposed to quality of life. Large-scale clinical trials investigating effects of inhibitors of RAAS and beta-blockers are conclusive about mortality benefits, but data about their impact on quality of life, symptom scores and exercise capacity are not as definitive.[1-3] One confounding issue about cardiac treatment objectives in most medical literature is the use of the words "mortality reduction" as a clinical imperative to prioritize those therapies that are backed up by evidence of mortality reduction from large randomized control trials (RCT's) and meta-analyses to be over and above other means of therapy. This issue needs clarification. The words "mortality reduction" is meaningless to patients because they know very well that everyone will eventually die and no doctor can prevent anyone from eventually dying. Moreover, publications which make such claims are also misleading readers because they convey only partial truths, because very few RCT's actually extend follow-ups of trial participants until everyone has died.[4] When all trial participants have died, then mortality reduction will be zero (100−100%=0).[5] The true benefit of a prognostically beneficial therapy is therefore an extension of survival. When the quantity of life is extended, a key question is therefore whether it represents a prolongation of life or a postponement of death. This depends on the quality of life of the patient. If the patients' quality of life is very poor, then the lengthening of survival may amount to a prolongation of suffering, rather than extension of life. From the patients' perspectives, if the quality of life is very poor, longevity may not necessarily be of paramount importance. In patients with advanced age, the primary concern is often not so much about years of life but rather life of years.

14.1.3
Principle of Verifiability of Therapeutic Benefits

The next issue is whether the clinical benefits conferred by the treatment can be perceived by or shown to patients or not. Much of the prognostic benefits demonstrated by RCT's are not verifiable to patients. The institution of any therapy for life extension is basically an act of faith, in that the prescriber believes by giving the same drug as the trial medication, one can expect the same prolongation of life as shown in the trial population. There is no direct way of proving or disproving that a certain prescription would definitely prolong the life of an individual patient undergoing treatment. Surrogate end-points are not reliable. For example, by the time a patient dies, it is impossible for anyone to claim categorically that the individual patient would have died 3 months or 1 year earlier if s/he had not taken that medication. Life-extending prognostic benefits can only be assumed from data collected in clinical trials conducted at a different time, in different places with different patient populations and healthcare systems. Quite often, the patient may not even fulfill the selection criteria for entry into the specific clinical trials. Whether the trial outcomes are translatable to the individual patient is often questionable. In other words, it is often through a large leap of faith that the therapeutic prognostic benefit of drugs shown in RCT's is believed to be applicable to an individual patient. The credibility of the clinician practitioner may become rather stretched if the drug side-effects or adverse reactions of the so-called prognostically beneficial agents are unfortunately troublesome, such as the coughs from ACE inhibitors or lethargy from beta-blockers.

In contrast, therapy to improve the quality of life can be adjusted and revised according to the feedback of symptoms obtained from the individual patient or through objective evaluation of exercise capacity. One may therefore argue that, despite the lack of data for positive survival benefits, prescribing diuretics, digoxin or other agents to improve symptoms and other aspects of quality of life is justifiable provided one pays due attention to the patient's well being. Patients would report back any symptomatic or functional benefits they derive from any new medication they take, although these subjective impressions may not be completely reliable. When in doubt, these subjective impressions can be verified through conducting objective tests or monitoring. For example, their claim of relief of congestive symptoms may be verified by resolution of pulmonary and/or lower limb oedema and reduction in body weight. Their claim of ability to walk more freely can be verified through pedometer monitoring before and after instituting the medication. Similarly, exercise tests can be conducted to verify improvements in exercise capacity or cardiac functional reserve. Claims of reduction in palpitations may be supported by reduction of arrhythmia episodes or severity during ambulatory ECG recordings. Resolution of postural hypotension may be confirmed by cessation of postural falls in blood pressure. By these means, the individual patients become "experimental" subjects in their own right, and their clinical benefits, subjective or objective, do not need to be assumed to be translatable from prior published claims but verified in each specific case. The clinicians and patients can therefore directly evaluate the evidence of clinical benefits. Empiricism is a hallmark of Western medicine, and if the patient can be the experimental subject himself, then it obviates the need to make belief that the benefits from distant trials are transferable to the particular individual patient. Moreover, unlike prognostic treatment, such medication can be adjusted in terms of dosages, frequency and ingestion time of day in order to minimize unwanted reactions and gain maximal benefits for the individuals.

14.1.4
Drugs for Prognostic or Symptomatic Benefits

Based on the overall objectives of treatment being primarily to improve the quality of life (through relieving symptoms, improving exercise intolerance and reducing hospitalization rates), and to improve longevity, although the latter is not necessarily of paramount importance if the quality of life is very poor,[1] we can classify the drugs according to these objectives, as shown in Table 14.1. Understanding the reasons behind instituting such therapies will aid clinicians in decision-making regarding which medication to continue or discontinue in daily practice. (Table 14.1)

Not infrequently, the agents for either treatment objects may produce contradictory outcomes. For example, beta-blockers especially administered acutely may worsen HF symptoms of dyspnoea and fatigue, but long-term may improve cardiac function which in turn

Table 14.1 Therapy for prognostic benefits or symptom relief

	Prophylactic	Symptom relief
Main objective of Rx	To improve prognosis	To improve symptoms and function
Liable to worsen or improve	Symptoms/function	Prognosis
Evidence of benefit established through RCTs showing the population given the test drug derived	Improved prognosis	Improved symptoms and/or function
Benefit	Through a belief that the individual being treated complies with the selection criteria of the RCT's and respond similarly	Can be established empirically on an individual patient basis
Verifiability in clinical practice	Impossible to establish in each patient whether the individual will actually gain prognostic benefit except indirectly (e.g., via improved organ function)	Individual patient can provide feedback whether symptomatically or functionally improved or not, and verifiable through objective tests (e.g., exercise tests)
Dosages	Therapy aimed to use the doses tested during the positive RCT's or highest tolerated doses	Dose adjustments can be made iteratively based on patient feedbacks or serial testing
Indication in late-stage HF	Indicated only to improve symptoms or if withdrawal results in symptomatic deterioration	Indicated to improve symptoms or if withdrawal results in symptomatic deterioration

RCT randomized controlled trials

would ameliorate symptoms. Similarly, diuretics are very effective in relieving congestive symptoms but activate the renin-angiotensin-aldosterone system (RAAS) that would worsen prognosis which can be ameliorated by ACE inhibitor or angiotensin receptor blocker therapy. However, rather than maximizing doses of the latter agents to trial-recommended "target" doses, optimization of dosage may be more conducive to improving exercise capacity as well, especially in patients with rather limited blood pressure reserve.[6]

14.1.5
Principle of Therapy Based on Pathophysiological Defects

A hallmark of Western medical practice is that it is grounded on scientific principles of cause and effect. Medical training has been built on detailed understanding of anatomy, physiology, pathology, biochemistry, pharmacology and applications of these bodies of knowledge into the diagnosis and treatment of diseases. In contrast, alternative medical practices based diagnosis and treatment, are based on no scientific grounds, and at times may even be contrary to science. However, an interesting modern development is the emergence of statistical medicine based on mega-trials which rank treatments according to significance tests rather than scientific mechanistic meanings. Quite often it has also been mooted that understanding why and how these drugs work is no longer important because the statistical significance of the benefits is so over-whelming and the means of prescribing the drugs have been established by how the RCT's were conducted. Such a philosophy is against the foundation of science-based Western medicine and is a hazardous trend. A more reliable approach is to take each RCT finding as an experimental data to establishing or falsify the validity of hypotheses which cumulatively will expand the total body of scientific knowledge which forms the bases of scientific medical practice. Known pharmacological therapies in modern practice are therefore presented with the background understanding of pathophysiological processes operative in HF. The strategy of medical therapy would therefore be to improve or preserve pump function, alleviate symptoms, prolong life and avoid iatrogenic complications.

14.1.5.1
Primary Defects

The initiating event causing the onset of HF is usually a damage or malfunction affecting component part(s) of the cardiac structure which results in the impairment of the entire cardiac pump function. The damage may affect the valve(s), the myocardium (through infarction, myocarditis), the intrinsic pacemaker and/or conducting tissues and the pericardium. Such malfunction constitutes the **primary defects** causing HF. The importance in considering this in clinical management is that once the presence of HF is established, a rational approach to management is critically dependent on the pathology. This is particularly so when the cause is remediable, through surgery or other interventions, such as coronary bypass surgery or angioplasty,[7] permanent pacemaker insertion, cardioverter/defibrillator implantation, valve repair or replacement, closure of septal defects, pericardiocentesis, pericardiectomy, or pharmacotherapy using antiarrhythmic, anti-ischemic or cardioprotective agents.

Not all primary defects are amenable to corrective intervention. HF secondary to myocardial infarction(s) is the most common cause in the West. Idiopathic dilated cardiomyopathy, which accounts for a smaller proportion of systolic dysfunction, is diagnosed once specific forms of heart muscle disease have been excluded. Diastolic ventricular dysfunction is often linked to left ventricular hypertrophy, most commonly as a result of chronic hypertension, but also secondary to rarer forms of infiltrative myocardial disease. Systolic and diastolic dysfunction frequently coexists, particularly with underlying ischemic heart disease. Patients with various systemic diseases, such as amyloidosis, sarcoidosis, haemochromatosis, beri-beri, thyroid disease, diabetes mellitus, also present with HF, and treatment objectives in these cases should be aimed at dealing with the underlying disease processes to prevent further damage and preserve cardiac pump function. Increasingly, clinicians are aware of the possibility of patients with silent myocardial ischemia[8] or hibernating myocardium[9,10] presenting with dyspnoea on exertion and diagnosed as having HF. Instead of commencing on standard therapy for HF such as diuretics and RAAS inhibitors, a more beneficial treatment option is the relief of myocardial ischemia and coronary revascularization.

14.1.5.2
Secondary Defects

The persistence of HF secondary to primary defects triggers compensatory mechanisms and neurohumoral activation that leads to secondary defects. More severe HF would trigger greater extents of neurohumoral activation. The sympathetic and RAAS are the key ones activated, although others, including vasopressin, endothelins, natriuretic peptides, are also released.[11] Initially these compensatory mechanisms tend to maintain cardiac output (through fluid retention and the Starling's effect) and systemic arterial pressure (through vasoconstriction), but they increase the preload and afterload of the failing heart. However, these agents also trigger detrimental effects, and the more important ones are arrhythmia and on-going myocardial apoptosis,[12] necrosis[13,14] and fibrosis.[15] The ability to suppress these detrimental effects is a major reason why ACE inhibitors, ARB's, aldosterone blockers and beta-blockers have been shown to be prognostically beneficial in trials on HF patients.

The congestion secondary to fluid retention would respond to diuretic therapy which is still the first line HF therapy despite absence of RCT data to confirm prognostic benefits. Loop diuretics have been shown in HF patients to improve their exercise ability by greater than 90%,[16] while none of the other therapeutic can achieve similar benefits.[17,18] The European Working Group Guidelines even went to the extent of using a trial of loop diuretic therapy as a guide to the diagnosis of HF.[19] Indeed, in all the clinical trials of HF therapy that showed survival benefits, the background therapy invariably included diuretics.[20-23]

Arterial vasoconstriction as a compensatory mechanism imposes higher afterload on the heart rendering it to pump less efficiently.[24] It can be treated by arterial vasodilators, but these agents have diverse effects. Alpha-adrenergic blockers, for instance, neither improve exercise tolerance[25] nor prognosis.[26] ACE inhibitors in general do not improve exercise tolerance[17] unless used at optimal doses,[27] but can improve prognosis most markedly in more severe failure.[18-20] Renal and splanchnic hypoperfusion may be helped by preferential vasodilation with dopaminergic (DA_1) agonism with low-dose dopamine or dopexamine to enhance renal function.[28,29] Venodilators such as nitrates are also effective in relieving excessive cardiac preload.[30] Great skill is required of the clinician to modulate the compensatory mechanisms without incurring undesirable detrimental effects.

When correction of the primary defects is considered impossible, or ruled out as being inappropriate, or delayed/awaited, then treatment of the secondary defects in order to relieve symptoms becomes a priority. Also, preventative/prophylactic therapies to slow the rates of progression of HF and avert sudden death would also benefit the patients, while avoiding iatrogenic complications if at all possible. Other secondary defects of HF would also require attention, such as ventricular overload which can be relieved by careful fluid balance management and venodilator therapy, hypoxia especially when pulmonary edema is severe by oxygen therapy or noninvasive or invasive ventilation, gut edema leading to malabsorption of nutrition and medication requiring parenteral administration of vital drugs, and cachexia which may be abated through nutritional supplementation.

14.1.5.3
Tertiary Defects

While therapy directed at counteracting secondary defects are crucial, these therapeutic endeavors are often not without complications which produce tertiary defects in HF, requiring significant clinical vigilance to avoid and skills to remedy. The impacts of these tertiary defects may even be more detrimental than the primary and secondary defects in HF, and if ignored might even dictate the patients' clinical outcomes. Listed in Table 14.2 are some common and serious complications of pharmacological agents regularly used in the treatment of HF.

While very effective in relieving congestion, powerful loop diuretics, especially in combination with metolazone or other thiazides, can produce detrimental electrolyte imbalances, such as hyponatraemia, hypokalemia and hypomagnesaemia – all of which are arrhythmogenic, excessive dehydration leading to hypovolemia and renal dysfunction, especially in combination with ACE inhibitors and further activation of the RAAS with its attendant hazards. Preservation of renal function in HF patients is extremely important, because without adequately functioning kidneys, medical therapy becomes almost impossible, as hemodialysis or hemofiltration are invasive and not well tolerated by such patients.

Hypokalaemia is a well known adverse reaction of diuretic therapy. Potassium supplementation is frequently prescribed, but this would not correct the concomitant diuretic-induced hypomagnesaemia which is also arrhythmogenic.[31] Moreover, measurement of serum magnesium levels does not reflect the more important intracellular hypomagnesaemia which is much more difficult to measure.[32] If serious arrhythmia arises as a consequence of such electrolyte imbalance, judicious replacement therapy is required. To prevent either, combination therapy with a potassium-sparing diuretics which are also magnesium sparing (such as spironolactone, eplerenone, amiloride) is indicated. In the presence of renal dysfunction, close monitoring of electrolytes and adjustments of dosages is essential.

There has been a common misconception that when an ACE inhibitor or ARB is added to loop diuretic therapy, then concurrent potassium-sparing diuretic therapy has to be stopped. However, ACE inhibitors and ARB's are relatively weakly potassium or magnesium sparing, and unlikely to be sufficient to counterbalance the potassium and magnesium

Table 14.2 Major complications of drug therapy in chronic heart failure

Drugs	Complications
ACEI	*Commonest*: coughs, hypotension *Serious*: worsening renal function, autonephrectomy in renal artery stenosis
Amiodarone	*Commonest*: skin sensitivity to sunlight, nausea, thyroid dysfunction *Serious*: thyrotoxic storm, rare proarrhythmia, pulmonary/hepatic fibrosis
Antiarrhythmics	*Commonest*: nausea *Serious*: negative inotropism (all, esp. disopyramide, verapamil, BB), proarrhythmia
ARB	*Commonest*: hypotension *Serious*: worsening renal function, autonephrectomy in renal artery stenosis
βB	*Commonest*: tiredness, bradycardia, coldness *Serious*: asthmatic attack, exacerbation of heart failure, heart block
Digoxin	*Commonest*: nausea *Serious*: life threatening arrhythmias, heart block
Diuretics	*Commonest*: postural hypotension, gout, urinary urgency *Serious*: Electrolyte imbalance (hypokalaemia, hypomagnesaemia, hyponatraemia); Arrhythmia
Dopamine	*Commonest*: nausea, palpitations *Serious*: arrhythmia, cardiotoxicity
Inotropes	*Commonest*: nausea, palpitations *Serious*: arrhythmia, vasoconstriction at high dose
Vasodilators	*Commonest*: headache, flushing, hypotension, edema *Serious*: heart block (verapamil, diltiazem)

losses by the more powerful loop diuretics, unless in renal dysfunction. It is therefore more sensible to continue the potassium sparing diuretics and adjust the dose to maintain the serum potassium at around 4.5 mmol/L by monitoring and empirical dose adjustments. The RALES II Study confirms that using spironolactone in addition to ACE inhibition confers a significant survival benefit of 27%.[33] Spironolactone, however, can cause gynecomastia and breast pain in men, in which case eplerenone or amiloride may be used instead.

While careful intravenous infusions can correct serious hypokalaemia and hypomagne-saemia, such infusion for hyponatraemia is trickier in HF. They often occur when the patients are still quite congested. Continuing high doses of diuretics usually exacerbates the hypona-traemia, and withholding diuretics or replacement of sodium worsens the congestion. Stringent fluid restriction may be necessary but is poorly tolerated. Treatment with a specific vasopressin (V_2) antagonist is required and will hopefully be widely available soon. Once serious hyponatraemia is present, dialysis or haemofiltration may be necessary to break the vicious cycle. If at all possible it is vital to avoid the onset of hyponatraemia by judicious use of diuretic therapy, avoid excessive fluid intake and by monitoring electrolytes assiduously.

Excessive diuresis leading to dehydration may reduce the preload too much; exacerbate systemic vasoconstriction and hypoperfusion of vital organs. One manifestation is raised serum urea and creatinine, which may if protracted progress to renal failure. Prompt treatment is required by stopping or reducing diuretics, and fluid replacement if necessary. In some patients, it may be in their interests to be more expedient to allow presence of minor edema to avoid over-diuresis and to preserve renal function.

Although the beneficial effects of ACE inhibitors and ARB's on prognosis are well known,[34] their impact on renal function and quality of life often feature less prominently.[3] In unilateral renal artery stenosis, ACE inhibitor and AT_1 blockade can cause chemical autonephrectomy which may be clinically undetectable by mere monitoring of serum urea and creatinine if the contralateral kidney is functioning satisfactorily and is able to compensate. In significant number of patients there are bilateral renal stenoses, these agents will cause renal failure which will render medical therapy of HF impracticable. In cases of suspected renal artery stenosis, prior investigation is required before initiating ACE inhibition or A II blockade to prevent such harm from occurring.

Since 1966, β-adrenoceptor inhibitors have been considered to be contraindicated in HF because of their negative inotropic and chronotropic effects.[35] Over the past decades, beta-blockers have now been established as a standard therapy for HF because on balance their cardioprotective properties prove to be evidently beneficial. Very slow introduction and careful upwards titration of dosages is essential. Readjustment of other concomitant medication may be necessary. However, it is important to be reminded that the potential of beta-blockers to exacerbate HF has not disappeared, and clinicians need to stay vigilant about patients, especially those with least cardiac contractile reserve, who might succumb to the detrimental effects of beta-blockers.

14.1.6
Acute vs. Chronic Heart Failure

Pathophysiologically, there is one crucial difference between acute and chronic HF that is relevant to management but often overlooked. In acute failure or cardiogenic shock, the circulation is inadequate to meet the requirements of metabolizing tissues at rest even when the compensatory mechanisms are fully activated and all cardiac reserves exhausted.[36] Therapy is therefore directed at elevating cardiac pumping performance to enhance the circulation in order to prevent hypoperfusion and maintain basal body metabolism. In contrast, in chronic HF ambulatory patients have adequate circulation at rest and become symptomatic during exertion when their cardiac reserve becomes exhausted. This important difference explains why certain treatment that proves effective in acute failure may not be beneficial in chronic failure, and vice versa. For instance, positive inotropic agents useful in acute failure and cardiogenic shock have not been shown to be beneficial in chronic failure.[37-42] Conversely, while ACE inhibition, angiotensin receptor blockade and beta blockade are beneficial in chronic HF, they are not helpful in cardiogenic shock or acute decompensation. It is therefore vitally important to apply specific therapy to appropriate subcategories of HF. Guidelines on overall management of acute HF have been published.[43] A summary of pharmacotherapeutic management of acute HF is shown in Table 14.3. Different categories of acute HF[24,44] would require specific approaches to therapy.

Table 14.3 Pharmacotherapeutic management of acute heart failure

Hypoxia	Oxygen therapy, CPAP/BiPAP, ventilate if $pCO_2 > 7$ kPa
Pain/anxiety	Analgesics, anxiolytics, beware respiratory depression of opiates
Congestion	iv diuretics, low-dose dopamine, dopexamine, (ultrafiltration)
Reduce preload	Transdermal patch or iv nitrates, loop diuretics, inodilators
Modulate afterload	Oral or iv Inodilators
Hypertension	Judicious lowering of BP; exclude acute renal stenosis if de novo
Monitoring	ECG, Filling pressures (RV and/or LV), Systemic ±pulmonary BP, CO
Treat causes	Accurate diagnosis and intervene to correct primary defect(s) if possible
Rate and rhythm	Treat arrhythmia, control heart rate, cardioversion if hemodynamically compromised
Heart/branch blocks	For serious heart blocks, atropine, isoproterenol, (pacing ± acute CRT)
Preshock syndrome	Recognition, prophylactic treatment, prevent deterioration into shock
Shock	Rule out or treat noncardiac causes of shock
Cardiogenic shock	iv inotropes, emergency correction of causal defects if possible
To avoid	Iatrogenic hypotension, negative inotropism or chronotropism

BP blood pressure; *CO* cardiac output; *ECG* electrocardiogram; *iv* intravenous; *LV* left ventricle; *PEEP* positive end-expiratory pressure; *RV* right ventricle

14.1.7
Systolic vs. Diastolic Heart Failure

The pathophysiology of systolic HF is much better understood than diastolic HF. The latter has generated so much confusion that many even counsel against using the term "diastolic HF" and adopt a more expedient but pathophysiologically less distinct entity of HF with preserved left ventricular ejection fraction (HFprEF) which consists of a phenotypic mix of conditions.[45] Therapy that is beneficial in systolic HF may not be effective in diastolic HF. Most of the large randomized controlled trials of therapeutic agents apply to systolic failure with low LV ejection fraction as an inclusion criterion. There is no data showing that ACE inhibition or beta blockade, are conclusively beneficial in patients with primarily diastolic HF. The only RCT recruiting large enough number is the CHARM-Preserve trial, but even in this, there was no unequivocal unadjusted benefits of candersartan over placebo.[46] The strategy of treatment should therefore be based on the above principles of HF therapy, targeting treatable underlying pathophysiological causes including tight control of hypertension and coronary revascularisation.[7] And symptom relief according to empirical approaches of therapy as described above.

14.2
Pharmacotherapy

Treatment of HF with pharmacological agents should not be dished out in similar manner to following a recipe book; for instance. After registering the presence of HF symptoms, patients are often prescribed evidence-based drugs such as ACE inhibitors and beta-blockers and the doses escalated in a formulaic way to target doses without regard to the etiology and cardiac defects. Such a rote-like approach may not be in the best interests of individual patients. Instead, considerations on initiating and maintaining patients on HF medication should at least be based on the following principles:-

- Treatment to relieve symptoms as a relative priority compared to improving prognosis.
- Treatment of primary cardiac defect(s) which are causative should be instituted first, followed by medication for secondary defects and avoiding precipitating undesirable iatrogenic complications.
- Drug therapy should be considered in parallel with other (life-style, surgical, interventional, device) options of therapy.
- Medication and doses should be instituted, adjusted, reviewed and revised/withdrawn according to variations in HF status.

In this section, pharmacological agents used in the treatment of HF are classified according to the objectives to improve quality or quantity of life or both, and according to the severity of HF. These are also put in the context of other nonpharmacological options of therapy. In Table 14.4, drugs used for improving symptoms and exercise capacity can be adjusted according to patient responses, but not prophylactic drugs for improving longevity or hospitalization rates. The indication for use of the latter drugs can only be established if there is clear statistically and clinically significant benefits shown in RCT's whereas the former drugs can be prescribed according to potential pharmacological benefits and adjusted according to responses. The prophylactic drugs are usually dose-escalated to a target dose but may need to be curtailed for reasons of intolerance or adverse reactions.

In Table 14.5, each therapeutic agent for HF is tabulated for use according to the severity of HF. This form of tabulation would empower clinicians to deliver treatment in a more rational way based on whether prophylactic therapies are paramount or whether symptom relief and improving quality of life are higher in the patients' agenda. Agents for prophylactic benefits (white lettering) are based on published reports of large-scale RCT's which show statistically significant benefits clearly summarized in various international guidelines[47,48] to which readers are referred for more details that cannot be included in this short chapter. However, since agents for improving elements of quality of life are less well publicized or understood, some salient practical points are included in this chapter.

14.2.1
Key Practical Points on Medication for Improving Quality of Life

The key drugs to improve symptoms specifically arising from HF are diuretics, digoxin, vasodilators and positive inotropic agents. Other cardioactive drugs not specifically for HF

Table 14.4 Treatments used to attain objectives of therapy in chronic heart failure

CONDITION	NYHA	DRUGS FOR IMPROVING:			
		Longevity	Quality of life		
			Symptoms	Exercise Capacity	Hospitalisation Rates
Asymptomatic LVD	I	only post-AMI ACEI, ARB, AldoA, βB	N/A	nil known	only post-AMI ACEI, ARB, AldoA, βB
mild HF	II	ACEI, ARB βB, ISDN+Hyd	ARB, Digx, Diur Vasodil	Diur, Digx ISDN+Hyd	ACEI, ARB, βB Digx, Diur
moderate HF	III	ACEI, ARB, AldoA βB, ISDN+Hyd	ARB, Digx, Diur Vasodil	Diur, Digx ISDN+Hyd	ACEI, ARB, AldoA, βB Digx, Diur
Severe HF	III+/IV	ACEI, ARB, AldoA βB, ISDN+Hyd	ARB, Digx, Diur Vasodil	Diur, Digx ISDN+Hyd	ACEI, ARB, AldoA, βB Digx, Diur
End-stage HF	IV+	(CTx, VAD)	Digx, Diur, pos-Inotr Vasodil	Diur, Digx Vasodil	Diur

Copyright Prof L B Tan

Key to table: White texts: for prophylactic treatment Black texts: for treating symptoms, exercise tolerance, with adjustments according to patient response.
ACEI: Angiotensin Converting Enzyme Inhibitors; *AldoA:* Aldosterone Antagonists; *AMI:* acute myocardial infarction; *ARB:* Angiotensin II Receptor Inhibitors; *βB:* beta blockers (only bisoprolol, carvedilol, nibivolol, metoprolol CR/XL); *CTx:* cardiac transplantation (not a drug therapy); *Digx:* Digoxin; *Diur:* Diuretics; *LVD:* left ventricular dysfunction; *N/A:* not applicable; *NYHA:* New York Heart Association Functional Class for Heart Failure; *pos-Inotr:* positive inotropes (e.g. iv dobutamine, enoximone, milrinone); *VAD:* ventricular assist device (not a drug therapy); *Vasodil:* Vasodilators (e.g. nitrates, calcium antagonists, K Channel openers)

can also be effective in improving symptoms and functional capacity such as antianginal medication to relieve myocardial ischaemia and exertional dyspnoea, antiarrhythmic and antihypertensive agents. Symptomatic arrhythmias (atrial fibrillation, supraventricular or ventricular tachyarrhythmias) may also precipitate or exacerbate HF symptoms and effective treatment can improve the quality of life.

14.2.1.1
Diuretics

Despite low numbers of RCT's of diuretic therapy,[49] these agents are still the first line therapy for congestive HF, most effective in relieving congestion and improve exercise ability.[16] Hitherto, all drugs shown through RCT's to be prognostically beneficial have been tested with trial participants given standard background therapy which included diuretics. However, probably because these drugs were first introduced for use about half a century ago and hardly the subject of recent original clinical studies, knowledge about their pharmacological properties, is highly variable amongst practicing clinicians. An excellent pharmacological review is an essential reading.[50] Some salient points for modern diuretic therapy are listed below:-

Table 14.5 Recommended therapy for chronic heart failure

Chronic HF NYHA	Asymptomatic LVD I	mild HF II	moderate HF III	Severe HF III+/IV	End-stage HF IV+
DRUG THERAPY for CHF					
Diuretics					
Loop D	O	+	+	+	+
K-Sparing	O	+ if K<4	+ if K<4	+ if K<4	+ if K<4
Metolazone/Thz	O	O	O	+ if olig/RefrEd	+ if olig/RefrEd
RAAS Inhibitors					
ACEI	+ if ↓EF - if RASt	+ if ↓EF - if RASt	+ if ↓EF - if RASt	+ if ↓EF - if RASt	O
ARB	+ post MI HF/ ↓EF - if RASt	+ if ↓EF - if RASt	+ if ↓EF - if RASt	+ if ↓EF - if RASt	O
AldoA	+ eple postMI HF - if K>5.5	+ if K<4	+ spironol - if K>5.5	+ spironol - if K>5.5	+ if K<4
β-Blockers	+ post-MI - if asthma	+ if ↓EF - if asthma	+ if ↓EF - if asthma	+ if ↓EF - if asthma	
Digoxin	+ if AF	+	+	+	+
Vasodilators					
ISDN+Hyd	O	+ if off ACEI	+ if off ACEI	+	+
alphaB	+ if Ht	+ if Ht	+ if Ht	+ if Ht	+ if Ht
CaA	+ if Ht / angina	+ if Ht / angina	+ if Ht / angina	+ if Ht / angina	+ if Ht / angina
Nesiritide	O	O	O	?+	?+
Nicorandil	+ if angina	+ if angina	+ if angina	+ if angina	+ if angina
Inotropes	O	O	O	O	+
LowD Dopamine	O	O	O	+ if oliguric	+ if oliguric
Anti-arrhythmics	O	+ if signif Arrhy	+ if signif Arrhy	+ if signif Arrhy	+ if signif Arrhy
Domiciliary O₂	O	O	O	?+	+
Anti-coag/platelet	+ if AF & *	+ if AF & *	+ if AF & *	+ if AF & *	+ if AF & *
Statins	+ if CAD	+ if CAD	+ if CAD	? + if CAD	? + if CAD
Non-drug Therapy					
CPAP / BiPAP	O	+ if CSA/OSA	+ if CSA/OSA	+ if CSA/OSA	+ if CSA/OSA
CSurg	O	+ if corrective	+ if corrective	+ if corrective	+ if corrective
CTx	O	O	O	O	+
VAD	O	O	O	O	+
Dialysis etc	O	O	O	+ if olig&RefrEd	+ if olig&RefrEd
DC Cardioversion	+ for AF	+ for AF	+ for AF	+ for AF	+ for AF

Table 14.5 (continued)

ExTr	+	+	+	+	O
CRT	O	+ if QRS>120ms	+ if QRS>120ms	+ if QRS>120ms	+ if QRS>120ms
CRT+ICD	O	+ if QRS>120ms	+ if QRS>120ms	+ if QRS>120ms	O
ICD	+ post MI HF&↓EF	+ if VT/VF&↓EF	+ if VT/VF&↓EF	+/– if VT/VF&↓EF	O
Pacing	+ if HB/Brady	+ if HB/Brady	+ if HB/Brady	+ if HB/Brady	+ if HB/Brady

copyright prof L B Tan

Key to table: White texts: for prophylactic treatment   **Black texts**: for treating symptoms, exercise tolerance, with adjustments according to patient response

'+' : indicated; 'O' : not indicated; '-' : contraindicated; * Intra-cardiac thrombus or history of thrombo-embolism; ACEI: Angiotensin Converting Enzyme Inhibitors; AF: Atrial fibrillation; AldoA: Aldosterone Antagonists; αB: Alpha blockers; ARB: Angiotensin II Receptor Inhibitors; βB: beta blockers (bisoprolol, carvedilol, metoprolol CR/XL, nebivolol); CaA: Calcium antagonists; CAD: Coronary artery disease; CPAP: Continuous positive airways pressure ventilation or bilevel PAP; CRT: Cardiac resynchronisation therapy through atrio-biventricular sequential pacing; CSA: Central Sleep Apnoea, Cheyne-Stokes respiration; CSurg: Corrective cardiac surgery (e.g. CABG, pericardiectomy, ASD/VSD repair, valve surgery); CTx: Cardiac transplantation; Dialysis etc: all forms of renal dialysis, ultrafiltration, or haemofiltration.; EF: Ejection fraction of the left ventricle; low = usually <40%; eple: eplerenone; ExTr: Exercise training; HB/Brady: heart block or haemodynamically significant bradycardia; HF: Heart failure; Ht = Hypertension; if K<4: If hypokalaemic; Aim to maintain serum K between 4.0 & 5.5; ISDN+Hyd: Isosorbide dinitrate + Hydralazine; K-Sparing: Potassium sparing diuretics (e.g. amiloride, triamterene, spironolactone); LowD Dopamine: low-dose dopamine (< 5 mcg/kg/min) for oliguria secondary to severe renal hypoperfusion; Loop D: Loop diuretics (e.g. furosemide, bumetanide); LVD: left ventricular dysfunction; NYHA: New York Heart Association Functional Class for Heart Failure; olig&RefrEd: Anuric or oliguric with refractory edema; RAAS Inhibitors: Inhibitors of the renin-angiotensin-aldosterone system; RASt: Renal artery stenosis; signif Arrhy: Haemodynamically significant arrhythmia; Thz: Thiazide diuretics (e.g. bendroflumethiazide, hydrochlorothiazide); VAD: Ventricular assist device, or artificial mechanical heart

The main reason why diuretics are necessary is to counteract a fundamental natural compensatory mechanism in HF which triggers retention of fluid.[51] The aim of diuretic therapy in HF is therefore to maintain fluid balance. In the state of impaired fluid homeostasis due to HF, diuretics are used to ensure fluid output is equal to intake. As either side of the equation can change independently, it is important to remember that diuretic dosages should always be reactive (to the amount of fluid intake). It is crucially important to decrease the dose when the fluid intake falls and never to allow the doses of diuretics to creep up so that it becomes necessary for the patient to drink excessively to keep up with the dehydration caused by over-diuresis.

Worthy of special mention is the risks of arrhythmias, secondary to electrolyte imbalance as a diuretic complication, which would paradoxically worsen the dyspnoea that the diuretic usage was aiming to alleviate. This can be avoided by judicious selection of diuretic combination (loop, thiazide, and K-sparing) for use, heeding the principles of therapy for congestion as outlined in the above sections.

The use of combination diuretics requires special mention:-

- Loop diuretics and metolazone combination is particularly potent and may be used sparingly to "kick-start" diuresis, esp. when IV administration is not an option. It is also particularly liable in upsetting electrolyte balance, esp. hyponatraemia which is the most harmful and difficult to treat.
- Loop and other thiazide diuretics combination is similar to the above but may not be as powerful.
- Loop or thiazide diuretics have propensity to induce severe hypokalaemia and hypo-magnesaemia. The use of K+ supplements does not address the hypomagnaesemia. The combined use with K+-sparing diuretics is more efficacious.

The frequency of diuretics dosing deserves some practical consideration:

- It is kinder to patients if nocturnal diuresis that will disturb sleep can be avoided, unless the patient already has in-dwelling urinary catheter, by avoiding late evening medication.
- Repeated split doses are more effective than the entire dose given once a day.
- For patients with stress incontinence and unable to reach toilets soon enough, the use of longer acting diuretics (e.g., torasemide) may be better tolerated and improve compliance.
- When intravenous therapy is indicated, there is suggestion that continuous infusion might be better than intermittent bolus injections.[52]

In HF patients with peripheral oedema, it is not always necessary to get rid of all traces of oedema by aggressive diuretic therapy. The margin between complete absence of peripheral oedema and dehydration (leading to renal dysfunction) is very narrow. Only symptomatic oedema or oedema associated complications (e.g., ulcerations, bedsores) requires more aggressive diuretic therapy.

To drown in one's own fluid (secondary to congestion) is one of the worst ways to experience the end of one's life. Hence diuretics are essential medication for late-stage HF therapy. If fluid intake were significantly diminished for whatever reasons (e.g., nausea, vomiting, swallowing difficulty, sedation) during late-stage HF, then the diuretics dosage should be concomitantly reduced. Features for hypovolaemia or dehydration include postural hypotension, dry mucosa, and reduction of skin turgor. In diuretic resistant late-stage HF with severe symptomatic congestion, it may be necessary to resort to temporary inotropic therapy or even dialysis or filtration to relieve the distressing congestive symptoms. Once the oedema has resolved, provided there is still adequate renal function, the patient may become responsive to and able to be maintained with oral diuretic therapy again. Worthy of special mention in late-stage palliative care for HF patients is that it is essential to keep treatments which maintain fluid balance and also preserve adequate renal function. Worsening of either could result in recurrence of troublesome congestion, with its attendant complications. Continuation of diuretic therapy may be necessary to achieve this objective, but the doses need to be carefully monitored and adjusted, because over-diuresis will result in hypovolaemia, and potential exacerbation of prerenal failure leading to deterioration in renal function. Without a functioning kidney, the alternative is dialysis or filtration, both of which are invasive and liable to induce ill-tolerated hypotensive symptoms thereby compromising the quality of life.

14.2.1.2
Digoxin

Many clinicians have been unfortunately confused by and misunderstood the academic debates surrounding the use of digoxin in the treatment of HF. Digoxin, which belongs to the class of drugs called digitalis, is the oldest drug that is still widely used in current cardiological practice. Digitalis is extracted from foxglove and was introduced into medical usage by William Withering, an eminent English physician from Birmingham, over 200 years ago. In 1785, he published the now famous book, "An Account of the Foxglove, and some of its Medical Uses."

There are two properties of digoxin which are useful therapeutically: (1) slowing the AV node conduction (e.g., for rate control of fast atrial fibrillation), and (2) positive inotropic effects to improve myocardial contractility. New-onset atrial fibrillation can be diagnosed clinically and an ECG would confirm it. The most important point to remember when facing a worsening HF patient is to determine whether the patient is haemodynamically compromised by the AF, which would warrant electrocardioversion, but maintaining the patient in sinus rhythms is a major challenge.

While the use of digoxin to control ventricular rates in fast AF is widely accepted, that for its positive inotropism has attracted much more controversies. One reason is that the positive inotropic effect of digoxin is difficult to detect in man at rest (hence the scientific confusion), but becomes manifest during exercise.[53] Because of this unusual property of digoxin, it rather approaches the characteristics of an ideal inotrope, because it is not desirable to flog the failing heart unnecessarily at rest, but it kicks in during exercise when the chronic HF patient really needs the extra inotropic support to ameliorate exercise intolerance.[54] In selected patients with severe systolic dysfunction, digoxin may improve symptoms and exercise capacity.[55] In a large-scale randomized placebo-controlled trial, it reduced hospitalization rates of HF patients and did not show any increase in overall mortality,[56] and with low-dose therapy, there is a suggestion that it would even improve survival.[57,58] That is why after centuries of research, digoxin is still the only orally active agent licensed for use as a positive inotropic agent to treat HF. The old dogma of having to push the dose as high as possible albeit within the therapeutic range has now been superseded by usage of low-dose digoxin (e.g., 62.5 μg/day) and dose titrate up if necessary according to response. Digoxin is therefore potentially helpful in sinus rhythm too and worth a therapeutic trial as it is often quite clear to the individual patient whether it has provided symptomatic benefit or not.

14.2.1.3
Vasodilators

Venodilators such as nitrates are helpful in relieving the symptoms of venous congestions, complementing the effects of diuretics. As the most widely used venodilator, nitrates are able to relieve symptoms and improve exercise capacity not only in ischemic HF patients, but also in nonischemic patients. Therapeutic trials of sublingual or oral nitrates are worthwhile in individual HF patients, either at the onset of dyspnea or before undertaking major exertions. The first ever RCT to show any prognostic benefits for any HF therapy was the combination nitrate and hydralazine treatment.[59] Arterial vasodilators such as hydralazine are particularly helpful in patients who are still relatively hypertensive, but the lowering of arterial pressure needs to be gradual to avoid symptoms of dizziness and postural hypotension. Most vasodilators (e.g., ACE inhibitors, ARB's) are combined venous and arterial vasodilators, and they may also improve symptoms. However, in most patients with late-stage HF, their arterial pressures are usually low, and they may have very little reserve to tolerate too much of vasodilatation. Symptoms may therefore improve with a low-dose vasodilator therapy and may paradoxically worsen with higher doses.[6, 18] Caution needs to be exercised when using vasodilators with negative inotropic effects such as verapamil and those with fluid-retentive properties such as dihydropyridine calcium antagonists (e.g., nifedipine, felodipine, amlodipine).

14.2.1.4
Inotropes

Having been mislead by pursuers of the concept that HF is distinctly a condition of impaired myocardial contractility and after decades of seeking the ideal positive inotropic agents,[60] it is now safe to conclude there is no place for such agents in the treatment of chronic HF for prognostic benefits.[61] However, on rare occasions, the symptoms of the patients may be so intractable despite all the best available medical therapy. For patients who desperately wish to improve quality of life even at the expense of quantity of life, there is still a place for empirical therapy using low-dose positive inotropic agents,[62] especially in the acute and subacute phases until more definitive treatment can be put in place.

References

1. Cohn JN, Johnson G, Ziesche S, et al. [V-HeFT II] A comparison of enalapril with hydralazine-isosorbide dinitrate in the treatment of chronic congestive heart failure. *N Engl J Med.* 1991;325:303-310.
2. Rector TS, Johnson G, Dunkman WB, et al. Evaluation by patients with heart failure of the effects of enalapril compared with hydralazine plus isosorbide dinitrate on quality of life. V-HeFT II. The V-HeFT VA Cooperative Studies Group. *Circulation.* 1993;87:VI71-VI77.
3. Bulpitt CJ. Quality of life with ACE inhibitors in chronic heart failure. *J Cardiovasc Pharmacol.* 1996;27(suppl 2):S31-S35.
4. Tan LB, Murphy R. Shifts in mortality curves: saving or extending lives? *Lancet.* 1999;354: 1378-1381.
5. Swedberg K, Kjekshus J, Snapinn S. Long-term survival in severe heart failure in patients with enalapril: ten year follow-up of CONSENSUS I. *Eur Heart J.* 1999;20:136-139.

6. Cooke GA, Williams SG, Marshall P, et al. A mechanistic investigation of ACE inhibitor dose effects on aerobic exercise capacity in heart failure patients. *Eur Heart J.* 2002;23: 1360-1368.

7. Carluccio E, Biagioli P, Alunni G, et al. Effect of revascularizing viable myocardium on left ventricular diastolic function in patients with ischaemic cardiomyopathy. *Eur Heart J.* 2009; 30(12):1501-1509.

8. Cohn PF. *Silent myocardial Ischemia and Infarction.* New York: Marcel Dekker; 1986.

9. Rahimtoola SH. The hibernating myocardium. *Am Heart J.* 1989;117(1):211-221.

10. Redwood SR, Ferrari R, Marber MS. Myocardial hibernation and stunning: from physiological principles to clinical practice. *Heart.* 1998;80:218-222.

11. Nicholls DP, Onuoha GN, McDowell G, et al. Neuroendocrine changes in chronic cardiac failure. *Basic Res Cardiol.* 1996;91(suppl 1):13-20.

12. Kajstura J, Cigola E, Malhotra A, et al. Angiotensin II induces apoptosis of adult ventricular myocytes in vitro. *J Mol Cell Cardiol.* 1997;29:859-870.

13. Tan LB, Jalil JE, Pick R, Janicki JS, Weber KT. Cardiac myocyte necrosis induced by angiotensin II. *Circ Res.* 1991;69:1185-1195.

14. Benjamin IJ, Jalil JE, Tan LB, Cho K, Weber KT, Clark WA. Isoproterenol-induced myocardial fibrosis in relation to myocyte necrosis. *Circ Res.* 1989;65:657-670.

15. Jalil JE, Doering CW, Janicki JS, Pick R, Shroff SG, Weber KT. Fibrillar collagen and myocardial stiffness in the intact hypertrophied rat left ventricle. *Circ Res.* 1989;64:1041-1050.

16. Bayliss J, Norell M, Canepa Anson R, Sutton G, Poole-Wilson PA. Untreated heart failure: clinical and neuroendocrine effects of introducing diuretics. *Br Heart J.* 1987;57:17-22.

17. Swedberg K, Gundersen T. The role of exercise testing in heart failure. [Review]. *J Cardiovasc Pharmacol.* 1993;22(suppl 9):S13-S17.

18. Williams SG, Cooke GA, Wright DJ, Tan LB. Disparate results of ACE inhibitor dosage on exercise capacity in heart failure: a reappraisal of vasodilator therapy and study design. *Int J Cardiol.* 2001;77:239-245.

19. The Task Force on Heart Failure of the European Society of Cardiology. Guidelines for the diagnosis of heart failure. *Eur Heart J.* 1995;16:741-751.

20. The CONSENSUS Trial Study Group. Effects of enalapril on mortality in severe congestive heart failure. Results of the Cooperative North Scandinavian Enalapril Survival Study (CONSENSUS). The CONSENSUS Trial Study Group. *N Engl J Med.* 1987;316:1429-1435.

21. SOLVD Investigators. Effect of enalapril on survival in patients with reduced left ventricular ejection fractions and congestive heart failure. *N Engl J Med.* 1991;325:293-302.

22. SOLVD Investigators. Effect of enalapril on mortality and the development of heart failure in asymptomatic patients with reduced left ventricular ejection fractions. *N Engl J Med.* 1992;327:685-691.

23. Packer M, Bristow MR, Cohn JN, et al.; for the US Carvedilol Heart Failure Study Group. The effect of carvedilol on morbidity and mortality in patients with chronic heart failure. *New Engl J Med.* 1996;334:1349-1355.

24. Tan LB, Williams SG, Wright DJ. Ventriculo-arterial function curves - a new dimension in characterising acute heart failure. *Eur J Heart Fail.* 2003;5:407-410.

25. Markham RV, Corbett JR, Gilmore A, Pettinger WA, Firth BG. Efficacy of prazosin in the management of chronic congestive heart failure: a six-month randomized, double-blind, placebo-controlled study. *Am J Cardiol.* 1983;51:1346-1352.

26. Cohn JN, Archibald DG, Phil M, et al. [V-HeFT I] Effect of vasodilator therapy on mortality in chronic congestive heart failure. Results of a Veterans Administration Cooperative Study. *N Engl J Med.* 1986;314:1547-1552.

27. Cooke GA, Williams SG, Marshall P, et al. A mechanistic investigation of ACE inhibitor dose effects on aerobic exercise capacity in heart failure patients. *Eur Heart J.* 2002;23:1360-1368.

28. Varriale P, Mossavi A. The benefit of low-dose dopamine during vigorous diuresis for congestive heart failure associated with renal insufficiency: does it protect renal function? *Clin Cardiol*. 1997;20:627-630.

29. Tan LB, Littler WA, Murray RG. Beneficial haemodynamic effects of intravenous dopexamine in patients with low-output heart failure. *J Cardiovasc Pharmacol*. 1987;10:280-286.

30. Franciosa JA. Isosorbide dinitrate and exercise performance in patients with congestive heart failure. *Am Heart J*. 1985;110(1 pt 2):245-250.

31. Douban S, Brodsky MA, Whang DD, Whang R. Significance of magnesium in congestive heart failure. *Am Heart J*. 1996;132:664-671.

32. Ng LL, Garrido MC, Davies JE, Brochwicz-Lewinski MJ, Tan LB. Intracellular free magnesium in lymphocytes from patients with congestive cardiac failure treated with loop diuretics with and without amiloride. *Br J Clin Pharmac*. 1992;33:329-332.

33. Pitt B, Zannad F, Remme WJ, et al. The effect of spironolactone on morbidity and mortality in patients with severe heart failure. Randomized Aldactone Evaluation Study Investigators. *N Engl J Med*. 1999;341(10):709-717.

34. Tan LB, Williams SG, Goldspink DF. From CONSENSUS to CHARM-how do ACEI and ARB produce clinical benefits in CHF? *Int J Cardiol*. 2004;94(2–3):137-141.

35. Epstein SE, Braunwald E. Beta-adrenergic receptor blocking drugs: mechanisms of action and clinical applications. *N Engl J Med*. 1966;275(1106–12):1175-1183.

36. Tan LB, Littler WA. Measurement of cardiac reserve in cardiogenic shock: implications for prognosis and management. *Br Heart J*. 1990;64:121-128.

37. Maskin CS, Forman R, Sonnenblick EH, Frishman WH, LeJemtel TH. Failure of dobutamine to increase exercise capacity despite hemodynamic improvement in severe chronic heart failure. *Am J Cardiol*. 1983;51:177-182.

38. Maskin CS, Kugler J, Sonnenblick EH, LeJemtel TH. Acute inotropic stimulation with dopamine in severe congestive heart failure: beneficial hemodynamic effect at rest but not during maximal exercise. *Am J Cardiol*. 1983;52:1028-1032.

39. Packer M, Carver JR, Rodeheffer RJ, et al.; for the PROMISE Study Research Group. Effect of oral milrinone on mortality in severe chronic heart failure. *N Engl J Med*. 1991;325: 1468-1475.

40. Packer M, Narahara KA, Elkayam U, et al.; Principle Investigators of REFLECT Study. Double-blind, placebo-controlled study of the efficacy of flosequinan in patients with chronic heart failure. *J Am Coll Cardiol*. 1993;22:65-72.

41. Xamoterol in Severe Heart Failure Study Group. Xamoterol in severe heart failure. *Lancet*. 1990;336:1-6.

42. Cohn JN, Goldstein SO, Greenberg BH, et al. A dose-dependent increase in mortality with vesnarinone among patients with severe heart failure. Vesnarinone Trial Investigators. *N Engl J Med*. 1998;339(25):1810-1816.

43. Nieminen MS, et al.; ESC Committee for Practice Guideline (CPG). Executive summary of the guidelines on the diagnosis and treatment of acute heart failure: the Task Force on Acute Heart Failure of the European Society of Cardiology. *Eur Heart J*. 2005;26(4):384-416. Epub 2005 Jan 28.

44. Cotter G, Moshkovitz Y, Kaluski E, et al. The role of cardiac power and systemic vascular resistance in the pathophysiology and diagnosis of patients with acute congestive heart failure. *Eur J Heart Fail*. 2003;5(4):443-451.

45. Brutsaert DL, De Keulenaer GW. Diastolic heart failure: a myth. *Curr Opin Cardiol*. 2006; 21(3):240-248.

46. Yusuf S, Pfeffer MA, Swedberg K, et al.; CHARM Investigators and Committees. Effects of candesartan in patients with chronic heart failure and preserved left-ventricular ejection fraction: the CHARM-Preserved Trial. *Lancet*. 2003;362(9386):777-781.

47. Task Force for Diagnosis and Treatment of Acute and Chronic Heart Failure 2008 of European Society of Cardiology; Dickstein K, Cohen-Solal A, Filippatos G, et al. ESC Guidelines for the diagnosis and treatment of acute and chronic heart failure 2008: the Task Force for the Diagnosis and Treatment of Acute and Chronic Heart Failure 2008 of the European Society of Cardiology. Developed in collaboration with the Heart Failure Association of the ESC (HFA) and endorsed by the European Society of Intensive Care Medicine (ESICM). *Eur Heart J.* 2008;29(19):2388-2442.

48. Hunt SA, et al.; American College of Cardiology; American Heart Association Task Force on Practice Guidelines; American College of Chest Physicians; International Society for Heart and Lung Transplantation; Heart Rhythm Society. ACC/AHA 2005 Guideline Update for the Diagnosis and Management of Chronic Heart Failure in the Adult: a report of the American College of Cardiology/American Heart Association Task Force on Practice Guidelines (Writing Committee to Update the 2001 Guidelines for the Evaluation and Management of Heart Failure): developed in collaboration with the American College of Chest Physicians and the International Society for Heart and Lung Transplantation: endorsed by the Heart Rhythm Society. *Circulation.* 2005;112(12):e154-e235.

49. Faris R, FlatherMD, PurcellH, Poole-Wilson PA, Coats AJS. Diuretics for heart failure. *Cochrane Database Syst Rev.* 2006;(1):CD003838. DOI: 10.1002/14651858.CD003838.pub2.

50. Brater DC. Diuretic therapy. *N Engl J Med.* 1998;339(6):387-395.

51. Harris P. Role of arterial pressure in the oedema of heart disease. *Lancet.* 1988;1(8593): 1036-1038.

52. Salvador DRK, Rey NR, Ramos GC, Punzalan FER. Continuous infusion versus bolus injection of loop diuretics in congestive heart failure. *Cochrane Database Syst Rev.* 2005; 3:CD003178. DOI: 10.1002/14651858.CD003178.pub3.

53. Tan LB, Murray RG, Tweddel AC, Hutton I. Cardiotonic effect of digitalis in sinus rhythm during exercise. In: Erdmann E, Greeff K, Skou JC, eds. *Cardiac Glycosides 1785–1985.* New York: Springer; 1986:455-460.

54. Tan LB. The search for an ideal oral positive inotropic agent. *Eur J Clin Pharmacol.* 1986;30: 509-512.

55. DiBianco R, Shabetai R, Kostuk W, Moran J, Schlant RC, Wright R. A comparison of oral milrinone, digoxin, and their combination in the treatment of patients with chronic heart failure. *N Engl J Med.* 1989;320(11):677-683.

56. The Digitalis Investigation Group. The effect of digoxin on mortality and morbidity in patients with heart failure. *N Engl J Med.* 1997;336(8):525-533.

57. Adams KF Jr, Patterson JH, Gattis WA, et al. Relationship of serum digoxin concentration to mortality and morbidity in women in the digitalis investigation group trial: a retrospective analysis. *J Am Coll Cardiol.* 2005;46(3):497-504.

58. Ahmed A, Pitt B, Rahimtoola SH, et al. Effects of digoxin at low serum concentrations on mortality and hospitalization in heart failure: a propensity-matched study of the DIG trial. *Int J Cardiol.* 2008;123(2):138-146.

59. Cohn JN, Archibald DG, Ziesche S, et al. Effect of vasodilator therapy on mortality in chronic congestive heart failure. Results of a Veterans Administration Cooperative Study. *N Engl J Med.* 1986;314(24):1547-1552.

60. Williams SG, Barker D, Goldspink DF, Tan LB. A reappraisal of concepts in heart failure: central role of cardiac power reserve. *Arch Med Sci.* 2005;1:65-74.

61. Cohn JN. Inotropic therapy for heart failure: paradise lost. *Eur Heart J.* 2009;30:2965-2966.

62. Metra M, Eichhorn E, Abraham WT, et al.; for the ESSENTIAL Investigators. Effects of low-dose oral enoximone administration on mortality, morbidity, and exercise capacity in patients with advanced heart failure: the randomized, double-blind, placebo-controlled, parallel group ESSENTIAL trials. *Eur Heart J.* 2009;30:3015-3026.

Nonpharmacological Therapies

15

Andrew J.S. Coats

15.1
Introduction

Chronic heart failure is both common and disabling. It predominantly affects older people and there is convincing evidence that it is increasing in prevalence with the aging population of developed societies. Heart failure is associated with a poor prognosis. What, as little as 30 years ago, was a condition of despair with no proven treatments that affected survival has changed with the advent of effective therapies. For a patient with a new diagnosis of heart failure the expectation of surviving 1 year has probably improved from about 60 to 80–90% with the advances in therapy that have become established over this period. These include ACE inhibitors, beta-blockers, aldosterone antagonists, cardiac resynchronization pacemakers and implantable defibrillators. Heart failure is, however, also associated with many debilitating symptoms for the sufferer. These can induce depression, withdrawal from society, an inability to work and even severe limitations on the ability to fulfill the needs of self-care and daily living. Exercise tolerance is particularly limited by a combination of dyspnoea, fatigue and a weakness of the peripheral musculature.

Here the modern therapies have been far less impressive. ACE inhibitors are only inconsistently associated with improved exercise tolerance and beta blockers may have paradoxical effects by reducing heart rate reserve at least transiently, before potential improvements in left ventricular function can overcome this limitation. Although at the most severe end diuretics can allow an acutely breathless patient to perform more work, the stable chronic patient cannot be said reliably to gain benefit in terms of functional capacity from any of our modern pharmaceutical interventions. In contrast the recent use of cardiac resynchronization therapies in selected patients does seem to be associated with an improvement in exercise tolerance.[1] One of the reasons the established treatments appear less effective in improving functional limitation may derive from the fact that recent research has suggested our fundamental understanding of the cause of these symptoms may have been misguided. It was for many years assumed that most of the dyspnoea of stable chronic heart failure was

A.J.S. Coats
University of East Anglia, Norwich Research Park, Norwich, Norfolk, UK
e-mail: ajscoats@aol.com

M.Y. Henein (ed.), *Heart Failure in Clinical Practice*,
DOI: 10.1007/978-1-84996-153-0_15, © Springer-Verlag London Limited 2010

due to congestion in the lungs and most of the muscular fatigue was related to impaired cardiac pumping capacity reducing muscular perfusion during exercise. This mind-set suggested that improving cardiac performance was the most likely way to improve the symptoms of exercise intolerance. Yet the evidence, scant as it was, was against this. Early after even cardiac transplantation exercise intolerance was hardly improved at all despite an entirely new cardiac pump. It appeared that secondary changes as diverse as skeletal muscle wasting and metabolic change, autonomic nervous system imbalance, breathing pattern changes and peripheral vascular and endothelial dysfunction may have become limiting factors in the patients' ability to exercise, induced by, but ultimately independent of the degree of left ventricular functional impairment. This new understanding produced a whole new discipline in the study of heart failure, that of studying the structural, muscular, ventilatory, immunological and metabolic sequelae of heart failure and the poorly understood condition of cardiac cachexia. It became realized that treatments needed to target the periphery as well as the heart to have any chance of improving exercise intolerance and decreasing symptoms. As a result attention focused on peripherally acting treatments such as the use of exercise rehabilitation to correct changes such as skeletal muscle wasting and muscle fiber type shift that were characteristic both of heart failure, and also of deconditioning. This led to an interest in training heart failure patients.

Nonpharmacologic treatment modalities play an important role alongside effective modern pharmaceutical, surgical and device therapies in many cardiovascular disorders. These treatments include those lifestyle measures that reduce the risk of underlying diseases such as coronary artery disease, diabetes, hypertension and hyperlipidemia and those life-style interventions that benefit either the symptoms or prognosis of established heart failure. The former will have formed a part of the management of the patients prior to the development of heart failure and should continue. Once chronic heart failure has become established nonpharmacologic treatments, including exercise prescriptions, may play an increasingly important role in management. Chronic Heart Failure has been the subject of over 100 randomized controlled trials (RCTs) that have assessed the effect of various pharmaceutical and device interventions on mortality and morbidity. These have formed the basis of one of the largest bodies of evidence to guide evidence-based therapeutics of all the chronic disorders in modern medicine. What has until recently been missing, however, is a similar evidence base for these nonpharmacological interventions for heart failure.

15.2
Patient and Care Education

For patients to get the optimum benefit from their therapy they, and their principal caregivers, need to have a good understanding of the nature and causes of chronic heart failure. Further information such as awareness of symptoms, diet, salt and fluid restriction, the nature and purpose of their drugs, and how to manage work and other physical activities, lifestyle changes, and measures of self-management of their disease is also important. Nonpharmacologic treatment should include dietary and other lifestyle advice, advice on appropriate levels of physical exercise, and health care education. The support engendered by learning these aspects with carers and other patients and their families can also be of major benefit. These educational programs should form part of a comprehensive multidisciplinary program organized by the treating physician in conjunction with other health care workers and primary care doctors, nurses, and, especially, the patients and their families. Other specialists including pharmacists dieticians, physiotherapists, psychologists, nurses, and social workers will play important supporting roles.[2]

15.3
Diet and Nutrition

Obesity is a well-known and well-studied risk factor for many of the known antecedents of heart failure, including coronary artery disease, diabetes, hypertension and hyperlipidemia. Adult obesity has been shown to increase the likelihood of later heart failure. Despite this, in what has been described as the "Obesity Paradox" once a patient has heart failure a higher body mass index (BMI) is actually protective, and weight loss is an ominous sign of worsening heart failure and a poor prognosis.[3,4] Described as cardiac cachexia this complication is a dramatic and catastrophic complication of heart failure, as it can be for other chronic disorders such as chronic renal failure, COPD, chronic liver disease and as a complication of cancer. This paradox means that as yet we do not know the optimum weight for a patient, let alone how to advise and ensure this is achieved and maintained in such patients. It also presents significant difficulties in public health messages, aiming for weight loss in many healthier people but a reversal of this advice in those who previously had most need to adhere to it. The challenge of the dietary management of the heart failure patient is to balance these conflicting needs, aiming for an optimal weight that may mean weight loss early in the natural history and strategies to prevent weight loss later in the clinical course. Data from 7,767 patients with stable HF enrolled in the Digitalis Investigation Group (DIG) trial showed crude all-cause mortality rates decreased in a near linear fashion across successively higher BMI groups, from 45.0% in the underweight group to 28.4% in the obese group (p for trend 0.001).[5] After multivariable adjustment, overweight and obese patients were at lower risk for death (hazard ratio [HR], 0.88; 95% confidence interval [CI], 0.80–0.96, and HR, 0.81; 95% CI, 0.72–0.92, respectively), compared with patients at an apparently healthier weight. Underweight patients with stable HF were at substantially increased risk for death (HR 1.21; 95% CI, 0.95–1.53).

Pasini et al have reported that CHF patients have on average a higher total energy expenditure (1,700±53 vs. 1,950±43 kcal/day; $p<0.01$), a negative calorie balance (104±35 vs. −186±40 kcal/day; $p<0.01$), a negative nitrogen balance (2.2±0.5 vs. −1.7±0.4 g/day; $p<0.01$), and a hypercatabolic hormonal status (cortisol/insulin ratio 32±1.7 vs. 65±5.1; $p<0.01$). This suggests a relatively inadequate calorie intake for daily activities, with consequent important protein breakdown that causes muscular wasting.[6] In another recent study the effects of nutritional supplementation were assessed. A supervised nutritional intervention was shown to improve clinical status and quality of life.[7] Sixty-five patients with heart failure were assigned to one of two groups: the intervention group (IG; $n=30$) who received a sodium-restricted diet (2,000–2,400 mg/day) with restriction of total fluids to 1.5 L/day, and the control group (CG; $n=35$) received traditional medical treatment and general nutritional recommendations. After 6 months kilocalories, macronutrients, and fluid intakes were significant lower in the IG than in the CG. Urinary excretion of sodium decreased significantly in the IG and increased in the CG (-7.9 vs. 29.4%, $p<0.05$). IG patients had significantly less frequent edema (37 vs. 7.4%, $p=0.008$) and fatigue (59.3 vs. 25.9%, $p=0.012$) at 6 months compared to baseline. Functional class also improved significantly. Physical activity increased $2.5\pm7.4\%$ in the IG and decreased -3.1 ± 12.0 in the CG ($p<0.05$). The IG had a greater increase in total quality of life compared with the CG (19.3 vs. 3.2%, $p=0.02$). These results suggest a more active approach to nutrition and weight may be appropriate for chronic heart failure patients. Kuehneman et al have demonstrated an important role for the dietician in a multidisciplinary heart failure program. Compared with the baseline, the quality of life scores improved by 6.7 points ($p<0.003$) at 3 months and by 5.9 points ($p<0.04$) at 6 months after dietician intervention.[8]

15.4
Psychological Support

Depression has been recognized as a common and adverse feature of CHF for some time.[9] Gottlieb has shown that in 155 patients with stable New York Heart Association functional class II, III, and IV HF patients with an ejection fraction <40, 48% of the patients could be considered depressed. Depressed patients tended to be younger than nondepressed patients. Women were more likely (64%) to be depressed than men (44%). Depressed patients scored significantly worse than nondepressed patients on all components of both the questionnaires measuring QoL. The authors suggested that pharmacologic or nonpharmacologic treatment of depression might have the capacity to improve the QoL of HF patients, although this presently has not been the subject of an adequately powered RCT.[10] The HART study[11] investigated the association of depression and social support in two subdomains of QoL, overall satisfaction and limitations in physical functioning in 695 heart failure patients. After adjustment for sociodemographic variables, depressive symptoms and social support were significantly associated with QoL scores ($p<0.001$) and accounted for 26% of the variance. The authors concluded that depression and social support play a substantially greater role in QoL than in perceived limitations in basic physical function and that targeting depression and low social support may be more important to improve overall QoL, whereas medical management of HF symptoms may have more impact on functional outcomes. This is consistent with a recent report on 2,322 patients from the HF-ACTION trials[12] in which symptoms of depression were seen to be minimally related to objective assessments of the severity of disease, but were more closely associated with patient (and clinician) perceptions of disease severity. The authors suggest that addressing depression might improve symptoms in patients with heart failure. These data support a more comprehensive rehabilitation approach than taking single elements in isolation, and this could include the use of antidepressant medication for coincident major depression in heart failure patients[13] and specific psychological interventions, such as mindfulness training.[14]

15.5
Sleep Disorders

Many patients with chronic heart failure complain of poor sleep. Historically this has been attributed to paroxysmal nocturnal dyspnoea, or to depression and anxiety. More recently it has been appreciated that many CHF patients also suffer from sleep disordered breathing (SDB) due to both obstructive and central sleep apnoea with frequent episodes of periodic breathing. One study reported 42% of patients with stable heart failure presenting to a heart failure clinic screened positive for SDB, despite receiving an optimal standard of care.[15] This is now recognized as a common condition and one which is believed to increase the risk of mortality. Treatment of SDB is considered an important part of the management of CHF. Improvements in SDB have been said to show a positive effect on cardiac output, on neurohormonal activity and quality of life. Continuous positive airway pressure has been the traditional method used to treat SDB in patients with CHF, but more recent devices such as a mandibular advancement device have also been shown to be effective.[16] Nocturnal, carbon dioxide inhalation by suppressing chemoreflex drive to ventilation (which is excessive in CHF[17]) has been shown to reduce the frequency of central sleep apnoea and improve quality of life.[18] Home oxygen therapy at night in heart failure patients with central sleep apnoea produced a greater reduction in apnoea and hypopnoea and greater increase in nocturnal oxygen saturation. These changes were associated with greater improvement in the Specific Activity Scale (0.82 ± 1.17 vs. -0.11 ± 0.73 Mets, $p=0.009$) in NYHA functional class ($p=0.007$) and in ejection fraction (5.45 ± 11.94 vs. $1.28 \pm 9.77\%$) compared to a control group. The authors concluded that 52-weeks of home oxygen therapy was both well tolerated and considered to be a valuable nonpharmacological therapeutic addition for heart failure patients with central sleep apnoea.[19]

For obstructive sleep apnoea CPAP has been shown to improve in cardiac function, sympathetic activity, and quality of life.[20] For nocturnal Cheyne–Stokes breathing nocturnal-assist servoventilation has been shown to improve daytime sleepiness compared with control. Significant falls also occurred in plasma brain natriuretic peptide and urinary metadrenaline excretion rates suggesting beneficial neurohormonal effects.[21] There remains, however, little evidence from RCTs to tell us whether it is cost-effective to screen routinely for SDB in CHF clinics and to treat all cases so detected.

15.6
Specialist Heart Failure Clinics and Nurses

In recent years the value of comprehensive hospital and community-based heart failure management programs has been accepted and they have become established as the standard of care in many countries. In the Netherlands for example 60% of hospitals support a HF management program. Most of the programs are organized as HF outpatient clinics. In all HF programs, cardiologists and nurses are involved. Other health care providers involved are, amongst others, general practitioners, dieticians, physical therapists, social workers and psychologists. All programs offer follow-up after discharge from the hospitals and in most of the programs patients have increased access to a health care provider. Behavioral interventions, psychosocial counseling, patient education and support of the informal caregivers are important components. In 90% of the programs, physical examination is the responsibility of the HF nurse and in 65% of the programs nurses are involved in optimizing medical treatment.[22]

After hospital discharge follow-up of CHF patients at a nurse-led heart failure clinic has been shown to be associated with fewer patients with events (death or admission) after 12 months (29 vs. 40, $p=0.03$) and fewer deaths after 12 months (7 vs. 20, $p=0.005$) in one study. The intervention group had fewer admissions (33 vs. 56, $p=0.047$) and days in hospital (350 vs. 592, $p=0.045$) during the first 3 months. After 12 months the intervention was associated with a 55% decrease in admissions/patient/month (0.18 vs. 0.40, $p=0.06$) and fewer days in hospital/patient/month (1.4 vs. 3.9, $p=0.02$). The intervention group had significantly higher self-care scores at 3 and 12 months compared to the control group ($p=0.02$ and $p=0.01$).[23]

Intensive home care of middle-aged patients with severe heart failure has been shown to result in improved quality of life and a decrease in hospital readmission rates.[24] A telephone-mediated nurse care management program for heart failure has also been shown to reduce the rate of rehospitalization for heart failure, although it has been suggested such programs may be less effective for patients at low risk compared to higher risk patients.[25, 26] Other reports of home health intervention programs have, however, reported less convincing benefits.[27] Success has also been reported of incorporating palliative care regimes into the management of end-stage CHF.[28]

The evidence to suggest that such CHF programs involving individualized multidisciplinary postdischarge healthcare, with a major focus on specialist nurse management are clinically and economically effective in CHF has been reviewed.[29] These programs appear to be most effective in "high-risk" patients who typically have recurrent readmissions in high-cost units. Overall, the literature suggests that these programs are able to reduce recurrent hospital stay by 30–50% relative to usual care (even in the presence of gold-standard treatment) in the short to medium term with comparable cost benefits.

15.7
Exercise Training

Despite the use of the established treatments CHF remains a common, lethal and disabling condition. From the late 1980s it was realized that many of the noncardiac changes that afflicted CHF patients including loss of skeletal muscle, impaired endothelial function, sympathetic overactivity and vagal withdrawal had become the major factors causing symptoms and limiting exercise tolerance.[30] Many were seen to be were similar, if admittedly more severe, to those seen in physical deconditioning. The earliest reports of a possible beneficial effect of training were seen in the late 1980s in nonrandomized retrospective reports of the benefits to exercise tolerance seen in some participants of cardiac rehabilitation programs that included an element of exercise training despite some having significantly impaired left ventricular systolic function or even a history of treatment for heart failure. The first RCT of exercise training in CHF patients was reported in 1990 and showed that in 11 patients with severe CHF exercise training could be tolerated and could improve patient reported symptoms.[31] In this first trial we showed that exercise training could increase exercise tolerance and improve the symptoms of dyspnoea and fatigue. In eleven patients with chronic heart failure secondary to ischemic heart disease (mean [SEM] age 63.0 [2.3] years; left ventricular ejection fraction (LVEF) 19%[8]) 8 weeks of home-based bicycle exercise training and 8 weeks of activity restriction were prescribed in random-order in a physician-blind, random-order, crossover trial. Training increased exercise duration from 14.2 (1.1) min to 16.8 (1.3) min and peak oxygen consumption from 14.3 (1.1) to 16.7 (1.3) mL/min kg. Heart rates at submaximum workloads and rate-pressure products were significantly reduced by training, and there was also a significant improvement in patient-rated symptom scores. No adverse events occurred during the training phase. This was a home-based physical training program that was shown to be feasible even in severe chronic heart failure.

Over the next 10 years multiple small and medium sized studies confirmed these early results and described a wide array of secondary benefits including improvements in skeletal muscle structure, biochemistry and function, improvements in endothelial function, partial restoration of impaired sympatho-vagal balance and improvement in respiratory control and breathing patterns. Improvements in myocardial performance and gross exercise hemodynamics were less consistent although improved peripheral vascular function was more consistently found.

The first trial to suggest a benefit in major outcomes such as death or heart failure hospitalization rates was performed by Belardinelli et al in Ancona, Italy and was published in 1999. In this trial Belardinelli randomized 99 stable CHF patients (59 ± 14 years of age; 88 men and 11 women) to exercise training at 60% of peak capacity, initially three times a week for 8 weeks, then twice a week for 1 year or control. Ninety-four patients completed the protocol (48 trained and 46 in control). Both quality of life and exercise tolerance were improved and mortality was lower after training ($n=9$ vs. $n=20$ for those with training vs. those without; relative risk (RR)=0.37; 95% CI, 0.17–0.84; $p=0.01$). Fewer hospital readmissions for heart failure were seen in the trained group (5 vs. 14; RR=0.29; 95% CI, 0.11–0.88; $p=0.02$). Although showing a significant reduction in mortality and morbidity, this was not a prospective trial powered and designed to evaluate this effect, so we should not consider this trial alone proved a mortality reducing benefit of exercise training in CHF.[32]

Later two meta-analyses suggested that in combining the results of all the small trials there was a significant 15–25% reduction in the combined endpoint of death or all-cause hospitalization.[33,34] While we waited for definitive evidence from a well powered major multicentre trial as to whether training has prognostic as well as symptomatic benefit, we performed the next-best thing, an individual patient data meta-analysis. This suggested a significant reduction in both the risk of death and in the number of hospitalizations for heart failure. We coordinated a collaborative meta-analysis with inclusion criteria of all randomized parallel group controlled trials of exercise training for at least 8 weeks with individual patient data on survival for at least 3 months. Nine datasets, totaling 801 patients were identified and analyzed; 395 patients received exercise training and 406 were controls. During a mean (SD) follow up of 705 (729) days there were 88 (22%) deaths in the exercise arm and 105 (26%) in the control arm. Exercise training significantly reduced mortality (HR 0.65, 95% CI, 0.46–0.92; log rank

$\chi^2 = 5.9$; $p = 0.015$). The secondary end point of death or admission to hospital was also reduced (0.72, 0.56–0.93; log rank $\chi^2 = 6.4$; $p = 0.011$). No statistically significant subgroup specific treatment effect was observed. We can summarize that training in selected CHF patients is beneficial and safe and can reduce mortality and morbidity.

In a second overview approach we searched the Cochrane Controlled Trials Register (*The Cochrane Library* Issue 2, 2001), MEDLINE (2000 to March 2001), EMBASE (1998 to March 2001), CINAHL (1984 to March 2001) and reference lists of articles, supplemented by direct enquiry of published experts. We selected all RCTs of exercise-based interventions for adults of all ages with chronic heart failure. The comparison group was the usual medical care as defined by the study, or placebo. Only those studies with criteria for diagnosis of heart failure (based on clinical findings or objective indices) were included. Studies were selected, and data were abstracted independently by two reviewers, supplemented by direct enquiry of authors where possible to obtain missing information. Twenty-nine studies were found to meet the inclusion criteria, with 1,126 patients randomized. The majority of studies included both patients with primary and secondary heart failure, NYHA class II or III. None of the studies specifically examined the effect of exercise training on mortality and morbidity as most were of short duration. Exercise training significantly increased VO_2 max by (WMD random effects model) 2.16 mL/kg/min (95% CI 2.82–1.49), exercise duration increased by 2.38 min (95% CI 2.85–1.9), work capacity by 15.1 W (95% CI 17.7–12.6) and distance on the 6-minute walk by 40.9 m (95% CI 64.7–17.1). Improvements in peak oxygen consumption were greater for training programs of greater intensity and duration. Health related quality of life (HRQoL) improved in the seven of nine trials that measured this outcome. We concluded that exercise training improves exercise capacity and quality of life in patients with mild to moderate heart failure in the short term.

The HF-ACTION trial, the largest ever intervention trial of a nonpharmacological treatment in chronic heart failure (CHF) randomized 2,331 stable NYHA class II–IV heart-failure patients with impaired systolic left ventricular function (ejection fraction ≤35%) to either a structured exercise program or to usual care. It assessed the effect of exercise training on mortality and morbidity and quality of life.[35, 36] Importantly the control group had a similar frequency of contact with the trial staff and expertise in heart failure management as the intervention group, receiving in the process advice on exercise and other heart failure care but without any specific exercise prescription. The exercise intervention started with supervised training sessions in hospital and after 18–36 weeks progressed to patient-initiated home-based training, predominantly aerobic training utilizing a bicycle or treadmill. Patients were followed up for a minimum of 1 year, a maximum of 4 and a median of 30 months. The primary end-point, the effect on all-cause mortality or all-cause hospitalization, was not reached at the prespecified significance level (−7%, $p = 0.13$). A prespecified baseline prognostic risk factor adjusted analysis, however, did show a significant 11% ($p = 0.03$) reduction in death or hospitalization in favor of training. On the basis of this trial result, combined with the prior evidence of two meta-analyses of the pre-HF-ACTION studies and the finding that training improves exercise tolerance and many aspects of pathophysiology[37] of the condition, it is the belief of most experts that exercise training should be recommended for all suitable heart failure patients.

HF-ACTION was designed to answer two related questions: would an exercise prescription reduce mortality and morbidity significantly when compared to usual care and is it safe for CHF patients to undertake such an intervention. Unlike a drug trial the treatment cannot be made double-blind and unlike tablets adherence to treatment requires active participation by the patients, who may be lazy, scared and/or easily fatigued or made short of breath by exercise. A much-enhanced dropout rate is to be expected, and compliance with exercise did fall significantly during the trial, as had been earlier seen in a Canadian trial of home-based training.[38]

The second report from HF-ACTION (Flynn et al) analyzed the results of a well-validated quality of life questionnaire (the Kansas City Cardiomyopathy Questionnaire). It showed significant improvements in both the global score and in all four subdimensions of the questionnaire (Physical limitations, Symptoms, Quality-of-life, and Social limitations) within 3 months of commencing training, improvements that were maintained for the duration of follow-up.

15.8
Questions and Controversies

Several questions remain unanswered about the best use of exercise training for chronic heart failure. We do not know the best and safest training regimens. Although the early trials used almost exclusively an aerobic training regimen (approximately 3 days a week for 20–60 min per session) other more recent trials have also looked at the efficacy and safety of exercise including resistance training. One study evaluated the effects of combined endurance/resistance training on NT-proBNP levels in patients with chronic heart failure (CHF). In this study, 27 consecutive patients with stable CHF and LVEF <35% were enrolled in a 4 months nonrandomized combined endurance/resistance training program. After 4 months, exercise training caused a significant reduction in circulating concentrations of NT-proBNP ($2,124 \pm 397$ pg/mL before, $1,635 \pm 304$ pg/mL after training, $p=0.046$, interaction), whereas no changes were observed in an untrained heart failure control group. This suggests that combined endurance/resistance training significantly reduced circulating levels of NT-proBNP in patients with CHF, arguing against any increase in adverse remodeling.[39] Other recent trials have shown an element of resistance as well as aerobic training to be beneficial, especially for improving muscle strength, bulk and endurance. The optimal mix of the two forms of exercise remains uncertain.[40]

Some supervised in-hospital training is necessary, especially at the commencement of a training program, and may well be beneficial for encouraging long term adherence at regular indefinite intervals. Home-based training can also be recommended in well-evaluated patients to make this a more practical treatment option for larger numbers of patients. McKelvie et al in the EXERT trial randomized 181 patients in New York Heart Association class I to III heart failure, (ejection fraction <40% and 6-minute walk distance <500 m) to 3 months of supervised training, then 9 months of home-based training or to usual care for 12 months. Training induced a significant increase in 6-minute walk distance at 3 and 12 months but no between-group differences. Incremental peak oxygen uptake increased in the exercise group compared with the control group at 3 months (0.104 ± 0.026 vs. 0.025 ± 0.023 L/min; $p=0.026$) and 12 months (0.154 ± 0.074 vs. 0.024 ± 0.027 L/min; $p=0.081$). Compared with the control group, significant increases were observed in the exercise group for arm and leg strength. No significant changes were observed in cardiac function or quality of life. Adherence to exercise was good during supervised training but reduced during home-based training. The authors noted that over the final 9 months of the study, there was little further improvement, suggesting that some in-hospital supervision of training may be necessary to continue to obtain benefit. In this regard it is interesting to note that the authors of the HF-ACTION trial did note that compliance with exercise did fall significantly during their trial as the patients entered the home-only phase of training. Others have gone further and advise against home-based exercise training in a community setting.[41] A Birmingham, UK group assessed the effectiveness of a home-based exercise program in addition to specialist heart failure nurse care in a RCT of a home-based walking and resistance exercise program plus specialist nurse care ($n=84$) compared with specialist nurse care alone ($n=85$) in a heart failure population in the West Midlands, UK. The Minnesota Living with Heart Failure Questionnaire (MLwHFQ) at 6 and 12 months was statistically significant and different between groups. There was, however, lower Hospital Anxiety and Depression Scale score (-1.07, -2.00 to -0.14) at 12 months, in favor of the exercise group. At 6 months, the control group showed a deterioration in physical activity, exercise capacity, and generic quality of life compared to the intervention group. Surprisingly given these results, the authors expressed the opinion that home-based exercise training programs may not be appropriate for community-based heart failure patients. In contrast a Canadian group examining the sustainability of training benefits in patients with heart failure 12 months after discharge from a RCT of 6 months of monitored home-based vs. supervised hospital-based in 198 patients, 102 previously randomized to "Hospital" training and 96 to "Home" training. At 12-months after discharge both groups had similar medical and socio-demographic characteristics, peak VO_2 declined in "Hospital" but was sustained in "Home" patients 12 months after discharge from CR ($p=0.002$) and physical HRQL was higher in the "Home" group at the 12-month follow-up. Twelve months after discharge "Home" patients had higher habitual physical activity scores compared to "Hospital" patients. They suggested that low-risk patients whose training is initiated in the home environment may be more likely to sustain positive physical and psychosocial changes over time than patients whose program is initially institution-based. The issue of optimal use of both the in-hospital and home-based training environment remains uncertain. It is my belief that the largest training effect can be produced by in-hospital training but that economic and resource concerns dictate that patients would then migrate to using more home-based training, whilst preserving a high participation rate in their exercise by regular refresher courses and the encouragement of some ongoing in-hospital training sessions.

References

1. Middlekauff HR. How does cardiac resynchronization therapy improve exercise capacity in chronic heart failure? *J Card Fail.* 2005;11(7):534-541 [review].
2. Colonna P, Sorino M, D'Agostino C, et al. Nonpharmacologic care of heart failure: counseling, dietary restriction, rehabilitation, treatment of sleep apnea, and ultrafiltration. *Am J Cardiol.* 2003;91(9A):41F-50F.

3. Anker SD, Ponikowski P, Varney S, et al. Wasting as independent risk factor for mortality in chronic heart failure. *Lancet*. 1997;349(9058):1050-1053.

4. Anker SD, Negassa A, Coats AJ, et al. Prognostic importance of weight loss in chronic heart failure and the effect of treatment with angiotensin-converting-enzyme inhibitors: an observational study. *Lancet*. 2003;361(9363):1077-1083.

5. Curtis JP, Selter JG, Wang Y, et al. Body mass index and outcomes in patients with heart failure. *Arch Intern Med*. 2005;165:55-61.

6. Pasini E, Opasich C, Pastoris O, Aquilani R. Inadequate nutritional intake for daily life activity of clinically stable patients with chronic heart failure. *Am J Cardiol*. 2004;93(8A):41A-43A.

7. Colin Ramirez E, Castillo Martinez L, Orea Tejeda A, Rebollar Gonzalez V, Narvaez David R, Asensio Lafuente E. Effects of a nutritional intervention on body composition, clinical status, and quality of life in patients with heart failure. *Nutrition*. 2004;20(10):890-895.

8. Kuehneman T, Saulsbury D, Splett P, Chapman DB. Demonstrating the impact of nutrition intervention in a heart failure program. *J Am Diet Assoc*. 2002;102(12):1790-1794.

9. Faris R, Purcell H, Henein MY, Coats AJ. Clinical depression is common and significantly associated with reduced survival in patients with non-ischaemic heart failure. *Eur J Heart Fail*. 2002;4(4):541-551.

10. Gottlieb SS, Khatta M, Friedmann E, et al. The influence of age, gender, and race on the prevalence of depression in heart failure patients. *J Am Coll Cardiol*. 2004;43(9):1542-1549.

11. de Leon CF, Grady KL, Eaton C, et al. Quality of life in a diverse population of patients with heart failure: baseline findings from The Heart Failure Adherence and Retention Trial (HART). *J Cardiopulm Rehabil Prev*. 2009;29(3):171-178.

12. Gottlieb SS, Kop WJ, Ellis SJ, et al.; HF-ACTION Investigators. Relation of depression to severity of illness in heart failure (from Heart Failure And a Controlled Trial Investigating Outcomes of Exercise Training [HF-ACTION]). *Am J Cardiol*. 2009;103(9):1285-1289.

13. Fraguas R, da Silva Telles RM, Alves TC, et al. A Double-blind, Placebo-controlled Treatment Trial of Citalopram for major depressive disorder in older patients with heart failure: the relevance of the placebo effect and psychological symptoms. *Contemp Clin Trials*. 2009;30:205-211.

14. Sullivan MJ, Wood L, Terry J, et al. The Support, Education, and Research in Chronic Heart Failure Study (SEARCH): a mindfulness-based psychoeducational intervention improves depression and clinical symptoms in patients with chronic heart failure. *Am Heart J*. 2009;157(1):84-90.

15. Trupp RJ, Hardesty P, Osborne J, et al. Prevalence of sleep disordered breathing in a heart failure program. *Congest Heart Fail*. 2004;10(5):217-220.

16. Eskafi M, Ekberg E, Cline C, Israelsson B, Nilner M. Use of a mandibular advancement device in patients with congestive heart failure and sleep apnoea. *Gerodontology*. 2004;21(2):100-107.

17. Chua TP, Clark AL, Amadi AA, Coats AJ. Relation between chemosensitivity and the ventilatory response to exercise in chronic heart failure. *J Am Coll Cardiol*. 1996;27(3):650-657.

18. Szollosi I, Jones M, Morrell MJ, Helfet K, Coats AJ, Simonds AK. Effect of CO_2 inhalation on central sleep apnea and arousals from sleep. *Respiration*. 2004;71(5):493-498.

19. Sasayama S, Izumi T, Matsuzaki M, et al.; The CHF-HOT Study Group. Improvement of quality of life with nocturnal oxygen therapy in heart failure patients with central sleep apnea. *Circ J*. 2009;73:1255-1262.

20. Mansfield DR, Gollogly NC, Kaye DM, Richardson M, Bergin P, Naughton MT. Controlled trial of continuous positive airway pressure in obstructive sleep apnea and heart failure. *Am J Respir Crit Care Med*. 2004;169(3):361-366.

21. Pepperell JC, Maskell NA, Jones DR, et al. A randomized controlled trial of adaptive ventilation for Cheyne-Stokes breathing in heart failure. *Am J Respir Crit Care Med*. 2003;168(9):1109-1114.

22. Jaarsma T, Tan B, Bos RJ, van Veldhuisen DJ. Heart failure clinics in the Netherlands in 2003. *Eur J Cardiovasc Nurs.* 2004;3(4):271-274.

23. Stromberg A, Martensson J, Fridlund B, Levin LA, Karlsson JE, Dahlstrom U. Nurse-led heart failure clinics improve survival and self-care behaviour in patients with heart failure: results from a prospective, randomised trial. *Eur Heart J.* 2003;24(11):1014-1023.

24. Vavouranakis I, Lambrogiannakis E, Markakis G, et al. Effect of home-based intervention on hospital readmission and quality of life in middle-aged patients with severe congestive heart failure: a 12-month follow up study. *Eur J Cardiovasc Nurs.* 2003;2(2):105-111.

25. Berg GD, Wadhwa S, Johnson AE. A matched-cohort study of health services utilization and financial outcomes for a heart failure disease-management program in elderly patients. *J Am Geriatr Soc.* 2004;52(10):1655-1661.

26. DeBusk RF, Miller NH, Parker KM, et al. Care management for low-risk patients with heart failure: a randomized, controlled trial. *Ann Intern Med.* 2004;141(8):606-613.

27. Feldman PH, Peng TR, Murtaugh CM, et al. A randomized intervention to improve heart failure outcomes in community-based home health care. *Home Health Care Serv Q.* 2004;23(1):1-23.

28. Davidson PM, Paull G, Introna K, et al. Integrated, collaborative palliative care in heart failure: the St. George Heart Failure Service experience 1999-2002. *J Cardiovasc Nurs.* 2004;19(1):68-75.

29. Stewart S, Horowitz JD. Specialist nurse management programmes: economic benefits in the management of heart failure. *Pharmacoeconomics.* 2003;21(4):225-240.

30. Clark AL, Poole-Wilson PA, Coats AJ. Exercise limitation in chronic heart failure: central role of the periphery. *J Am Coll Cardiol.* 1996;28(5):1092-1102 [review].

31. Coats AJ, Adamopoulos S, Meyer TE, Conway J, Sleight P. Effects of physical training in chronic heart failure. *Lancet.* 1990;335(8681):63-66.

32. Belardinelli R, Georgiou D, Cianci G, Purcaro A. Randomized, controlled trial of long-term moderate exercise training in chronic heart failure: effects on functional capacity, quality of life, and clinical outcome. *Circulation.* 1999;99(9):1173-1182.

33. Piepoli MF, Davos C, Francis DP, Coats AJ; ExTraMATCH Collaborative. Exercise training meta-analysis of trials in patients with chronic heart failure (ExTraMATCH). *BMJ.* 2004;328(7433):189.

34. Taylor RS, Brown A, Ebrahim S, et al. Exercise-based rehabilitation for patients with coronary heart disease: systematic review and meta-analysis of randomized controlled trials. *Am J Med.* 2004;116(10):682-692.

35. O'Connor CM, Whellan DJ, Lee KL, et al.; HF-ACTION Investigators. Efficacy and safety of exercise training in patients with chronic heart failure: HF-ACTION randomized controlled trial. *JAMA.* 2009;301(14):1439-1450.

36. Flynn KE, Piña IL, Whellan DJ, et al. Effects of exercise training on health status in patients with chronic heart failure: HF-ACTION randomized controlled trial. *JAMA.* 2009;301(14):1451-1459.

37. Crimi E, Ignarro LJ, Cacciatore F, Napoli C. Mechanisms by which exercise training benefits patients with heart failure. *Nat Rev Cardiol.* 2009;6(4):292-300.

38. McKelvie RS, Teo KK, Roberts R, et al. Effects of exercise training in patients with heart failure: the Exercise Rehabilitation Trial (EXERT). *Am Heart J.* 2002;144(1):23-30.

39. Conraads VM, Beckers P, Vaes J, et al. Combined endurance/resistance training reduces NT-proBNP levels in patients with chronic heart failure. *Eur Heart J.* 2004;25(20):1797-1805.

40. Gunn E, Smith KM, McKelvie RS, Arthur HM. Exercise and the heart failure patient: aerobic vs strength training–is there a need for both? *Prog Cardiovasc Nurs.* 2006 Summer;21(3):146-150 [review].

41. Jolly K, Taylor RS, Lip GY, et al. A randomized trial of the addition of home-based exercise to specialist heart failure nurse care: the Birmingham Rehabilitation Uptake Maximisation study for patients with Congestive Heart Failure (BRUM-CHF) study. *Eur J Heart Fail.* 2009;11(2):205-213.

Atrial Fibrillation and Heart Failure Syndromes

16

Lynne Williams, Gregory Y. H. Lip, and Robert J. MacFadyen

Heart failure syndromes are characterized by acute and chronic symptomatic clinical presentations of variable etiology. Definitions of heart failure in many studies and surveys vary enormously. Most heart failures involve failure of cardiac mechanics resulting in reduced stroke volume or cardiac work, which in turn occur as a consequence of several processes. Heart failure syndromes are frequently characterized as primarily linked to either systolic or diastolic ventricular dysfunction but most often involve combinations of both to result in elevated pulmonary pressure and pulmonary edema causing breathlessness and exercise limitation.

Changes in cardiac rhythm and conduction are integral to many patients presentation or the evolution of their disease. The impact of atrial fibrillation (AF), while a relatively straightforward ECG diagnosis, in contrast occurs by a variety of mechanisms, and its impact depends critically on the setting in which it occurs. AF has a key role to play in heart failure syndromes and in some cases in the presentation and the evolution of ventricular dysfunction. The detection of and integration of AF into heart failure pathobiology is complex, and the presence of AF cannot be viewed as an isolated phenomenon within HF.

In most cases, the evolution of AF in HF can be expected if not predicted individually. It often appears due to a failure to recognize evolving changes in cardiac conduction (most often sinus node disease) with progressive HF, advancing age; poor treatment choices (prominently uncontrolled hypertension and worsening hypertensive heart disease) or failure to control an etiological process linked to AF such as recurrent ischemia; primary or secondary valve dysfunction (most often mitral regurgitation and atrial dilatation); atherosclerosis; progressive renal dysfunction; structural cardiac remodeling or neurohormonal suppression. Ultimately the evolution of AF in a HF syndrome in most cases results in a significant worsening of symptom control, marks a poorer prognosis, and is associated with important changes in management strategy.

R.J. MacFadyen (✉)
University Department of Medicine, City Hospital, Dudley Road, Birmingham, UK
e-mail: robert.macfadyen@swbh.nhs.uk

M.Y. Henein (ed.), *Heart Failure in Clinical Practice*,
DOI: 10.1007/978-1-84996-153-0_16, © Springer-Verlag London Limited 2010

16.1
Epidemiology

First, interpreting the epidemiology of AF in heart failure symptoms is unfortunately complicated by frequent failure to separate the etiology of AF in HF. Secondly, data are often selected from population studies of AF where there is poor definition of HF and overlapping samples with patients whose AF links to entirely separate processes. Most AF epidemiology relevant to HF is therefore an inadequate summary of prevalence and detailed linkages present and gives an incomplete or overly simplified image of the biology behind clinical practice.

16.1.1
Prevalence

AF is frequently cited as "the most common arrhythmia" whose overall prevalence is approximately 1.5% of the population. A nominal HF diagnosis is suggested to be relevant to 15–20 million people worldwide, linked to increasing age, and the consequence of improved therapies for coronary artery disease resulting in nonfatal infarction in place of fatal infarction. Thus HF has become a dominant association with the development of AF in surveys from many developed countries.

Superficially, AF and HF presentations share many similar statistically independent "clinical risk factors" (Table 16.1). In some population samples, two thirds of HF patients are over the age of 65 and on this ground alone are likely to have AF as a coexistent condition. The complication of whether this is as a consequence of aging and/or HF or that AF causes a HF diagnosis to emerge is much harder to define from these associations. Data from the Framingham study suggest that the presence of a HF diagnosis increases the risk of AF appearing by 4.5-fold in men and 5.9-fold in women.[1] The EuroHeart Failure survey conducted in 2000–2001 reported the presence of AF (either as a

Table 16.1 Risk factors common to atrial fibrillation (AF) and congestive heart failure (CHF)

Risk factor	Odds ratio for AF (Male / Female)	Hazard ratio for CHF (Both sexes)
Hypertension	1.4 / 1.5	1.32
Myocardial infarction (STEMI of NSTEMI)	1.4 / 1.2	1.63
Diabetes	1.4 / 1.6	1.31
Age	2.1 / 2.2	1.77
Smoking	1.1 / 1.4	1.28
Valvular heart disease	1.8 / 3.4	1.96
Heart failure	4.5 / 5.9	NA

STEMI: ST-elevation myocardial infarction; NSTEMI: non ST-elevation myocardial infarction. Adapted from Morrison et al[98]

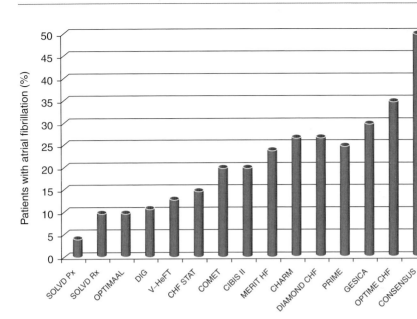

Fig. 16.1 Prevalence of atrial fibrillation in clinical studies of heart failure. Adapted from Ref[97]

paroxysmal or permanent rhythm change) in up to 45% of patients,[2] with an overall prevalence of new onset AF in patients hospitalized for heart failure ranging from 8 to 36% in different regions of Europe. The prevalence of AF has been shown to correlate with the severity of systolic heart failure and underlying left ventricular dysfunction, with rates of 10–20% in mild to moderate disease, but estimates of up to 50% with advanced disease (Fig. 16.1).[3]

16.1.2
Prognosis

The prognostic importance of emergent AF in any heart failure patient is clearly linked to the origins of the rhythm change and its potential for reversibility. Whether this reflects a temporary change producing an acute decompensation and provoked by a reversible stimulus such as acute reversible ischemia, transient mitral valve dysfunction; treatable sepsis, intoxication, hormone imbalance or drug interaction remains poorly defined in epidemiological studies. Population level analyses from clinical trials samples in HF patients are less rewarding as they frequently contain inadequate patient diagnostic detail with respect to AF. However, broad subgroup analysis of the large clinical trials such as SOLVD,[4] VAL-HeFT,[5] and serial community observations from the Framingham Heart Study[6] demonstrate the obvious fact that the presence or development of AF at any time, and by any means, is associated with higher mortality. In the SOLVD study, the 1.34-fold increase in all-cause mortality conferred by AF appeared to be related to death from progressive pump failure rather than changes in sudden cardiac death.[4] In the setting of the Framingham study, the definition of AF was suggested to show a gender specific difference in prognosis with a 2.7-fold increase in mortality in women but only a 1.6-fold increase in men. Why this should occur was not clear.[6] The DIG study, examining primarily the impact of digoxin in HF patients in sinus rhythm, revealed that the emergence of an atrial tachyarrhythmia (predominantly AF) predicted a 2.5-fold risk of subsequent mortality and an threefold risk of hospitalizations for worsening heart failure symptoms.[7] Finally, data from the Italian Network on Congestive Heart Failure cohort study[8] confirmed that chronic AF was an independent predictor of both all-cause mortality and sudden death, with a hazard ratio similar to those associated with factors such as age, NHYA class, systolic blood pressure, presence of ventricular arrhythmias, and the presence of a left bundle branch block (LBBB). In those patients with both chronic AF and a LBBB on surface ECG (3.3% of the entire cohort), the risk of death was particularly high, as was the rehospitalization rate for heart failure.[9]

The impact of underlying cardiac contraction on the prognostic significance of AF is interesting. AF appears to have variable effects on 5-year survival in patients with heart failure symptoms dependent on the integrity of underlying left ventricular contraction. When compared with patients in sinus rhythm and preserved LVEF, survival is significantly reduced in patients with AF and a left ventricular ejection fraction >55%. Milder reductions in systolic LVEF (between 41 and 55%) are challenging to interpret but in these patients also there appears to be a reduction in survival where AF is present. Perhaps in contrast the appearance of AF in cases with more significant systolic ventricular dysfunction appears to make no difference to survival. The most likely explanation for this anomaly is that the impact of AF in these cases is overwhelmed by the significant mortality impact of the severity of the underlying systolic ventricular dysfunction as the dominant factor in survival.[10]

Fundamentally, the documentation of AF is problematic in studies of patients with HF syndromes. Population surveys of prevalence depend critically on the sample frame and size and more importantly the technique used to define AF. AF is frequently paroxysmal and even in patients with significant ventricular dysfunction, where the hemodynamic impact of the loss of atrial systole and diastolic filling is greatest, these patients need not always be symptomatic to rhythm change, which might be needed to facilitate detection of AF by ECG recording. What is clear is that dependent on the etiology of paroxysmal atrial fibrillation (PAF) and whether symptomatic or not, PAF leading to permanent rhythm change and permanent AF is far more likely to be documented that PAF. Whether underlying HF syndromes causally facilitate the progression of AF from paroxysmal to permanent AF,[11] with progression to permanent AF in turn resulting in an adverse effect on mortality compared with PAF has been suggested but is not clearly defined.[12]

16.2
Pathophysiology

In a point population survey of patients with a diagnosis of both a heart failure syndrome and coexistent AF, it is impossible to separate the primary underlying condition. For example in the Framingham Heart Study, as many as 20% of the participants who went on to develop heart failure or AF were "diagnosed" with both conditions on the same day implying simultaneous recognition rather than sequential appearance of one or the other.[6] In clinical practice, however, we appreciate that in the majority of patients, one condition is recognized prior to the development of the other, implying causality as opposed to consequence. Fundamental to this is an appreciation that a better understanding of the etiology of individual cases and the interaction between AF and heart failure syndromes is essential to target therapies aimed at either interrupting the development of either AF in heart failure or vice versa, and preventing disease progression of either in established cases.

Approximately, 15–25% of patients with known AF go on to develop a heart failure syndrome.[6,13] Loss of sinus rhythm and permanent AF can influence ventricular function via a number of mechanisms including its association with increased sympathetic tone, secondary ventricular dilatation and wall thinning (through tachycardiomyopathy), and impaired systolic ventricular contraction or contractile synchrony.[14] Upon resolution of tachycardia, pathologic changes of the ventricle lead to diastolic dysfunction.[14-16] Just as AF can lead to impaired ventricular function, abnormal ventricular function, either systolic or diastolic in origin, can lead to the development of AF.

Animal studies and experimental models have contributed to identifying the pathophysiological mechanisms by which patients with heart failure syndromes go on to develop AF. Most of these focus on changes to the underlying electrophysiological properties of the atria with the net effect being to lower the arrhythmia threshold and increase susceptibility to the development of AF.[17] Systolic heart failure results in abnormalities of multiple ion channels, including a decrease in the density of L-type Ca^{2+} (I_{Ca}), transient outward K^+ (IK_o), and slow, delayed rectifier currents (IK_s), as well as an increased transient inward Na^+/Ca^{2+} exchanger current, resulted in an increased risk of AF and an increase AF duration.[18] In animal experiments, paroxysms of AF have been shown to result in an increase in atrial interstitial fibrosis, which in turn promotes heterogeneous atrial conduction and an increase in the duration of AF.[19] Thus the underlying clinical paradigm of "AF begets AF." Changes in atrial structure seen in systolic heart failure, such as atrial stretch and fibrosis, also contribute to the predisposition to AF. Changes in ventricular dimensions and or mitral valve function (predominantly ischemic but also functional valvular regurgitation due to torsional change in papillary muscle mechanics) equally can contribute to altering atrial electro mechanical remodeling in systolic heart failure.

Diastolic dysfunction and its linkage to AF in HF syndromes is more complex and confounded frequently by the role of arterial hypertension and its control (or more often lack of adequate control and the prevalence of left ventricular hypertrophy). In hypertensive heart disease, increased diastolic ventricular filling pressures can directly lead to atrial stretch, which in turn results in increased left atrial size and, subsequently, increased risk for AF.[20] Additionally, progressive diastolic dysfunction, independent of left atrial size, is associated with an increasing risk of AF over 5 years, from 1% in patients with normal diastolic function to 21% in those with evidence of restrictive ventricular diastolic filling.[21] Additional mechanisms may play a role in this setting, and patients with diastolic heart failure and hypertension who carry a variant of the aldosterone synthase gene (and subsequently have nominally increased aldosterone levels) have a small increased risk of developing AF.[22]

16.3
Management

16.3.1
Prevention

16.3.1.1
ACE-I/ARB

The role of blocking the renin angiotensin aldosterone system (RAAS) using angiotensin converting enzyme inhibitors (ACE-i) in the prevention of morbidity and mortality in systolic heart failure and in patients with hypertensive heart disease is well accepted. Any vasodilator decreasing after load could potentially slow the progression of left ventricular diastolic dysfunction and potentially result in beneficial effects on left atrial remodeling.[23] However, drugs that modify activity of the RAAS appear to have effects on left atrial remodeling over and above the effect on after load reduction. In animal models of systolic dysfunction or experimental LVH, ACE inhibitor treatment reduces cardiac fibrosis and in particular results in a decrease in atrial fibrosis and AF episode duration.[24] ACE inhibition has been shown to have beneficial effects on atrial stretch,[25,26] interstitial fibrosis,[27-29] inflammation,[30-32] bioenergetics,[33] and electrical remodeling,[34,35] and has been shown to delay or defer first and recurrent AF in patients with hypertension[36] and left ventricular dysfunction.[5,36-39]

Two large meta-analyses have suggested that inhibition of the RAAS in humans may also show evidence for deferred emergence of AF. A meta-analysis of 11 randomized clinical trials with 56, 308 patients demonstrated a significantly reduced incidence of AF in patients with systolic heart failure (relative risk reduction of 44%).[40] A second meta-analysis of nine randomized controlled trials demonstrated a 18% risk reduction in new-onset AF across the trials and a 43% risk reduction in patients with heart failure.[41] It must be clear that this evidence is not conclusive and does not suggest that these important treatments prevent AF appearing altogether but merely that on balance there is perhaps a specific benefit in deferring this rhythm change by these treatments compared to the alternatives.

16.3.2
Pharmacologic Therapies

Managing AF in heart failure syndromes is complex. Despite the adverse hemodynamic effect of the onset of permanent AF in systolic dysfunction available data from AF as a whole does not support attempts to restore sinus conduction at all costs.[42,43] However, only a small minority of participants enrolled in these studies of AF had documented systolic dysfunction. In fact the main causal pathology in these studies was hypertensive heart disease. In the AFFIRM trial only 23% of patients had a prior heart failure diagnosis, and the mean LVEF for the group was typically well preserved at 55%.[42] The recent atrial fibrillation and congestive heart failure (AF-CHF) trial was a prospective, multi-center, randomized trial of 1,376 patients with paroxysmal or persistent AF and an LVEF <35% associated with NYHA Class III/IV symptoms.[44] Patients were randomized to either a rate-control strategy (using beta-blockers and/or digoxin with AV nodal ablation if drugs were ineffective) or a rhythm-control approach (amiodarone along with electrical cardioversion as needed). Death from cardiovascular causes, adjusted for baseline differences, was similar in both groups. Secondary outcomes, including death from any cause, stroke, and worsening heart failure, were also similar in both groups. Thus, it would appear that despite the logic and hemodynamic benefits of sinus rhythm, strategies to maintain or restore it in systolic heart failure patients are not effective in terms of hard outcomes.

16.3.2.1
Rate Control

Rate control of AF is based mainly on pharmacologic depression of atrio-ventricular nodal conduction, and there are a large range of drug therapies to achieve this end. However, in the presence of HF, this strategy requires cautious clinical assessment to avoid iatrogenic injury induced by coexistent negative inotropic effects of some drug treatments (e.g., Verapamil or Diltiazem) or interaction with occult AV or ventricular conduction disease. These may cause symptomatic bradycardia or unprovoked syncope with injury leading to a need for permanent pacemaker therapy. Equally any rate control strategy must be seen to give adequate rate control to optimize ventricular cardiac output particularly in the absence of atrial systole.

Consensus suggests a preference for the use of beta-blockers, with additional benefit derived from a combination with digoxin (in contrast to the poor efficacy of digoxin monotherapy). The former strategy is likely to provide adequate rate control both at rest and on exertion, in addition to the overall documented beneficial effects of both agents in systolic heart failure. Although calcium channel blockers are effective for rate-control in patients with AF alone, they should be used with caution in patients with both AF and systolic ventricular dysfunction due to their documented negative inotropic effects.[45] In the AFFIRM substudy, long-term rate control was achieved with beta-blockers alone in 58%, and when used in combination with digoxin, in 70% of patients.[46] The retrospective analysis of the US Carvedilol study demonstrated a greater survival benefit of Carvedilol in heart failure patients when used concurrently with digoxin, the combination being superior to either agent alone.[47] Amiodarone is also clearly effective for rate control, but due to its adverse side-effect profile should be reserved for those cases where other medications have failed to control symptoms attributable to poor rate control.[48,49]

AV nodal ablation may be an alternative treatment in the presence of intolerable symptoms and poor rate control despite pharmacologic therapies. Studies have shown no significant difference between pharmacologic and nonpharmacologic strategies for rate control in terms of quality of life, cardiac performance, or mortality. However, limited trials of patients assigned to an "ablate and pace" strategy have been shown to have fewer symptoms of palpitation and better control of exertional dyspnoea.[50,51]

16.3.2.2
Rhythm Control

The effect of rhythm control (attempts to restore or preserve sinus rhythm in those HF patients who have converted to AF) with pharmacologic therapies has been evaluated in several clinical trials. The main treatment tested in these strategies has been the class III anti-arrhythmic agent amiodarone. These have shown no significant effect on mortality, hospitalization, or symptom class despite successfully increasing the probability of conversion to, and maintenance of, sinus rhythm. The presence of sinus rhythm in HF, by whatever method it is achieved, is clearly a favorable prognostic factor[42,49,52] but clearly the loss of sinus rhythm and subsequent restoration is not an equivalent state in terms of prognosis. Notwithstanding this the potential of amiodarone to maintain sinus rhythm in patients with HF has been demonstrated repeatedly in several studies, including the Canadian Trial of Atrial Fibrillation (CTAF)[53] and the Congestive Heart Failure Survival Trial of Antiarrhythmic Therapy (CHF-STAT).[54] Given its neutral effect on all-cause mortality, amiodarone is the drug of choice for rhythm control in heart failure patients.

A newer class III drug, Dronedarone, shares many electrophysiological effects with amiodarone. Several randomized studies in differing populations of patients with AF have shown its ability prolong time to recurrence of AF after electrical cardioversion in the DAFNE trial,[55] and prevent recurrences of AF in the EURIDIS and ADONIS trials (unpublished data). However, these early efficacy trials excluded patients with significant left ventricular dysfunction. Although the subsequent ATHENA (a trial with dronedarone to prevent hospitalization or death in patients with atrial fibrillation) trial in HF patients suggested a reduction in cardiovascular mortality and hospitalisations,[56] these results were not reproducible in the ANDROMEDA (antiarrhythmic trial with Dronedarone to moderate to severe CHF evaluating morbidity decrease) trial. The latter, larger, trial was halted prematurely as interim analysis suggested a significantly increased mortality in patients on active Dronedarone treatment, mostly related to worsening heart failure in patients with NYHA Class III/IV functional status.[57]

Dofetilide, a class III antiarrhythmic agent which is the d-stereoisomer of d/l sotalol, is considered safe for the treatment of AF in patients with underlying heart disease. Treatment has been shown to increase the likelihood of maintaining sinus rhythm at 1 year, as well as preventing new cases of AF in patients with symptomatic heart failure. The restoration and maintenance of sinus rhythm was also associated with a significant survival benefit and reduced hospitalisations.[58,59] However, use of dofetilide in HF, similar to the profile seen with sotalol, is pro arrhythmogenic. Treatment is associated with an increased risk of torsades de pointes ventricular tachycardia and the long-term risk benefit of this drug is largely unknown.

In a meta-analysis of four randomized controlled trials of 1,380 patients, a further class III agent, azimilide, at high doses (100 and 125 mg/day) has been shown to prolong time to symptomatic recurrence of AF, with the impact being greatest in those with a history of coronary artery disease or heart failure.[60] In the ALIVE (AzimiLide post-infarct survival evaluation) trial of this agent, there was a lower incidence of new cases of AF and a trend toward higher conversion rates to sinus rhythm in 3,000 patients with recent infarcts and evidence of left ventricular systolic dysfunction.[61] There was no effect on all-cause mortality.[62]

The balance of use of anti-arrhythmic drug therapy for AF in HF is complex. Many treatments aimed at rhythm control and restoration of sinus rhythm, while conceptually attractive do not guarantee better outcome and some have a cost in terms of iatrogenic injury. Anti-arrhythmic therapy designed to restore or retain sinus rhythm continues to have a role in the management of AF in heart failure, in those patients intolerant to rate control, when this strategy is ineffective, or particularly when the onset of AF results in acute decompensated heart failure (as is often the case in hypertensive heart disease). The potential hazards associated with these agents have led to much of the interest in nonpharmacologic strategies for rhythm control.

16.4
Nonpharmacologic Therapies

16.4.1
Catheter Ablation

In most consensus guidelines, nonpharmacologic therapies for AF in HF syndromes are considered second-line strategies, used when drugs have failed or are limited by unacceptable side effects. Trials with drug therapy in impaired ventricular function and a lowered arrhythmia threshold such as the AFFIRM study have also highlighted the potential of maintaining sinus rhythm, if achievable avoiding the adverse effects of antiarrhythmic agents.[63] The development of catheter ablation of atrial arrhythmias has been developed over many years. In some settings, this has been established for AF management as an effective therapeutic option usually in cases resistant to pharmacologic rate or rhythm control. Generally, repeated procedures can create successful long-term maintenance of sinus rhythm without a need for adjunct anti-arrhythmic therapy in the majority of patients.[64,65] Catheter ablation has been shown to improve left ventricular function, exercise capacity, quality of life, and symptoms related to both arrhythmia and heart failure.[66,67] In the study by Hsu et al., these benefits were demonstrated even in patients who had concurrent structural heart disease and adequate rate control prior to ablation, with an increase in left ventricular ejection fraction of around 21% in patients with heart failure.[67] Although the success rates associated with newer technologies have been improving (>80% success in cases of PAF), catheter-based ablation of permanent AF is more technically challenging, requiring extensive ablation, prolonged procedure times, and often multiple procedures. The cost effectiveness of these procedures and their impact on longer term morbidity and mortality has hardly been addressed.

Less sophisticated, more radical, and cheaper options such as atrio-ventricular nodal ablation and permanent pacemaker implantation have been outlined.[50,68,69] Although this strategy provides effective rate limitation and a regular ventricular rhythm, there is also a resultant loss of coordinated atrial contraction, and the real potential of an adverse effect of right ventricular pacing in patients with systolic dysfunction.[50] Nodal ablation after biventricular pacemaker insertion is, however, now a routine adjunct procedure to ensure adequate paced cycles in patients with systolic heart failure and left conduction block receiving cardiac resynchronization therapy. In the PAVE study, patients undergoing AV nodal ablation were randomized to either biventricular or right ventricular pacing, and at 6-months biventricular pacing resulted in a significant increase in left ventricular ejection fraction and exercise tolerance.[70] Results from the PABA-CHF study, which compares pulmonary vein isolation (PVI) with AV node ablation and biventricular pacing (AVNA/BVP), has demonstrated significant improvements in quality of life, LVEF, and exercise tolerance with PVI when compared with the AVNA/BVP strategy.[71] Further substudy analysis has found that patients treated with PVI were likely to experience an improvement in AF severity, often regressing from persistent or permanent AF to PAF, while treatment with AVNA/BVP was more likely to result in a worsening of AF severity.[72]

16.4.2
Anticoagulation

The population prothrombotic risk of cardiac embolism in patients with AF is well accepted. This risk of thrombosis and thrombo-embolism is not uniform across all patients in AF. The presence of atrial stretch and dilatation, a lack of organized mechanical atrial contraction, and a subsequent increase in atrial pressure all lead to conditions for blood stasis and thrombus formation. The presence of AF is linked to abnormalities of the haemostatic system, endothelial dysfunction, and platelet activation that increase the risk of thrombo-embolic events.[73] However, it is equally clear that these linkages may be due to the confounding effects of concomitant disease rather than the change in cardiac rhythm per se as they are not evident in persistent lone AF devoid of structural heart disease or risk factors for atherosclerosis.

In general terms, metaanalyses of patients with AF derived from five clinical trials for primary prevention and one for secondary prevention in patients with AF demonstrate a five to sixfold increase in the risk of stroke, with an annual risk of 6%.[74] In the absence of systolic ventricular dysfunction, Warfarin, in doses maintaining an INR between 2.0 and 2.6, results in a 62% risk reduction of stroke, compared with a 22% risk reduction in those treated with aspirin alone. The number needed to treat to prevent 1 stroke was 37 patients, and the overall risk of bleeding complications was 0.3% per year for major intracranial hemorrhage and 0.6% per year for major hemorrhage.

The interpretation of thromboembolism in heart failure is indeed complex and is confounded by the nature of the events that might be regarded as thrombotic, the conventional risk factors for VENOUS thromboembolism, which are obviously distinct from those linked to arterial thrombosis, or from the cardiac thrombo-embolism most commonly linked to AF. Some assessments suggest that a heart failure diagnosis with sinus rhythm predisposes to arterial or venous thrombo-embolism, with the systemic event rate ranging from 0.9 to 5.5/100 patient years.[75] Systematic reviews indicate an increased risk of venous thromboembolism, cardio-embolic stroke, and sudden death due to new coronary occlusions.[76] Population samples are hard to interpret as these do not easily distinguish confounding factors in the analysis to address causality for individual cases of stroke. Many patients presenting with stroke or peripheral thromboembolism have underlying left ventricular systolic impairment, as evidenced by population surveys such as the Framingham study.[77] In the Framingham Heart Study, the risk of stroke was 4.1% per year for men and

2.8% per year for women with heart failure. Many of these cases had coexistent AF yet the individual origins of the rhythm change the timing of recognition and management strategies linked to this are obscure.[78] Not every case of stroke in a patient with AF is cardio embolic in origin. Equally in the Northern Manhattan study (NOMAS), the presence of a reduced left ventricular systolic ejection fraction was strongly associated with ischemic stroke, but this persists after adjusting for risk factors such as AF and therefore this association is not simply explicable by AF alone.[79]

The risk of stroke in systolic heart failure patients has been shown to be directly related to the degree of underlying left ventricular impairment. In a subgroup analysis of the SAVE study (survival and ventricular enlargement),[80] the overall risk of stroke was 8.1% at 5 years, with a twofold increase in stroke risk in those patients with an LVEF <28%, and an inverse relationship between stroke and LVEF (with an 18% increase in stroke risk for every 5% reduction in LVEF). This risk is predictably greater in the presence of AF, with the AF Investigators reporting an annual risk of stroke of 1.3%, rising to 3.6% in the presence of heart failure. Subsequent analysis demonstrated a 2.5-fold greater risk of stroke in the presence of moderate to severe left ventricular dysfunction.[81] These associations do not consistently integrate recognition and treatment strategies for known stroke disease far less the presence of AF in individual patients, and may thus over state the risk attributed to impaired systolic ventricular dysfunction of multiple etiology.

However, it is clear that whole body anticoagulation, as in patients with AF and normal ventricular function and conventional stroke risk factors, is an imperative consideration for heart failure patients with AF. On the basis of current evidence, the presence of a left ventricular ejection fraction less than 50% and AF carries an annual stroke risk of 6–10% depending on age and comorbid conditions, and it is in these patients Warfarin should be considered unless contraindicated by individual circumstances (Table 16.2).

Table 16.2 Annual stroke risk and recommendations for anticoagulation

Annual stroke risk	Risk factors	Recommendation
Low (1%)	Age<65 years No major risk factors[a]	Aspirin
Low moderate (1.5%)	Age 65–74 years No major risk factors[a]	Aspirin
High moderate (2.5%)	Age 65–74 years No major risk factors[a] But either diabetes mellitus or coronary artery disease	Warfarin
High (6%)	Age<75 years and either hypertension, heart failure or LVEF<50%; or age>75 years in the absence of other risk factors[a]	Warfarin
Very high (10%)	Age>75 years and either hypertension, heart failure, or LVEF<50%; or any age and prior stroke, TIA, or systemic thromboembolism	Warfarin

[a]Major risk factors include: prior stroke, transient ischemic attack, systemic thromboembolism, hypertension, heart failure, LVEF<50%. Adapted from Hart et al[74]

The population linkage of partly thrombotic disease processes such as cerebral, coronary, or peripheral artery disease and HF syndromes has provoked consideration of the use of whole body anticoagulation in HF associated with sinus rhythm. In contrast to patients with HF syndromes and AF, subgroup analyses of several large heart failure trials failed to demonstrate any beneficial effect of anticoagulation in heart failure.[82] Specific trials of anticoagulation with Warfarin showed no net benefit of this treatment in any sub group of HF with sinus rhythm. A retrospective analysis of the SOLVD trials[83] showed a small reduction in all cause mortality, death, or hospitalization for heart failure associated with warfarin use, suggesting that warfarin was a predictor of favorable outcome. However, there was no reduction in stroke, pulmonary embolism, or other vascular events following warfarin administration. In the SAVE trial,[80] warfarin use was associated with an 81% reduction in stroke risk, although no direct comparison with aspirin use was made. In contrast, analysis from the V-HeFT trials[84] did not show any significant difference in thrombo-embolic events amongst patients on anticoagulation, and surprisingly, the incidence of thrombo-embolic events in the V-HeFT II trial was higher in the warfarin group than in those without anticoagulation. In the PROMISE trial,[85] patients anticoagulated with warfarin showed a significant reduction in stroke rate, but the effect was most marked in those with severe heart failure (as defined by an LVEF <20%). In summary, while the benefits of antithrombotic treatment in established AF to prevent stroke in the context of systolic HF syndromes are unquestioned, the role for this in HF with sinus rhythm is unproven. Further trials examining this issue in systolic HF are currently underway (see below).

16.5
Problem Areas

16.5.1
Atrial Fibrillation and Heart Failure with Preserved Ejection Fraction (HFpEF)

The focus of heart failure research has traditionally been aimed at those patients with evidence of left ventricular systolic impairment. However, approximately 40–50% of patients presenting with heart failure symptoms have a preserved left ventricular ejection fraction.[86,87] These patients are typically elderly, female, obese, and hypertensive. Changing population demography and age distribution implies that this clinical group of heart failure patients is likely to increase dramatically. While the prognosis of patients with HFpEF is clearly worse than an age-matched population,[87] the exact mechanisms for this are unclear. However, the levels of hospitalization and use of resources do approach those of patients with impaired systolic function.

The presence of diastolic ventricular dysfunction (most commonly due to hypertensive left ventricular hypertrophy) results in a rise in filling pressures, mediates atrial remodeling, and is associated with a 5.2-fold increased risk for the development of AF.[21] It is well established that concentric left ventricular hypertrophy is the dominant association for the development of AF. It is therefore of little surprise that AF occurs in HFpEF with a similar incidence to that seen in heart failure with reduced left ventricular function. AF was recorded in 29% of patients with an LVEF >40% in the CHARM-Preserved trial,[88] and in 23% of patients with an LVEF >50% in the New York Heart Failure Consortium Registry.[89] As mentioned earlier, the impact of AF on 5-year survival and events varies in patients with heart failure symptoms dependent on the integrity of underlying left ventricular function. The impact is greater in those patients with more severe systolic ventricular impairment. Equally and predictably when compared with patients in sinus rhythm, survival was significantly reduced in patients with AF and a left ventricular ejection fraction >55%, as well as in those patients with a mildly reduced ejection fraction of between 41 and 55%. The emergence of AF therefore has an adverse population effect regardless of ventricular impairment but its impact increases with systolic ventricular dysfunction compared to sinus rhythm.

16.5.2
Aspirin in Heart Failure

Currently antiplatelet therapy (predominantly aspirin) is widespread in the population treatment of atherosclerotic vascular disease yet its evidence base is frequently incomplete. The evidence for benefit of antiplatelet therapy in heart failure syndromes is limited. In the SAVE study,[80] patients treated with aspirin had a 56% lower incidence of stroke following myocardial infarction, with the greatest benefit seen in those with an LVEF <28% (in whom the reduction in stroke was 66%). Results from the SOLVD trial were similar,[83] with the risk reduction being greater in female than male patients. In addition, antiplatelet use in the SOLVD trials was associated with a significant decrease in all-cause mortality, as well as the risk of death or hospitalization for heart failure, but this survival benefit was likely to be due to the beneficial effects of Enalapril in the active treatment group. In the V-HeFT I study, there was a nonsignificant trend toward reduction in thrombo-embolic events with antiplatelet therapy.[84] However, in V-HeFT II, no benefit could be demonstrated where concomitant aspirin use was evident.

Three randomized controlled trials to date have attempted to identify the optimal regime in patients with heart failure for the prevention of systemic thrombo-embolic events. These trials compare the predominantly antithrombotic effect of warfarin to the antiplatelet effect of aspirin. The Warfarin/Aspirin Study in Heart failure (WASH) was a small study comparing warfarin (target INR of 2.5) to aspirin (300 mg daily) or neither therapy in 279 patients with left ventricular systolic dysfunction (LVEF < 35%).[90] This study demonstrated no difference in the combined primary end-points of all-cause mortality, nonfatal myocardial infarction, and nonfatal stroke between the three treatment arms. Patients on warfarin had a nonsignificant trend to fewer cardiovascular hospitalizations than those on aspirin or no therapy. In the Warfarin and Antiplatelet Therapy in Chronic Heart Failure (WATCH) study,[91] the results of which have never been published fully, 1,587 patients with an LVEF < 30% were randomized to receive either warfarin (INR 2.5) or blinded antiplatelet therapy (aspirin 162 mg daily or clopidogrel 75 mg daily). No difference was seen in the composite endpoint of death or nonfatal myocardial infarction or stroke in the three treatment arms. However, similar to the WASH study, there were fewer hospitalizations for heart failure in the warfarin group. Warfarin use in WATCH showed a beneficial trend in nonfatal stroke (0.7 vs. 2.1%) compared to aspirin, but this was offset by a significantly higher bleeding rate in the warfarin group in comparison to the antiplatelet drugs (5.56, 3.6, and 2.48% with warfarin, aspirin and clopidogrel, respectively). Unfortunately, this trial was terminated early due to poor recruitment and the final reported sample was statistically underpowered.

The HELAS (efficacy of antithrombotic therapy in chronic heart failure) study[92] was a small double blind, placebo controlled trial, randomizing 197 patients with heart failure (NYHA II–IV) and an LVEF<35% to either aspirin 325 mg vs. warfarin in patients with ischemic heart disease or warfarin vs. placebo in patients with idiopathic dilated cardiomyopathy. No difference was seen between the treatments in the ischemic cardiomyopathy group in terms of primary end points (nonfatal stroke, peripheral or pulmonary embolism, myocardial infarction, rehospitalization with heart failure, or death due to heart failure). Importantly in this study patients who developed new AF were withdrawn from the analysis. However, this study was again terminated early due to poor recruitment and affected by inadequate statistical power. Interestingly, the overall thromboembolic event rate was low at 2.2/100 patient years.

In summary, aspirin has little evidence to support its routine use in heart failure with or without AF to prevent potential thrombo-embolic events. There is a possible risk of worsening heart failure and hospitalizations. The major randomized controlled trials above have all been plagued by poor recruitment, early termination, and poor statistical power. It is hoped that the ongoing Warfarin Aspirin Reduced Cardiac Ejection Fraction trial (WARCEF) might add to the current knowledge base. This is a double-blinded, multi-center study of patients with left ventricular ejection fraction <35% (who have no past documented AF) comparing all cause mortality, stroke, and intracranial hemorrhage in patients randomized to receive aspirin 325 mg or warfarin (INR 2.5–3.0).

16.5.3
Atrial Fibrillation Recognized by Implanted Cardiac Devices: A New Challenge

Contemporary management of systolic ventricular dysfunction has been extended dramatically in recent years by the impact of cardiac resynchronisation therapy.[93] Currently this is focused on those symptomatic patients with significant left ventricular systolic dysfunction on optimized therapy with left conduction block linked clearly with improvements in electromechanical ventricular dyssynchrony. The impact of this therapy on symptoms, mortality and morbidity, and cardiac mechanics has been substantial. Although the exact mechanism of benefit are multifactorial, they clearly extend to patients with systolic ventricular dysfunction who have established AF[94] provided high percentages (>96%) of biventricular pacing can be achieved. The indications for such electromechanical treatment to induce cardiac remodeling are currently being explored in patients with less severe symptomatic classes, narrow complex ventricular conduction, patients with HF symptoms and hypertrophic cardiomyopathy (and preserved ventricular contraction) and in future may extend to larger proportions of HF patients.[95]

One interesting side effect of these device programs relevant to AF and HF interactions has been the increased capacity to document occult cardiac rhythm change, such as atrial or ventricular arrhythmia, not associated with symptoms. Modern devices with appropriate electrode positioning and algorithms can reliably identify and document abnormal atrial arrhythmias such as AF not only for the purpose of adjusting therapies intended for ventricular arrhythmia but also to document these per se. These episodes can be notified automatically in regular centralized daily data monitoring.[96] These episodes would not have been documented in other circumstances and due to the unique shift in the sample frame of this form of observation, to an asymptomatic often transient arrhythmia, its clinical significance and appropriate therapeutic responses have not been established.

Initial reports of the prevalence of AF detected by this means are surprising with much lower prevalence than might otherwise have been predicted. In the TRENDS registry of 2,486 patients, around 60% were suggested to have HF syndromes and in which half had pacemaker and half ICD detected atrial tachyarrhythmia detection (99). The mean CHADS2 score, a stroke risk score that awards a point value to each of five risk factors, including a history of HF, hypertension, age, diabetes, and prior stroke or TIA, was 2.2 in this population. The arrhythmia burden estimates provided during follow up showed that 76% had zero burden of AT/AF; 12% had low burden (episodes lasting <5.5 h) and 12% had high burden (≥5.5 h). During an average follow-up of 1.4 years, (3,382 patient-years), there were only 40 events regarded as thrombo embolic comprising 20 strokes, 17 clinical TIAs, and three systemic embolisms. The annualized rate of these events was therefore only 1.2% and lower than other sample frames that might have predicted. However, around 20% of the sample of patients was on warfarin and 60% on aspirin. More controlled observations are required.

Currently, there are two major trials (ASSIST; IMPACT) of home monitored asymptomatic detection of AF (as atrial high rate events confirmed by electrogram verification) whereby given arrhythmia burden is linked to a therapy either with pacing algorithms (ASSIST) or with warfarin (IMPACT) for the arrhythmia. In the case of IMPACT, this is keyed on confirmed arrhythmia and duration and conventional thrombotic risk scoring (CHADS-2). These results are awaited with interest and will better define this new era of automated arrhythmia detection and management.

16.6
Summary

The impact of AF in heart failure syndromes is complex. The setting of this rhythm change is key to its significance both as a primary cause of an acute HF presentation or merely an epiphenomenon of significance in a process of evolving cardiac dysfunction. Current epidemiology gives little insight into this complexity and new techniques to recognize and define AF earlier in the process of individual patients illness present new research challenges as to how best manage this arrhythmia, its interaction with cardiac function and both cardiac and systemic consequences such as cardiogenic thromboembolism. The expanding research field in this well recognized clinical association can only provide a better basis for individualized patient care.

References

1. Benjamin EJ, Levy D, Vaziri SM, et al. Independent risk factors for atrial fibrillation in a population-based cohort: the Framingham Heart Study. *JAMA*. 1994;271:840-844.
2. Cleland JGF, Swedberg K, Follath F, et al. The Euro Heart Failure survey programme – a survey on the quality of care among patients with heart failure in Europe. Part 1: patient characteristics and diagnosis. *Eur Heart J*. 2003;24:442-463.
3. Camm AJ, Savalieva I. Atrial fibrillation: advances and perspectives. *Dialog Cardiovasc Med*. 2003;8:183-202.
4. Dries DL, Exner DV, Gersch BJ, et al. Atrial fibrillation is associated with an increased risk for mortality in patients with asymptomatic and symptomatic left ventricular systolic dysfunction: a retrospective analysis of the SOLVD trials. *J Am Coll Cardiol*. 1998;32:695-703.
5. Maggioni AP, Latini R, Carson PE, et al. Valsartan reduces the incidence of atrial fibrillatio n in patients with heart failure: results from the Valsartan Heart Failure Trial (Val-HeFT). *Am Heart J*. 2005;149:548-557.
6. Wang TJ, Larson MG, Levy D, et al. Temporal relations of atrial fibrillation and congestive heart failure and their joint influence on mortality: the Framingham Heart Study. *Circulation*. 2003;107:2920-2925.
7. Mathew J, Hunsberger S, Fleg J, et al. Incidence, predictive factors, and prognostic significance of supraventricular tachyarrhythmias in congestive heart failure. *Chest*. 2000;2000:914-922.
8. Baldasseroni S, Opasisch C, Giorni M, et al. Left bundle branch block is associated with increased 1-year sudden and total mortality rate in 5517 outpatients withcongestive heart failure. *Am Heart J*. 2002;143:398-405.
9. Baldasseroni S, De Biase L, Fresco C, et al. Italian Network on Congestive Heart Failure. Cumulative effect of complete left bundle-branch block and chronic atrial fibrillation on 1-year mortality and hospitalization in patients with congestive heart failure. A report from the Italian network on congestive heart failure (in-CHF database). *Eur Heart J*. 2002;23: 1692-1698.
10. Pai RG, Varadarajan P. Prognostic significance of atrial fibrillation is a function of left ventricular ejection fraction. *Clin Cardiol*. 2007;30:349-354.
11. Santinelli V, et al. Atrial fibrillation progression in patients with and without lone atrial fibrillation. A Five Year Prospective Follow-Up Study (abstr). *J Am Coll Cardiol*. 2008;51(suppl A):A6.
12. Keating RJ, Gersh B, Hodge D. Effect of atrial fibrillation pattern on survival in a community-based cohort. *Am J Cardiol*. 2005;96:1420-1424.
13. Miyasaka Y, Barnes ME, Gersh BJ, et al. Incidence and mortality risk of congestive heart failure in atrial fibrillation patients: a community-based study over two decades. *Eur Heart J*. 2006;27:936-941.
14. Shinbane JS, Wood MA, Jensen DN, et al. Tachycardia-induced cardiomyopathy: a review of animal models and clinical studies. *J Am Coll Cardiol*. 1997;29:709-715.
15. Spinale FG, Tomita M, Zellner JL, Cook JC, Crawford FA, Zile MR. Collagen remodeling and changes in LV function during development and recovery from supraventricular tachycardia. *Am J Physiol Heart Circ Physiol*. 1991;261:H301-H318.
16. Tomita M et al. Changes in left ventricular volume, mass, and function during the development and regression of supraventricular tachycardia-induced cardiomyopathy. *Disparity between recovery of systolic versus diastolic function Circulation*. 1991;83:635-644.
17. Ehrlich JR et al. Atrial fibrillation and congestive heart failure: specific considerations at the intersection of the two common and important cardiac disease sets. *J Cardiovasc Electrophysiol*. 2002;13:399-405.
18. Li D et al. Effects of experimental heart failure on atrial cellular and ionic electrophysiology. *Circulation*. 2000;101:2631-2638.

19. Li D et al. Promotion of atrial fibrillation by heart failure in dogs: atrial remodeling of a different sort. *Circulation.* 1999;100:87-95.

20. Tsang TS et al. Left atrial volume: important risk marker of incident atrial fibrillation in 1,655 older men and women. *Mayo Clin Proc.* 2001;76:467-475.

21. Tsang TS et al. Left ventricular diastolic dysfunction as a predictor of the first diagnosed nonvalvular atrial fibrillation in 840 elderly men and women. *J Am Coll Cardiol.* 2002;40:1636-1644.

22. Amir O et al. Aldosterone synthase gene polymorphism as a determinant of atrial fibrillation in patients with heart failure. *Am J Cardiol.* 2008;102:326-329.

23. Tsang TS et al. Left atrial volume as a morphophysiologic expression of left ventricular diastolic dysfunction and relation to cardiovascular risk burden. *Am J Cardiol.* 2002;90:1284-1289.

24. Li D et al. Effects of angiotensin-converting enzyme inhibition on the development of the atrial fibrillation substrate in dogs with ventricular tachypacing-induced congestive heart failure. *Circulation.* 2001;104:2608-2614.

25. Mattioli AV, Bonatti S, Monopoli D, Zennaro M, Mattioli G. Influence of regression of left ventricular hypertrophy on left atrial size and function in patients with moderate hypertension. *Blood Press.* 2005;14:273-278.

26. Tsang TS, Barnes ME, Abhayaratna WP, et al. Effects of quinapril on left atrial structural remodeling and arterial stiffness. *Am J Cardiol.* 2006;97:916-920.

27. Brilla CG, Funck RC, Rupp H. Lisinopril-mediated regression of myocardial fibrosis in patients with hypertensive heart disease. *Circulation.* 2000;102:1388-1393.

28. Brooks WW, Bing OH, Robinson KG, Slawsky MT, Chaletsky DM, Conrad CH. Effect of angiotensin-converting enzyme inhibition on myocardial fibrosis and function in hypertrophied and failing myocardium from the spontaneously hypertensive rat. *Circulation.* 1997;96:4002-4010.

29. Weber KT, Brilla CG, Campbell SE, Guarda E, Zhou G, Sriram K. Myocardial fibrosis: role of angiotensin II and aldosterone. *Basic Res Cardiol.* 1993;88(suppl 1):107-124.

30. Anand IS, Latini R, Florea VG, et al. C-reactive protein in heart failure: prognostic value and the effect of valsartan. *Circulation.* 2005;112:1428-1434.

31. Fliser D, Buchholz K, Haller H. Antiinflammatory effects of angiotensin II subtype 1 receptor blockade in hypertensive patients with microinflammation. *Circulation.* 2004;110:1103-1107.

32. Xu ZG, Lanting L, Vaziri ND, et al. Upregulation of angiotensin II type 1 receptor, inflammatory mediators, and enzymes of arachidonate metabolism in obese Zucker rat kidney: reversal by angiotensin II type 1 receptor blockade. *Circulation.* 2005;111:1962-1969.

33. Ferrari R, Cicchitelli G, Merli E, Andreadou I, Guardigli G. Metabolic modulation and optimization of energy consumption in heart failure. *Med Clin North Am.* 2003;87:493; xiii.

34. Kumagai K, Nakashima H, Urata H, Gondo N, Arakawa K, Saku K. Effects of angiotensin II type 1 receptor antagonist on electrical and structural remodeling in atrial fibrillation. *J Am Coll Cardiol.* 2003;41:2197-2204.

35. Nakashima H, Kumagai K, Urata H, Gondo N, Ideishi M, Arakawa K. Angiotensin II antagonist prevents electrical remodeling in atrial fibrillation. *Circulation.* 2000;101:2612-2617.

36. Wachtell K, Lehto M, Gerdts E, et al. Angiotensin II receptor blockade reduces new-onset atrial fibrillation and subsequent stroke compared to atenolol: the Losartan Intervention For End Point Reduction in Hypertension (LIFE) study. *J Am Coll Cardiol.* 2005;45:712-719.

37. Ducharme A, Swedberg K, Pfeffer MA, et al. Prevention of atrial fibrillation in patients with symptomatic chronic heart failure by candesartan in the Candesartan in Heart failure: Assessment of Reduction in Mortality and morbidity (CHARM) program. *Am Heart J.* 2006;152:86-92.

38. Pedersen OD, Bagger H, Kober L, Torp-Pedersen C. Trandolapril reduces the incidence of atrial fibrillation after acute myocardial infarction in patients with left ventricular dysfunction. *Circulation.* 1999;100:376-380.

39. Vermes E, Tardif JC, Bourassa MG, et al. Enalapril decreases the incidence of atrial fibrillation in patients with left ventricular dysfunction: insight from the Studies Of Left Ventricular Dysfunction (SOLVD) trials. *Circulation.* 2003;107:2926-2931.

40. Healey JS, Baranchuk A, Crystal E, et al. Prevention of atrial fibrillation with angiotensin-converting enzyme inhibitors and angiotensin receptor blockers: a meta-analysis. *J Am Coll Cardiol.* 2005;45:1832-1839.

41. Anand K, Mooss AN, Hee TT, Mohiuddin SM. Meta-analysis: inhibition of renin-angiotensin system prevents new-onset atrial fibrillation. *Am Heart J.* 2006;152:217-222. '

42. The Atrial Fibrillation Follow-up Investigation of Rhythm Management (AFFIRM) Investigators. A comparison of rate control and rhythm control in patients with atrial fibrillation. *N Eng J Med.* 2002;347:1825-1833.

43. Van Gelder IC et al. A comparison of rate control and rhythm control in patients with recurrent persistent atrial fibrillation. *N Eng J Med.* 2002;347:1834-1840.

44. Roy D et al. Rhythm control versus rate control for atrial fibrillation and heart failure. *N Eng J Med.* 2008;358:2667-2777.

45. Hunt SA et al. ACC/AHA 2005 Guideline Update for the Diagnosis and Management of Chronic Heart Failure in the Adult: a report of the American College ofCardiology/American Heart Association Task Force on Practice Guidelines (Writing Committee to Update the 2001 Guidelines for the Evaluation and Management of Heart Failure): developed in collaboration with the American College of Chest Physicians and theInternational Society for Heart and Lung Transplantation: endorsed by the Heart Rhythm Society. *Circulation.* 2005;112: e154-e235.

46. Olshansky B, et al.; The AFFIRM investigators. The Atrial Fibrillation Follow-up Investigation of Rhythm Management (AFFIRM) study: approaches to control rate in atrial fibrillation. *J Am Coll Cardiol.* 2004;43:1201-1208.

47. Khand AU et al. Carvedilol alone or in combination with digoxin for the management of atrial fibrillation in patients with heart failure? *J Am Coll Cardiol.* 2003;42:1944-1951.

48. Delle Karth G et al. Amiodarone versus diltiazem for rate control in critically ill patients with tachyarrhythmias. *Crit Care Med.* 2001;29:1149-1153.

49. Fuster V et al. ACC/AHA/ESC 2006 Guidelines for the Management of Patients with Atrial Fibrillation: a report of the American College of Cardiology/AmericanHeart Association Task Force on Practice Guidelines and the European Society of Cardiology Committee for Practice Guidelines (Writing Committee to Revise the 2001 Guidelines for the Management of Patients With Atrial Fibrillation): developed in collaboration with the European Heart Rhythm Association and the Heart Rhythm Society. *Circulation.* 2006;114:e354.

50. Brignole M et al. Assessment of atrioventricular junction ablation and VVIR pacemaker versus pharmacological treatment in patients with heart failure and chronic atrial fibrillation: a randomized, controlled study. *Circulation.* 1998;98:953-960.

51. Weerasooriya R et al. The Australian Intervention Randomized Control of Rate in Atrial Fibrillation Trial (AIRCRAFT). *J Am Coll Cardiol.* 2003;41:1697-1702.

52. The AFFIRM investigators. Relationships between sinus rhythm, treatment, and survival in the Atrial Fibrillation Follow-up Investigation of Rhythm Management (AFFIRM) study. *Circulation.* 2004;109:1509-1513.

53. Roy D et al. Amiodarone to prevent recurrence of atrial fibrillation. *N Eng J Med.* 2000;342: 913-920.

54. Deedwania PC et al. Spontaneous conversion and maintenance of sinus rhythm by amiodarone in patients with heart failure and atrial fibrillation: observations from the Veterans Affairs Congestive Heart Failure Survival Trial of Antiarrhythmic Therapy (CHFSTAT). *Circulation.* 1998;98:2574-2579.

55. Touboul P et al. Dronedarone for prevention of atrial fibrillation: a dose-ranging study. *Eur Heart J.* 2003;24:1481-1487.

56. Hohnloser SH, et al. A placebo-controlled, double-blind, parallel arm trial to assess the efficacy of dronedarone 400 mg bid for the prevention of cardiovascular hospitalization or death from any cause in patients with atrial fibrillation/ atrial flutter (AF/AFL). Heart Rhythm Society 2008 Scientific Sessions: 2008. Heart Rhythm Society 2008 Scientific Sessions; 2008.

57. Kober L et al. Increased mortality after dronedarone therapy for severe heart failure. *N Eng J Med.* 2008;358:2678-2687.
58. Pedersen OD et al. Efficacy of dofetilide in the treatment of atrial fibrillation–flutter in patients with reduced left ventricular function: a Danish Investigations of Arrhythmia and Mortality On Dofetilide (DIAMOND) substudy. *Cicrulation.* 2001;104:292-296.
59. Torp-Pedersen C et al. Dofetilide in patients with congestive heart failure and left ventricular dysfunction. Danish Investigations of Arrhythmia and Mortality on Dofetilide Study Group. *N Eng J Med.* 1999;341:857-865.
60. Connolly SJ et al. Doseeresponse relations of azimilide in the management of symptomatic, recurrent atrial fibrillation. *Am J Cardiol.* 2001;88:974-979.
61. Pratt CM et al. The efficacy of azimilide in the treatment of atrial fibrillation in the presence of left ventricular systolic dysfunction: results from the Azimilide Postinfarct Survival Evaluation (ALIVE) trial. *J Am Coll Cardiol.* 2004;43:1211-1216.
62. Camm AJ et al. Azimilide Post Infarct Evaluation (ALIVE): azimilide does not affect mortality in post-myocardial infarction patients. *Circulation.* 2004;109:990-996.
63. Corley SD et al. Relationships between sinus rhythm, treatment, and survival in the Atrial Fibrillation Follow-Up Investigation of Rhythm Management (AFFIRM) Study. *Cicrulation.* 2004;109:1509-1513.
64. Oral H et al. Pulmonary vein isolation for paroxysmal and persistent atrial fibrillation. *Circulation.* 2002;105:1077-1081.
65. Pappone C et al. Atrial electroanatomic remodeling after circumferential radiofrequency pulmonary vein ablation: efficacy of an anatomic approach in a large cohort of patients with atrial fibrillation. *Circulation.* 2001;104:2539-2544.
66. Gentlesk PJ et al. Reversal of left ventricular dysfunction following ablation of atrial fibrillation. *J Cardiovasc Electrophysiol.* 2007;18:9-14.
67. Hsu LF et al. Catheter ablation for atrial fibrillation in congestive heart failure. *N Eng J Med.* 2004;351:2373-2383.
68. Kay GN et al. The Ablate and Pace Trial: a prospective study of catheter ablation of the AV conduction system and permanent pacemaker implantation for treatment of atrial fibrillation. *J Interv Card Electrophysiol.* 1998;2:121-135.
69. Ozcan C et al. Significant effects of atrioventricular node ablation and pacemaker implantation on left ventricular function and long-term survival in patients with atrial fibrillation and left ventricular dysfunction. *Am J Cardiol.* 2003;92:33-37.
70. Doshi RN et al. Left ventricular-based cardiac stimulation post AV nodal ablation evaluation (the PAVE study). *J Cardiovasc Electrophysiol.* 2005;16:1160-1165.
71. Khan MN, et al. Late-Breaking Clinical Trial abstracts from the American Heart Association's Scientific Sessions 2006: Randomized Controlled Trial of pulmonary vein antrum isolation vs. AV node ablation with bi-ventricular pacing for treatment of atrial fibrillation in patients with congestive heart failure (PABA CHF). *Circulation.* 2006;114:abstract.
72. Khan MN, et al. Progression of atrial fibrillation in the pulmonary vein antrum isolation vs. AV node ablation with biventricular pacing for treatment of atrial fibrillation patients with Congestive Heart Failure Trial (PABA-CHF). *Heart Rhythm.* 2006;3:abstract.
73. Kamath S et al. Platelet activation, haemorheology and thrombogenesis in acute atrial fibrillation: a comparison with permanent atrial fibrillation. *Heart.* 2003;89:1903-1905.
74. Hart RG et al. Antithrombotic therapy to prevent stroke in patients with atrial fibrillation: a meta-analysis. *Ann Intern Med.* 1999;131:492-501.
75. Baker DW, et al. Management of heart failure. IV. Anticoagulation for patients with heart failure due to left ventricular systolic dysfunction. *J Am Med Assoc.* 1994;272:1614-1618.
76. Lip GYL, Gibbs CR. Antiplatelet agents versus control or anticoagulation for heart failure in sinus rhythm: a Cochrane systematic review. *QJM.* 2002;95:461-468.
77. Wolf PA, Kannel WB, McNamara PM. Occult impaired cardiac function, congestive heart failure and risk of thrombotic stroke: The Framingham Study. *Neurology.* 1970;20:373.

78. Kannel WB, Wolf PA, Verter J. Manifestations of coronary disease predisposing to stroke. The Framingham Study. *JAMA*. 1983;250:2942-2946.
79. Hays AG, Sacco RL, Rundek T, et al. Left ventricular systolic dysfunction and the risk of ischemic stroke in a multiethnic population. *Stroke*. 2006;37:1715-1719.
80. Loh E, Sutton MS, Wun CC, et al. Ventricular dysfunction and the risk of stroke after myocardial infarction. *N Eng J Med*. 1997;336:251-257.
81. Atrial Fibrillation Investigators. Echocardiographic predictors of stroke in patients with atrial fibrillation: a prospective study of 1066 patients from three clinical trials. *Arch Intern Med*. 1998;158:1316-1320.
82. The CONSENSUS Trial Study Group. Effect of Enalapril on mortality in severe congestive heart failure. Results of the Cooperative North Scandinavian Enalapril Survival Study (CONSENSUS). *N Eng J Med*. 1987;316:1429-1435.
83. Al-Khadra AS, Salem DN, Rand WM, et al. Warfarin anticoagulation and survival: a cohort analysis from the studies of left ventricular dysfunction. *J Am Coll Cardiol*. 1998;31:749-753.
84. Dunkman DB, Johnson GR, Carson PE, et al. Incidence of thromboembolic events in congestive heart failure. *Circulation*. 1993;87(suppl 6):94-101.
85. Falk RH, Pollak A, Tandon PK, et al. The effect of warfarin on prevalence of stroke in patients with severe heart failure. *J Am Coll Cardiol*. 1993;21:218.
86. Redfield MM. Burden of systolic and diastolic ventricular dysfunction in the community: appreciating the scope of the heart failure epidemic. *JAMA*. 2003;289:194-202.
87. Vasan RS, Larson MG, Benjamin EJ, et al. Congestive heart failure in subjects with normal versus reduced left ventricular ejection fraction: prevalence and mortality in a population-based cohort. *J Am Coll Cardiol*. 1999;33:1948-1955.
88. Yusuf S, Pfeffer MA, Swedberg K, et al. Effects of candesartan in patients with chronic heart failure and preserved left ventricular ejection fraction: the CHARM-Preserved Trial. *Lancet*. 2003;362:777-781.
89. Klapholz M, Maurer M, Lowe AM, et al. Hospitalization for heart failure in the presence of a normal left ventricular ejection fraction: results of the New York Heart Failure Registry. *J Am Coll Cardiol*. 2004;43:1432-1438.
90. Cleland JG, Findlay I, Jafri S, et al. The Warfarin/Aspirin Study in Heart failure (WASH): a randomised trial comparing antithrombotic strategies for patients with heart failure. *Am Heart J*. 2004;148:157-164.
91. Massie BM, Krol WF, Ammon SE, et al. The Warfarin and Antiplatelet Therapy in Heart Failure trial (WATCH): rationale, design, and baseline patient characteristics. *J Card Fail*. 2004;10:101-112.
92. Cokkinos DV, Haralabopoulos GC, Kostis JB, et al. Efficacy of antithrombotic therapy in chronic heart failure: the HELAS study. *Eur J Heart Fail*. 2006;8:428-432.
93. Freemantle N, Tharmanathan P, Calvert MJ, et al. Cardiac resynchronisation for patients with heart failure due to left ventricular systolic dysfunction – a systematic review and meta analysis. *Eur J Heart Fail*. 2006;8:433-440.
94. Gasparini M, Regoli F. Trials of CRT in atrial fibrillation and atrial rhythm management issues. In: Yu C-M, Hayes DL, Auricchio A, eds. *Cardiac Resynchronization Therapy*. 2nd ed. London: Blackwell; 2008:277-289 [chapter 15].
95. Hayes DL, Yu C-M. Ongoing trials to further shape the future of CRT. In: Yu C-M, Hayes DL, Auricchio A, eds. *Cardiac Resynchronization Therapy*, 2nd ed. London: Blackwell; 2008:290-300 [chapter 16].
96. Braunschweig F, Mortensen PT, Gras D, et al. Monitoring of physical activity and heart rate variability in patients with chronic heart failure using cardiac resynchronization devices. *Am J Cardiol*. 2005;95:1104-1107.
97. Savelieva I, Camm AJ. Atrial fibrillation and heart failure: natural history and pharmacological treatment. *Europace*. 2004;5:S5-S19.
98. Morrison TB, Bunch TJ, Gersch BJ. Pathophysiology of concomitant atrial fibrillation and heart failure: implications for management. *Nature Clin Prac Cardiovasc Med*. 2009;6:46-56.

Natriuretic Peptides

17

Krister Lindmark and Kurt Boman

17.1
Introduction

Natriuretic peptides are clinically used as biomarkers of heart failure and have in recent years become more and more valuable in the diagnosis of heart failure. B-type natriuretic peptide (BNP) and N-terminal pro-BNP (NT-pro-BNP) have become commercially available, their accurate assays have been made, and their most widespread use has been achieved, although other natriuretic peptides can be of interest as well. The body of data supporting the use of BNP and NT-pro-BNP is steadily increasing. Low levels of BNP and NT-pro-BNP can, because of their high negative predictive values, be used to rule out heart failure, and high levels of these peptides predict a poor prognosis. There are, however, several pitfalls in the use of natriuretic peptides that one has to be aware of when using them in routine clinical practice. Many unanswered questions also remain to be resolved.

The natriuretic peptides have very potent physiological and pharmacological effects and are naturally very interesting for pharmaceutical companies. Several naturally occurring and chemically altered natriuretic peptides have been the subject of clinical trials. This chapter will, however, focus on the use of natriuretic peptides as a diagnostic tool rather than a therapeutic one.

17.2
Natriuretic Peptides

The natriuretic peptides are a family of peptides with similarities in structure but somewhat different biologic properties, mostly affecting sodium and water balance. The basic structure of the natriuretic peptides is a ring with one or two tails. The ring structure is responsible for most of the biologic effects which may be systemic, autocrine or paracrine

K. Lindmark (✉)
Department of Cardiology, Heart Center, Umeå University Hospital, Umeå, Sweden
e-mail: krister.lindmark@ull.se

M.Y. Henein (ed.), *Heart Failure in Clinical Practice*,
DOI: 10.1007/978-1-84996-153-0_17, © Springer-Verlag London Limited 2010

according to type of natriuretic peptide.[1] A-type natriuretic peptide (ANP) is produced by the cardiac myocytes and has mostly systemic effects with diuresis and natriuresis. B-type natriuretic peptide (BNP) is produced by both atrial and ventricular cardiomyocytes and has mostly systemic effects. It was first identified in the porcine brain and was initially called brain natriuretic peptide.[2] When it was discovered that the left ventricle is the principle source, the name changed to B-type natriuretic peptide. C-type natriuretic peptide (CNP) is expressed in the central nervous system and endothelial cells. It acts as an autocrine and paracrine factor on vascular tone and cell growth.[3] D-type natriuretic peptide (DNP) is found in snake venom but has also been detected in human plasma.[4] V-type natriuretic peptide (VNP) is a chimera of CNP and ANP but has not been detected in humans. Urodilatin has a local role in the renal distal tubules.[5] Guanylin and uroguanylin are involved in salt and water metabolism in the gastrointestinal system.[6]

The rest of the chapter will focus on BNP as this is the only natriuretic peptide that is routinely used for clinical purposes.

17.3
Physiology of BNP

The main effects of BNP are reducing peripheral vascular resistance, natrieuresis and diuresis thus opposing the pathophysiological hormonal responses of heart failure. Secretion of BNP is regulated by cardiomyocyte wall tension and is proportional to the degree of myocardial stretch.[7] The effects of BNP are mediated by cell surface receptors, natriuretic peptide receptors (NPRs), that are widely expressed not only in the cardiovascular system but also in the lungs, kidneys, skin, platelets and within the CNS.[8]

BNP is produced in the cardiac myocytes. The production is regulated at the level of gene expression.[9] The initial molecule is a 134 amino acid protein, pre-pro-BNP. After cleavage of a signal peptide, a 108 amino acid prehormone, pro-BNP, remains. Before release into the blood stream, pro-BNP is cleaved into the biologically inert NT-pro-BNP and the biologically active BNP.[10] Some pro-BNP is released into the blood without being cleaved. The biological importance of this is unclear.

Clearance and half life of BNP and NT-pro-BNP differ. Clearance of BNP is mediated by specific receptors, as well as by endopeptidases and by direct renal clearance. NT-pro-BNP is cleared mostly by direct glomerular filtration. Half life of BNP in healthy subjects is estimated to be 21 min and is 70 min for NT-pro-BNP.[11]

17.3.1
Measurements

Measurements of peptide levels are made by immunoassay methods. A number of methods are described and many are commercially available both for automatic use and outpatient clinical assessment. The latter gives an answer within 15 min, which is an advantage in clinical management of the patients but might have slightly less precision.[12]

The stability of BNP in the blood sample is a central problem when measuring BNP, but the breakdown of BNP can be counteracted by adding EDTA to the tube, or by adding a protease inhibitor.[13] NT-pro-BNP has been found to be a stable molecule with regard to precision, sample stability, and correlation between sample types.[14] It is important to be aware of the type of methods used for assessing peptide levels, the specificity of the method, as well as the type of analytic interference. Significant differences in measurements, up to eight times, have been found for two commercially available methods for NT-pro-BNP.[15] This is especially important when cut-off values are determined for NT-pro-BNP and BNP as differences between NT-pro-BNP and BNP are even greater.[16]

17.3.2
Units

It is also important to recognize what units are used. Both units for mass concentration (ng/L or pg/mL), which is recommended,[17] and substance concentration (pmol/L) are used. For converting pmol/L to ng/L the following equations are used:

For BNP, ng/L = pmol/L × 3,47 and for NT-pro-BNP, ng/L = pmol/L × 8,457.

17.3.3
NT-pro-BNP vs. BNP

NT-pro-BNP and BNP are reasonably correlated and either can be used in clinical care. Their clinical performances are in general rather similar for various clinical conditions. However, two studies have directly compared BNP and NT-pro-BNP[18,19] and found that NT-pro-BNP is slightly superior to BNP for predicting death and morbidity or rehospitalization for heart failure. Most importantly, clinicians must understand the differences between NT-pro-BNP and BNP, especially as their absolute levels are not interchangeable.

17.4
Clinical Usefulness

17.4.1
Rule-Out Heart Failure

Heart failure is a condition that leads to increased filling pressures which, in turn, causes increased cavity wall stress, and hence, increased levels of BNP and NT-pro-BNP. Consequently, normal levels indicate the absence of systolic heart failure. Current guidelines advocate the use of BNP/NT-pro-BNP to rule out heart failure. Normal values of BNP/NT-pro-BNP can with a high negative predictive value exclude heart failure in untreated patients.[20] This is especially useful in the primary care setting where a simple laboratory test can reduce the need for an expensive and time consuming echocardiogram.[21]

In the emergency setting, BNP/NT-pro-BNP measurements lead to a more rapid and confident exclusion of heart failure than without using BNP or NT-pro-BNP. Several studies have demonstrated the efficacy of BNP/NT-pro-BNP to rule out heart failure in dyspnoeic patients[22-25] although higher cut-off-values have to be used, in this setting, than in the primary care setting. In a blinded emergency room study, the use of NT-pro-BNP was associated with shorter patient stay and a lower rate of rehospitalizations.[26]

17.4.2
Rule-In Heart Failure

The value of predicting heart failure with an increased level of BNP/NT-pro-BNP has been less well studied, and its use is not as good as the possibility of excluding heart failure. As BNP/NT-pro-BNP is released in response to increased left ventricular wall stress, it is not exclusive to heart failure but can result from any other condition that leads to increased wall stress. Conditions that can lead to increased levels of BNP/NT-pro-BNP are listed in Table 17.1.

17.4.3
Prognostication

High levels of BNP/NT-pro-BNP are associated with a worse prognosis in patients admitted to the hospital with decompensated heart failure. There is a stronger association between BNP/NT-pro-BNP and short term survival than established risk markers in heart failure, such as troponin-T, hemoglobin and NYHA-class. In a study of 720 patients, the group with an NT-pro-BNP-value of less than 5,180 pg/mL at admission had an 80-day mortality of 5%, whereas the group with NT-pro-BNP above 5,180 pg/mL had an 80 day mortality of 19%.[27] In a long-term study of 1 year, patients presenting with acute decompensated heart failure and NT-pro-BNP above 986 pg/mL had a remarkable increase in 1-year mortality with a hazard ratio of 2.88 in a multivariate analysis. In the same study, it was shown that NT-pro-BNP is equally valuable in the prediction of death in patients with dyspnoea from other causes than heart failure.[28] A study of 182 patients also showed that a 30% decrease of NT-pro-BNP from admission to discharge was associated with a better prognosis.[29] On the other hand, the predischarge value was a strong independent predictor of postdischarge outcomes.[30] Hence, special attention should be paid to patients with high predischarge values for a need of intensified treatment.

In chronic heart failure, substudies of several large multicenter trials have shown that single determinations of BNP/NT-pro-BNP are strong predictors of survival. Baseline concentrations are linearly related to death.[18,31] In contrast, studies that examine changes over time are few and provide conflicting results. Before more decisive studies are conducted, the clinical value of repeated measurements in stable patients is limited.

In heart failure with preserved systolic function or diastolic heart failure, BNP/NT-pro-BNP levels are elevated,[32] but the levels of natriuretic peptides are dependent on the underlying type of diastolic abnormality. Patients with relaxation abnormalities usually do

Table 17.1 Differential diagnosis of elevated BNP/NT-pro-BNP

COPD
Asthma
Pneumonia
Bronchitis
Lung cancer
Acute coronary syndrome
Hypertrophic cardiomyopathy
Takutsubo cardiomyopathy
Congenital heart disease
Myocarditis
Pericarditis
Atrial fibrillation
Ventricular tachycardia
Supraventricular tachycardia
Bradycardia
Aortic stenosis
Aortic regurgitation
Mitral stenosis
Mitral regurgitation
Pulmonary embolism
Pulmonary arterial hypertension
Sepsis
Renal insufficiency
Anemia
Burns
ARDS
Sleep apnoea
Heart failure

not have elevated levels in contrast to those with pseudo-normalization or restrictive filling patterns.[33] As diastolic function increases in severity as assed by Doppler filling patterns of mitral inflow, natriuretic peptides rise as a reflection of increased wall stress.[34] Even in heart failure with preserved systolic function or diastolic heart failure, the BNP/NT-pro-BNP levels have a clear prognostic significance.[35]

17.4.4
BNP/NT-pro-BNP-Based Treatment

Since the arrival of these biomarkers, there has been hope that they can be helpful in the treatment of individual patients. Large multicenter studies have shown benefits of angiotensinogen converting enzyme (ACE)-inhibitors, beta-blockers, angiotensin II receptor blockers (ARB), and aldosterone antagonists, and in all these studies, all doses have been titrated to a fixed level. All patients may not have maximum benefit with the study-chosen doses. Some may benefit from higher doses than others. Several studies have been conducted on these premises to titrate the medications according to BNP/NT-pro-BNP levels. The first study with 69 patients showed promising results[36] and so did the following STARS-BNP,[37] but subsequent larger studies have failed to show any clear benefit of a BNP/NT-pro-BNP-based therapy.[38-40]

17.5
Cost-Effectiveness

A number of studies have been performed to assess cost-effectiveness of using peptides in heart failure management. In a small study, it was found that BNP measurement appeared to be significantly cost-effective for the selection of patients for echocardiography.[41] In a meta analysis by Davenport et al[42] ECG, BNP and NT-pro-BNP were found to be useful in excluding a diagnosis of left ventricular systolic function (good sensitivity). However, they concluded that there was no evidence to justify the use of tests in combination or the use of one test over another. The additional cost of BNP was not self-evidently justified by improved test accuracy. In a report from the Swedish Council on Technology Assessment in Health Care,[42] it was concluded that the knowledge of the cost-effectiveness of natriuretic peptides assay in relation to other methods of diagnosing heart failure is still insufficient.

17.6
Kidneys and BNP/NTproBNP

The relationship between BNP/NT-pro-BNP and renal function is complex. Severe renal insufficiency can lead to water retention and increased cardiac wall stress, and hence, increased release of BNP/NT-pro-BNP. In addition, there is a strong comorbidity with a high percentage of heart failure patients having renal insufficiency and vice versa. NT-pro-BNP is almost solely cleared from the blood stream by glomerular filtration, whereas BNP is cleared by means of specific receptors and endopeptidases.[43] Therefore, there is a stronger correlation between glomerular filtration rate (GFR) and NT-pro-BNP-levels than between GFR and BNP-levels, even though the difference is not very large. It is important to remember that increased levels of BNP/NT-pro-BNP in patients with renal disease do not just indicate a decreased elimination but can predict heart failure and also have prognostic implications.[44] In a study of patients with stage 5 renal failure on haemodialysis, NT-pro-BNP had an inverse relation to ejection fraction (EF), and a cut-off value of NT-pro-BNP above 7.200 pg/mL correlated with a decreased left ventricular function.[45]

17.7
Other Pitfalls and Controversies

What is the "normal value" for natriuretic peptides?

"Normal values" are not well defined. It depends on the clinical setting and the prevalence of the condition being tested. A number of clinical conditions, outlined in Table 17.1, are associated with elevated level of natriuretic peptides. In primary care practice, for example, it is very difficult to establish accurate normal values in view of the variety of patients presenting, i.e., should it be healthy people or those with symptoms similar to heart failure but without heart failure. It is also important to recognize the prevalence of disease when negative or positive predictive values are established. This is often overlooked and not always presented. Assessment of BNP/NT-pro-BNP in the elderly with various degrees of breathlessness needs careful consideration as their levels normally increase with age. It can be argued that this is more of a pathological than a physiological change with age-dependent changes in the heart and renal function as well as changes in the metabolism of BNP. In the elderly, increased levels can be observed without apparent heart disease.[46]

Levels of BNP/NT-pro-BNP are clearly lower in obese patients with heart failure.[47] Several potential mechanisms have been proposed to explain this, but the reasons are still not clear. Several authors have suggested lower cut-off values for obese patients, but it has not yet affected the guidelines.

Several antihypertensive drugs are effective in reducing the filling pressures, i.e., ACE-inhibitors, ARBs, and aldosterone antagonists. For beta-blockers, there is an initial rise in the concentration of natriuretic peptides followed by decreasing levels. The use of these drugs can, as a result, mask an overt heart failure. It is not uncommon for well-treated heart failure patients to drop to normal BNP/NT-pro-BNP levels on an optimum medication despite still having a reduced left ventricular function.

BNP/NT-pro-BNP-levels are also higher in women than in men, but differences are usually small. This should not make a problem in individual patients but could have consequences if larger populations are screened.

Finally, it must be remembered that natriuretic peptides should always be evaluated from a perspective that considers clinical symptoms, underlying heart disease and pretest probability. This will be even more important in elderly patients with multiple clinical comorbidities. Today, there are few studies with patients above the age of 80 in whom the prevalence of heart failure is around 10–15% and managed mainly in primary health care. The higher prevalence of the disease will impact both the negative and positive predictive values of natriuretic peptides and the cut-off levels in these patients have still not been settled satisfactorily.

References

1. Levin ER, Gardner DG, Samson WK. Natriuretic peptides. *N Engl J Med.* 1998;339(5): 321-328.
2. Sudoh T, Kangawa K, Minamino N, Matsuo H. A new natriuretic peptide in porcine brain. *Nature.* 1988;332(6159):78-81.
3. Minamino N, Makino Y, Tateyama H, Kangawa K, Matsuo H. Characterization of immunoreactive human C-type natriuretic peptide in brain and heart. *Biochem Biophys Res Commun.* 1991;179(1):535-542.
4. Schirger JA, Heublein DM, Chen HH, et al. Presence of Dendroaspis natriuretic peptide-like immunoreactivity in human plasma and its increase during human heart failure. *Mayo Clin Proc.* 1999;74(2):126-130.
5. Gunning M, Brenner BM. Urodilatin: a potent natriuretic peptide of renal origin. *Curr Opin Nephrol Hypertens.* 1993;2(6):857-862.
6. Forte LR, Currie MG. Guanylin: a peptide regulator of epithelial transport. *Faseb J.* 1995;9(8): 643-650.
7. Daniels LB, Maisel AS. Natriuretic peptides. *J Am Coll Cardiol.* 2007;50(25):2357-2368.
8. Koller KJ, Goeddel DV. Molecular biology of the natriuretic peptides and their receptors. *Circulation.* 1992;86(4):1081-1088.
9. Yasue H, Yoshimura M, Sumida H, et al. Localization and mechanism of secretion of B-type natriuretic peptide in comparison with those of A-type natriuretic peptide in normal subjects and patients with heart failure. *Circulation.* 1994;90(1):195-203.
10. Schellenberger U, O'Rear J, Guzzetta A, Jue RA, Protter AA, Pollitt NS. The precursor to B-type natriuretic peptide is an O-linked glycoprotein. *Arch Biochem Biophys.* 2006;451(2):160- 166.
11. Pemberton CJ, Johnson ML, Yandle TG, Espiner EA. Deconvolution analysis of cardiac natriuretic peptides during acute volume overload. *Hypertension.* 2000;36(3):355-359.
12. Yeo KT, Wu AH, Apple FS, et al. Multicenter evaluation of the Roche NT-proBNP assay and comparison to the Biosite Triage BNP assay. *Clin Chim Acta.* 2003;338(1–2):107-115.
13. Belenky A, Smith A, Zhang B, et al. The effect of class-specific protease inhibitors on the stabilization of B-type natriuretic peptide in human plasma. *Clin Chim Acta.* 2004;340 (1–2):163-172.
14. Barnes SC, Collinson PO, Galasko G, Lahiri A, Senior R. Evaluation of N-terminal pro-B type natriuretic peptide analysis on the Elecsys 1010 and 2010 analysers. *Ann Clin Biochem.* 2004;41(Pt 6):459-463.
15. Mueller T, Gegenhuber A, Poelz W, Haltmayer M. Comparison of the Biomedica NT-proBNP enzyme immunoassay and the Roche NT-proBNP chemiluminescence immunoassay: implications for the prediction of symptomatic and asymptomatic structural heart disease. *Clin Chem.* 2003;49(6 pt 1):976-979.
16. Olofsson M, Boman K. Usefulness of natriuretic peptides in primary health care – an explorative study in elderly patients. Submitted. *Scand J Prim Health Care.* 2009;28:29-35.
17. Apple FS, Panteghini M, Ravkilde J, et al. Quality specifications for B-type natriuretic peptide assays. *Clin Chem.* 2005;51(3):486-493.
18. Masson S, Latini R, Anand IS, et al. Direct comparison of B-type natriuretic peptide (BNP) and amino-terminal proBNP in a large population of patients with chronic and symptomatic heart failure: the Valsartan Heart Failure (Val-HeFT) data. *Clin Chem.* 2006;52(8): 1528-1538.
19. Omland T, Sabatine MS, Jablonski KA, et al. Prognostic value of B-Type natriuretic peptides in patients with stable coronary artery disease: the PEACE Trial. *J Am Coll Cardiol.* 2007; 50(3):205-214.

20. Dickstein K, Cohen-Solal A, Filippatos G, et al. ESC Guidelines for the diagnosis and treatment of acute and chronic heart failure 2008: the Task Force for the Diagnosis and Treatment of Acute and Chronic Heart Failure 2008 of the European Society of Cardiology. Developed in collaboration with the Heart Failure Association of the ESC (HFA) and endorsed by the European Society of Intensive Care Medicine (ESICM). *Eur Heart J.* 2008;29(19): 2388-2442.

21. Zaphiriou A, Robb S, Murray-Thomas T, et al. The diagnostic accuracy of plasma BNP and NTproBNP in patients referred from primary care with suspected heart failure: results of the UK natriuretic peptide study. *Eur J Heart Fail.* 2005;7(4):537-541.

22. Januzzi JL Jr, Camargo CA, Anwaruddin S, et al. The N-terminal Pro-BNP investigation of dyspnea in the emergency department (PRIDE) study. *Am J Cardiol.* 2005;95(8):948-954.

23. Mueller T, Gegenhuber A, Poelz W, Haltmayer M. Diagnostic accuracy of B type natriuretic peptide and amino terminal proBNP in the emergency diagnosis of heart failure. *Heart.* 2005;91(5):606-612.

24. Bayes-Genis A, Santalo-Bel M, Zapico-Muniz E, et al. N-terminal probrain natriuretic peptide (NT-proBNP) in the emergency diagnosis and in-hospital monitoring of patients with dyspnoea and ventricular dysfunction. *Eur J Heart Fail.* 2004;6(3):301-308.

25. Lainchbury JG, Campbell E, Frampton CM, Yandle TG, Nicholls MG, Richards AM. Brain natriuretic peptide and n-terminal brain natriuretic peptide in the diagnosis of heart failure in patients with acute shortness of breath. *J Am Coll Cardiol.* 2003;42(4):728-735.

26. Moe GW, Howlett J, Januzzi JL, Zowall H. N-terminal pro-B-type natriuretic peptide testing improves the management of patients with suspected acute heart failure: primary results of the Canadian prospective randomized multicenter IMPROVE-CHF study. *Circulation.* 2007;115 (24):3103-3110.

27. Goetze JP, Mogelvang R, Maage L, et al. Plasma pro-B-type natriuretic peptide in the general population: screening for left ventricular hypertrophy and systolic dysfunction. *Eur Heart J.* 2006;27(24):3004-3010.

28. Januzzi JL Jr, Sakhuja R, O'Donoghue M, et al. Utility of amino-terminal pro-brain natriuretic peptide testing for prediction of 1-year mortality in patients with dyspnea treated in the emergency department. *Arch Intern Med.* 2006;166(3):315-320.

29. Bettencourt P, Azevedo A, Pimenta J, Frioes F, Ferreira S, Ferreira A. N-terminal-pro-brain natriuretic peptide predicts outcome after hospital discharge in heart failure patients. *Circulation.* 2004;110(15):2168-2174.

30. Logeart D, Thabut G, Jourdain P, et al. Predischarge B-type natriuretic peptide assay for identifying patients at high risk of re-admission after decompensated heart failure. *J Am Coll Cardiol.* 2004;43(4):635-641.

31. Olsson LG, Swedberg K, Cleland JG, et al. Prognostic importance of plasma NT-pro BNP in chronic heart failure in patients treated with a beta-blocker: results from the Carvedilol Or Metoprolol European Trial (COMET) trial. *Eur J Heart Fail.* 2007;9(8):795-801.

32. Lubien E, DeMaria A, Krishnaswamy P, et al. Utility of B-natriuretic peptide in detecting diastolic dysfunction: comparison with Doppler velocity recordings. *Circulation.* 2002;105(5): 595-601.

33. Alehagen U, Lindstedt G, Eriksson H, Dahlstrom U. Utility of the amino-terminal fragment of pro-brain natriuretic peptide in plasma for the evaluation of cardiac dysfunction in elderly patients in primary health care. *Clin Chem.* 2003;49(8):1337-1346.

34. Iwanaga Y, Nishi I, Furuichi S, et al. B-type natriuretic peptide strongly reflects diastolic wall stress in patients with chronic heart failure: comparison between systolic and diastolic heart failure. *J Am Coll Cardiol.* 2006;47(4):742-748.

35. Bettencourt P, Azevedo A, Fonseca L, et al. Prognosis of decompensated heart failure patients with preserved systolic function is predicted by NT-proBNP variations during hospitalization. *Int J Cardiol.* 2007;117(1):75-79.

36. Troughton RW, Frampton CM, Yandle TG, Espiner EA, Nicholls MG, Richards AM. Treatment of heart failure guided by plasma aminoterminal brain natriuretic peptide (N-BNP) concentrations. *Lancet*. 2000;355(9210):1126-1130.

37. Jourdain P, Jondeau G, Funck F, et al. Plasma brain natriuretic peptide-guided therapy to improve outcome in heart failure: the STARS-BNP Multicenter Study. *J Am Coll Cardiol*. 2007;49(16):1733-1739.

38. Pfisterer M, Buser P, Rickli H, et al. BNP-guided vs symptom-guided heart failure therapy: the Trial of Intensified vs Standard Medical Therapy in Elderly Patients With Congestive Heart Failure (TIME-CHF) randomized trial. PRIMA-study, presentation ACC Orlando March-2009, SIGNAL-HF-study, presentation Heart Failure Nice, *JAMA*. 2009;301(4):383-392.

39. Eurlings, L. et al. Can pro-brain natriuretic peptide-guided therapy of heart failure improve heart failure morbidity and mortality? Main outcome of the PRIMA study [abstract 402-14]. Presented at the ACC 58th Annual Scientific Session (Orlando, USA; 29–31 March 2009).

40. Persson H et al. SIGNAL-HF Study. Presented at the European Heart Failure Association Annual Meeting; June 1, 2009; Nice, France. *Eur J Heart Fail*. Suppl (2009) 8(suppl 2)

41. Sim V, Hampton D, Phillips C, et al. The use of brain natriuretic peptide as a screening test for left ventricular systolic dysfunction- cost-effectiveness in relation to open access echocardiography. *Fam Pract*. 2003;20(5):570-574.

42. Davenport C, Cheng EY, Kwok YT, et al. Assessing the diagnostic test accuracy of natriuretic peptides and ECG in the diagnosis of left ventricular systolic dysfunction: a systematic review and meta-analysis. *Br J Gen Pract*. 2006;56(522):48-56.

43. Goetze JP, Jensen G, Moller S, Bendtsen F, Rehfeld JF, Henriksen JH. BNP and N-terminal proBNP are both extracted in the normal kidney. *Eur J Clin Invest*. 2006;36(1):8-15.

44. DeFilippi C, van Kimmenade RR, Pinto YM. Amino-terminal pro-B-type natriuretic peptide testing in renal disease. *Am J Cardiol*. 2008;101(3A):82-88.

45. David S, Kumpers P, Seidler V, Biertz F, Haller H, Fliser D. Diagnostic value of N-terminal pro-B-type natriuretic peptide (NT-proBNP) for left ventricular dysfunction in patients with chronic kidney disease stage 5 on haemodialysis. *Nephrol Dial Transplant*. 2008;23(4):1370-1377.

46. Raymond I, Groenning BA, Hildebrandt PR, et al. The influence of age, sex and other variables on the plasma level of N-terminal pro brain natriuretic peptide in a large sample of the general population. *Heart*. 2003;89(7):745-751.

47. Horwich TB, Hamilton MA, Fonarow GC. B-type natriuretic peptide levels in obese patients with advanced heart failure. *J Am Coll Cardiol*. 2006;47(1):85-90.

Cardiac Resynchronization Therapy

18

Jeffrey Wing-Hong Fung and Cheuk-Man Yu

Cardiac resynchronization therapy (CRT), or biventricular pacing therapy, is the first approved nonsurgical treatment of advanced heart failure (HF) employing implantable device. This therapy is characterized by the implantation of an additional left ventricular (LV) lead, usually through the coronary sinus, to reach the lateral or postero-lateral vein in order to pace the LV free wall.[1] The conventional right ventricular lead is usually needed to pace the septal region while the right atrial lead is placed to provide sensing and back-up pacing when necessary. CRT can be delivered by implantation of a pacemaker (CRT-P) or a defibrillator (CRT-D). In HF population, about one-quarter will exhibit features of prolongation of QRS duration, which is also a marker of poor prognosis.[2] Because of the presence of electrical activation delay within the LV, these patients will develop electromechanical delay in the form of systolic dyssynchrony (i.e., uncoordinated contraction in different regions of the LV). This will accelerate the pathophysiologic process of LV adverse remodeling with cavity dilatation, deterioration of systolic function, elevation of filling pressure and mitral regurgitation. The current guidelines recommend CRT for HF patients with New York Heart Association (NYHA) class III or IV symptoms despite optimal medical therapy, reduced ejection fraction of <35%, and a prolonged QRS duration of >120 or 130 ms.[3,4]

18.1
Clinical Benefits of CRT

Since the first case report of biventricular pacing, to date, more than 4,000 patients have been included in completed randomized clinical trials of CRT.[5] These studies confirmed the clinical benefits of CRT which included improvement of NYHA class and Minnesota Living With Heart Failure Quality of life (MLHFQ) score and exercise capacity (peak VO_2 consumption and 6-Minute Hall Walk distance).[6–15] A few large randomized trials also

J. Wing-Hong Fung (✉)
Medicine and Therapeutics, Prince of Wales Hospital,
The Chinese University of Hong Kong, Shatin, Hong Kong, China
e-mail: jwhfung@cuhk.edu.hk

M.Y. Henein (ed.), *Heart Failure in Clinical Practice*,
DOI: 10.1007/978-1-84996-153-0_18, © Springer-Verlag London Limited 2010

reported a lower mortality and/or HF hospitalization in the CRT treatment arm.[6, 10, 14, 15] Table 18.1 summaries the clinical design and results of major multicenter clinical trials of CRT. Several reviews and meta-analysis of CRT trial data have been published.[16, 17] As similar to the finding of CArdiac REsynchronization in Heart Failure (CARE-HF) study, the meta-analysis confirmed a reduction of all-cause mortality by 21–22% and hospitalization for worsening HF by 29–32%.[16–18] Furthermore, the MLHFQ score reduced by a mean difference of 7.6 points, and 6-Minute Hall Walk distance increased by a mean difference of 28 m for all symptomatic patients, and by 30 m when limited to NYHA functional class III and IV HF. The NYHA functional class was improved by one class in 58% of patients who received CRT when compared with 37% of controls.[16, 17]

18.2
Cardiac Structural and Functional Benefits of CRT

Favorable changes in LV structure and function form another major and unequivocal benefit of CRT. These changes included LV reverse remodeling, improvement of LV systolic function (ejection fraction, cardiac output) and contractility (+dp/dt), reduction of mitral regurgitation, as well as improvement of intra- and inter-ventricular systolic dyssynchrony.[19] Furthermore, atrial reverse remodeling with increase in atrial contractility and better compliance was also evident after CRT,[20] while right ventricular systolic function was reported to be increased.[21] Most of these changes can be detected by various cardiac imaging technologies, in particular echocardiography.

LV reverse remodeling is described in HF patients in whom progressive LV dilatation and deterioration in contractile function are not simply arrested, but are partially reversed. Clinical trials of CRT observed that after CRT for 3–6 months, LV end-systolic volume decreased by about 18% while LV ejection fraction increased by 5–7% (absolute unit).[15, 22] There is progressive reduction in LV volumes over time and even beyond 2 years. In CARE-HF study, the LV end-systolic volume decreased by 36%, while the LV ejection fraction increased by 11%.[15] In fact, LV reverse remodeling is accompanied not only by increase in systolic function but also by favorable change of LV geometry, which becomes less spherical in shape,[19, 23] regression of LV mass,[24] decrease in natriuretic peptide levels,[25–27] as well as favorable myocardial gene expression.[26] Of note, these favorable changes almost exclusively occurred only in responders of LV reverse remodeling (usually defined by ≥15% reduction of LV end-systolic volume), but not in the nonresponders. Furthermore, patients who exhibited LV reverse remodeling response after CRT for 3–6 months were associated with highly favorable long-term clinical outcome, including a lower all-cause mortality (6.9% vs. 30.6%, Log-rank $\chi^2 = 13.26$, $p = 0.0003$), cardiovascular mortality (2.3% vs. 24.1%, Log-rank $\chi^2 = 17.1$, $p < 0.0001$) and HF events (11.5% vs. 33.3%, Log-rank $\chi^2 = 8.71$, $p = 0.0032$) (Fig. 18.1).[28] Whether patients who received CRT are likely to show LV reverse remodeling response appears to be largely dependent on the amount of pretreatment intraventricular systolic dyssynchrony.[22, 29–33] Interestingly, cessation of CRT even for 4 weeks will abolish the beneficial echocardiographic changes of LV reverse remodeling in which LV will enlarge again while systolic function deteriorates.

Table 18.1 Summary of major multicenter clinical trials of CRT

Study (no. of patients) (reference)	No. of patients	NYHA class	QRS width by criteria, ms	Actual QRS duration, mean±SD (inter-quartile range)	Underlying rhythm	Design	ICD indica-tion	Primary end-point	Results
MUSTIC-SR[6]	58	III	>150	174±20	SR	Crossover	No	6MHW	Improvement in 6MWH, NYHA class, QOL and peak VO$_2$; and reduced hospita-lizations
MUSTIC-AF[7]	43	III	>200	206±19	AF	Crossover	No	6MHW	Improvement in 6MWH, NYHA class, QOL and peak VO$_2$, and fewer hospita-lizations
PATH-CHF[8]	41	III, IV	≥120	175±32	SR	Crossover	No	Peak VO$_2$, 6MHW	Improvement in 6MWH, QOL, and NYHA class
PATH-CHF II[9]	86	III, IV	≥120	155±20	SR	Crossover ± (no pacing vs. LV pacing)	Both	Peak VO$_2$, anaerobic VO$_2$, 6MWH	Exercise tolerance, 6MWH, and QOL improved

(continued)

Table 18.1 (continued)

Study (no. of patients) (reference)	No. of patients	NYHA class	QRS width by criteria, ms	Actual QRS duration, mean ± SD (interquartile range)	Underlying rhythm	Design	ICD indication	Primary end-point	Results
MIRACLE[10]	453	III, IV	≥130	165±20	SR	Randomized, parallel arms	No	6MHW, NYHA class, QOL	Improvement in all three primary end points
MIRACLE-ICD[11]	369	III, IV	≥130	162±22	SR	Randomized, parallel arms	Yes	6MHW, NYHA class, QOL	Improvement in QOL and functional class; no improvement in 6MWH
MIRACLE-ICD II[12]	186	II	≥130	166±25	SR	Randomized, parallel arms	Yes	VO$_2$	Improvement in QOL, functional status, and exercise capacity
CONTAK-CD[13]	490	II–IV	≥120	160±27	SR	Randomized, crossover and parallel controlled	Yes	6MHW, NYHA class, QOL	Slightly decreased morbidity and mortality end point; improvement in exercise capacity, QOL, and NYHA class

COMPANION[14]	1,520	III, IV	≥120	160±??	SR	Randomized, parallel arms	No	Composite: time to death from or hospitalization for any cause	CRT and CRT-D reduced the risk of the primary end point
CARE-HF[15]	813	III, IV	≥120	160±??(152–180)	SR	Open-label randomization to control vs. CRT device	No	Composite: death from any cause and hospitalization for a major cardiovascular event	CRT reduced complications and risk of death; and improved symptoms and QOL

Modified from Chap. 14 of Ref. 1

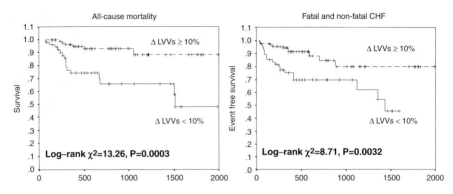

Fig. 18.1 Patients who achieved early LV reverse remodeling between 3 and 6 months after CRT predicts a lower long term all-cause mortality and cardiovascular event rate (reproduced from ref. 28)

18.3
Other Benefits of CRT

In patients who received CRT, favorable decrease in natriuretic peptide levels (both BNP and NT-proBNP) has been reported.[25-27] Interestingly, those who had reduction of NT-proBNP of ≥50% after CRT for 3 months were associated with lower mortality (Log-rank $\chi^2 = 4.01, p = 0.04$) and composite end-point of mortality or hospitalization for cardiovascular causes (Log-rank $\chi^2 = 4.31, p = 0.02$).[27]

Another important benefit of CRT is related to its impact on atrial fibrillation (AF). For patients with known paroxysmal AF, CRT has been shown to reduce AF burden in terms of shorter duration in AF as well as lesser patients with recurrent AF episodes.[34] Similar benefits were observed for HF patients who were upgraded to CRT-D from a conventional pacemaker or defibrillator.[35] For patients who are AF naïve, a lower annual incidence of new-onset AF of 2.8% was reported when compared with the control group of 10.2% ($p = 0.025$).[36] Furthermore, in another study of 97 HF patients who received CRT and were without history of AF, reduction of new-onset AF was more likely to occur in patients who showed improvement of left atrial contractile function after a mean follow up of 1,200±705 days (12.8% vs. 40%, $p = 0.002$).[37] In fact, this group was also associated with a lower mortality (17% vs. 44%, $p = 0.004$). Interestingly, CRT will not increase the vulnerability of ventricular tachyarrhythmias, but rather reduce the chance of sudden cardiac death even with CRT-P.[38] Furthermore, improvement of heart rate variability (HRV), after CRT, has been reported in large clinical studies. Patients who remained in persistently low HRV (standard deviation of 5-min median atrial–atrial intervals, or SDAAM <50 ms) were associated with a higher mortality.[39]

18.4
CRT Device Based Diagnostics for Monitoring of HF Decompensation

With the increasing use of CRT, it is now possible to incorporate HF monitoring capabilities into implantable devices. In HF patients, despite receiving optimal medical therapy, repeated hospitalization due to acute HF decompensation remains common, in particular in those with NYHA Class III and IV symptoms. Therefore, an additional objective of incorporating implantable device is not only to reduce dyssynchrony and its associated benefits but also to provide a platform to closely monitor HF on a continuous basis so as to predict and prevent HF exacerbation and improve clinical outcome. Currently, a few monitoring parameters designed for HF has been described in the literature, which included intrathoracic impedance, HRV and right ventricular pressure. However, additional monitoring parameters have been incorporated into CRT, pacemaker, and defibrillator platforms, such as heart rate, night heart rate, activity, arrhythmia log, as well as peak endocardial acceleration sensor.

18.4.1
Intrathoracic Impedance

Intrathoracic impedance monitoring is on the basis of the concept that when there is pulmonary congestion and alveolar edema with increasing left-sided chamber filling pressure, the impedance in the lung will decrease. This concept was confirmed first in canine model of overdrive pacing-induced HF where elevation of LV end-diastolic pressure correlated linearly and negatively with reduction of intrathoracic impedance.[40] In the first human study, 34 patients who were in NYHA functional class III or IV HF were studied for 1 year. A conventional ICD lead was inserted transvenously to the RV apex and was connected to a modified pacemaker.[41] A constant current was sent through the tissue between the RV coil electrode and device case and the voltage was then measured to calculate the intrathoracic impedance. To eliminate the effect of cardiac and respiratory movements, more than two thousand impedance measurements were averaged over 2 min to provide a mean impedance value. The key observations were that a decrease in intrathoracic impedance provided early HF warning with a mean lead time of 18 days prior to admission and that symptom of dyspnoea occurred only 3 days prior to hospital admission (Fig. 18.2). During the hospitalization period, the intrathoracic impedance demonstrated a significant correlation with the pulmonary capillary wedge pressure ($r=-0.61$, $p<0.001$) and net fluid loss with diuretic therapy ($r=-0.70$, $p<0.001$) (Fig. 18.3). A special algorithm of prediction of HF based on the reduction of intrathoracic impedance was developed, and by using 60 Ω-day as the nominal threshold, it had a sensitivity of 77% for prediction of HF hospitalization at the cost of

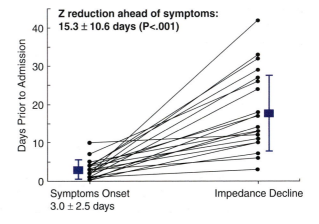

Fig. 18.2 Intrathoracic impedance decrease compared with onset of symptoms before hospitalization for decompensated heart failure. Impedance reduction ahead of symptoms for 15 days on average

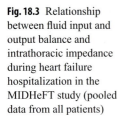

Fig. 18.3 Relationship between fluid input and output balance and intrathoracic impedance during heart failure hospitalization in the MIDHeFT study (pooled data from all patients)

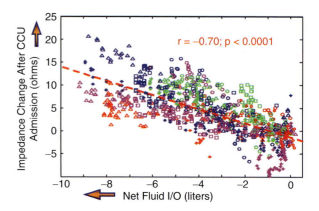

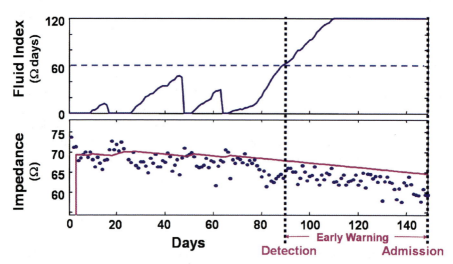

Fig. 18.4 Prediction of heart failure decompensation by intrathoracic impedance monitoring. The algorithm of OptiVol™ consists of measurement of daily impedance (*blue dots*), the establishment of reference impedance (*pink line*), the record of cumulative sum of impedance value that fall below the reference impedance value as fluid index (*blue line*), and the alert threshold value set at 60 Ω day (*blue dotted line*). When the fluid index rises above the threshold value, alert can be set and appropriate action can then taken at the early warning period so as to avoid heart failure hospitalization

1.5 false-positives per patient–year of monitoring, and gave an early warning of 13.4 ± 6.2 days before HF hospitalization (Fig. 18.4). Intrathoracic impedance measurement is currently incorporated into CRT-D pulse generator (The OptiVol® fluid index, Medtronic Inc., Minneapolis, MN). The recent results of the European Insync Sentry Observational Study showed that, with the same threshold of 60 Ω-day for HF deterioration alert, an adjusted sensitivity and positive predictive value of 60% was observed among 373 patients after a median follow up of 4.2 months.[42] One important solution of applying HF monitoring capabilities into practice is the ability of setting up an alert system. This can be done through device interrogation at clinic follow up, the use of audible alert build inside the device, the use of additional portable device for self-monitoring by patients, as well as wireless telemetry monitoring system, which transmits information to the dedicated server while physicians can retrieve information through internet-based systems. Further clinical trials to confirm the clinical utility of intrathoracic impedance is ongoing, which include SENSE-HF study.[43]

18.4.2
Heart Rate Variability

Clinical trials conducted in patients with chronic HF or following myocardial infarction demonstrated that reduced RR interval variability, or HRV, is associated with increased mortality risk.[44] Continuous monitoring of HRV is now possible when measured from the signals generated from the atrial lead of CRT system. Typically, HRV is quantified by measuring the standard deviation of the 5 min median A–A interval (SDAAM) continuously.[39,45] Clinical study on HF patients who received CRT demonstrated that the therapy improved long-term HRV when compared with the control group who had the device programmed to "off" mode.[45] This reflects that the favorable improvement of LV systolic function resulted in less sympathetic activation and better vagal control of the heart over time. In the MIRACLE study, patients with SDAAM <50 ms had significantly higher all-cause and cardiovascular mortality with a hazard ratio of 3.2 and 4.43, respectively, when compared to those with SDAAM >100 ms, when followed for a mean duration of 18 months.[39] With a threshold of 200 ms-days, the sensitivity for predicting HF hospitalization is 70% at a cost of 2.4 false positive events per patient–year follow up.[39]

18.4.3
Hemodynamic and Activity Sensors

Hemodynamic sensor requires a specialized transvenous lead positioned in the RV outflow tract that measures the RV systolic and diastolic pressures. The device estimates pulmonary artery diastolic pressure and maximum change in RV pressure over time. In the Chronicle Offers Management to Patients with Advanced Signs and Symptoms of Heart Failure (COMPASS-HF) trial, 274 patients were randomized to Chronicle-guided treatment group or to a control group where clinicians were blinded to device-based hemodynamic measurements. Patients were followed for 6 months.[46] Although the primary end-point of cumulative HF related hospitalization, emergency department visit or urgent clinic visit requiring intravenous HF therapy, had only an insignificant 21% reduction in the Chronicle group ($p=0.33$), subgroup analysis of NYHA class III patients (85% of the study population) showed a significant reduction in the primary end-point by 41% ($p=0.03$). During the randomized period, there was also 36% reduction in the relative risk of HF-related hospitalizations in the Chronicle group when compared with the control group ($p=0.03$).[46]

Mean daily physical activity (MDPA) index measured by pedometers have been shown to predict mortality in HF.[47] There was significant and sustained improvement in MDPA irrespective of baseline NYHA class after CRT in one study.[48] The MDPA index retrieved from the device may then have the potential to monitor patients' response to the therapy received. The role of MDPA index to predict HF exacerbation has been evaluated and compared with SDAAM and the night heart rate changes in one study.[39] However, the sensitivity of MDPA was lower than that of SDAAM to predict hospitalization over the entire range of false-positive rates. Its role in predicting HF exacerbation is probably complementary to other parameters, e.g., HRV and/or intrathoracic impedance.

18.5
Evolving and Potentially New Indications of CRT

18.5.1
Patients with Atrial Fibrillation

The prevalence of AF in patients with moderate to advanced HF was 15–30% and increases as the severity of HF increases.[49] Currently, CRT can be recommended to patients with AF and wide QRS complex only as Class IIa indication because of the fact that most of the randomized clinical trials have excluded patients with permanent AF. Two interesting but interlinked questions emerge when considering CRT for patients with AF. One is whether CRT has any favorable impact on AF development and the other is whether CRT is beneficial in patients with AF and HF. The former issue remains controversial and is still under debate. Post-hoc analysis of CARE-HF trial suggested that the device had no favorable impact on AF incidence when compared to medical therapy alone.[50] However, favorable structural changes and improvement in contractile function in both atria were observed after CRT especially among the responders.[20, 51] In addition, such improvement was associated with lower incidence of AF in an observational study.[37] A randomized CRT trial with device switches on and off together with monitoring of asymptomatic atrial high rate episodes would clarify the controversy about the effect of CRT on AF development.

The latter issue about the beneficial role of CRT in patients who have already developed AF appears to be even more crucial as the prevalence of AF in advanced HF was high and the combination was associated with high mortality. The irregular and intermittently high ventricular rate via native atrioventricular (AV) conduction may limit the percentage of biventricular pacing in CRT recipients who are in permanent AF. Some device algorithms may help to solve the issues but at the expense of higher pacing rate. On the basis of several observational studies,[52–56] comparable beneficial effects to those in sinus rhythm by CRT were consistently observed in AF patients. In a recent meta-analysis involving more than 1,000 patients, similar clinical and echocardiographic benefits between patients in AF and sinus rhythm were observed.[57] However, conflicting results were observed with regard to the need of AV junction ablation in AF patients receiving CRT.[58] In a prospective but nonrandomized study, the benefit of CRT was only observed in AF patients with AV junction ablation but not in those without it even though the percentage of pacing was more than 85%.[59] On the other hand, the necessity of AV junction ablation in patients with permanent AF was not reproducibly demonstrated in two recent studies.[53, 54] Such controversy leads to another interesting issue which is the optimal pacing dosage in CRT patients. In a retrospective analysis, the greatest magnitude of benefit was observed in those with >92% of biventricular pacing.[60] It seems that 100% biventricular pacing may not be absolutely necessary for all CRT patients.

In summary, CRT can be considered particularly for those AF patients with refractory symptom despite optimal medical therapy. ß blockers and digoxin should be gradually titrated to target doses after CRT, if they were limited by bradycardia beforehand, as optimal drug therapy was shown to be necessary for maximal CRT response.[61] AV junction ablation may not be absolutely necessary for every patient after CRT but can be considered in those with very low percentage of pacing despite optimal pharmacotherapy. A properly designed randomized trial is imminently necessary to clarify the role of AV junction ablation in patients with permanent AF receiving CRT.

18.5.2
Patients with Mild Heart Failure Symptom or Moderate LV Dysfunction

From mechanistic point of view, the primary benefit of CRT is to correct underlying electromechanical abnormality in those with wide QRS complex and impaired LV systolic function. It may be reasonable to postulate that CRT may also be potentially beneficial to those less symptomatic patients (NYHA class I or II) or those with only moderately impaired LV systolic function (LV ejection fraction 35–50%), provided electromechanical abnormality is the main culprit of the LV systolic dysfunction. In an early randomized controlled clinical study, it was shown that CRT had significant impact on disease progression and promoted LV reverse remodeling even in patients with mildly symptomatic chronic HF (NYHA class II and LV ejection fraction <35%).[62] Recently, a large scale randomized controlled trial has addressed this important clinical question of whether CRT will be of any benefit in those with only mild HF symptom. More than 600 patients with wide QRS complex and LV EF <40% were randomized in a 2 to 1 ratio to CRT-ON and CRT-OFF with a follow up duration of 12 months.[63] Although there was no statistical difference in the primary end-point of HF composite response, patients in CRT-ON arm had significantly better LV reverse remodeling and delayed time to HF hospitalization. Information about the role of CRT in patients with moderately impaired LV systolic function is scarce. A small nonrandomized study has attempted to address the issue in 15 HF patients with LV ejection fraction between 35 and 50% and wide QRS complex and compared the clinical and echocardiographic changes to 30 patients with standard CRT indication (LV ejection fraction <35%).[64] Significant improvement in LV ejection fraction, reverse remodeling and NYHA class was observed in both groups, suggesting that CRT may be useful in HF patients with LV dyssynchrony even at early stage of HF. Preliminary results from these studies provide evidence to support the beneficial role of CRT in these HF patients with mild symptoms or moderately impaired LV systolic function though large scale study is still necessary to confirm the definitive role of the device in early stage of HF.

18.5.3
Patients with Standard Pacing Indication

Right ventricular apical pacing is associated with adverse effect on LV systolic function and development of HF.[65] The concept of ventricular desynchronization by right ventricular apical pacing has been proposed and CRT may also play a role in reversing the desynchronization effect by device upgrading to biventricular pacing. Twenty HF patients with LV ejection fraction <35%, permanent AF, AV junction ablation and right ventricular pacing were upgraded to biventricular pacing.[66] Dramatic improvements in both clinical and echocardiographic parameters were observed after the upgrade, together with reduction in HF hospitalization.

Special attention is required when considering permanent pacing for those with severe HF. In Dual Chamber and VVI Implantable Defibrillator (DAVID) trial, patients with low ejection fraction receiving DDDR with high percentage of right ventricular pacing were associated with adverse clinical outcomes.[67] The decision of pacing mode and sites became a critical issue in those with systolic HF and standard pacing indication. It is of great clinical interest to examine whether CRT would be of any benefit in those with both heart block and HF. The Homburg Biventricular Pacing Evaluation study was the first randomized controlled study that compared the biventricular pacing approach with conventional right ventricular pacing in patients with LV dysfunction and a standard pacing indication.[68] It was shown that biventricular pacing was superior to right ventricular pacing in improving HF status and LV ejection fraction. Similar results were also observed in PAVE study.[69] Greatest improvement in 6 min walking distance, which was the primary endpoint of the study, was observed in those with LV ejection fraction <45% or NYHA class II/III receiving biventricular pacing after AV junction ablation for ventricular rate control in AF patients. Based on these clinical studies, it appears that CRT has a promising role in those patients with HF and requires ventricular pacing support instead of right ventricular pacing, which is nowadays a class IIA indication under the current recommendation guidelines.

Despite the tremendous research effort in recent decades, the optimal pacing modes and sites for patients with normal LV ejection fraction and standard pacing indication remain unclear. In fact, early animal and acute human studies have already demonstrated the beneficial effect of CRT over conventional right ventricular pacing in preserving LV systolic function.[70-72] Such hypothesis has recently been tested in a randomized study.[73] Two hundred patients with normal LV ejection fraction and standard pacing indication will be randomized to either biventricular or right ventricular apical pacing for 12 months. The primary endpoints are LV ejection fraction and end-systolic volume. The definitive role of CRT in patients with standard pacing indication may become clearer then.

18.5.4
Narrow QRS Complex with Mechanical Dyssynchrony

It was reported that systolic asynchrony detected by echocardiography existed in 27–43% of patients with HF but narrow QRS complex.[74-77] Therefore, a therapeutic opportunity is to consider CRT for HF patients with narrow QRS complexes who have evidence of systolic asynchrony by echocardiography. Early nonrandomized studies do provide encouraging results in supporting CRT in these HF patients. The first study examined 14 HF patients with narrow QRS complexes.[78] The investigators reported the improvement of NYHA class and 6-Minute Hall Walk distance in the narrow QRS group. However, there were no data provided on the change in maximal exercise capacity and quality of life score. Another pilot study examined eight HF patients with narrow QRS duration and reported an insignificant increase in ejection fraction by 4.7% when CRT was commenced acutely.[79] However, these two studies were limited by a small sample size. The potential benefit of CRT was evaluated in 51 narrow complex patients and compared to 51 wide complex patients in one study.[80] There was a significant reduction of LV end-systolic volume in both narrow and wide QRS groups. Improvement of NYHA class, maximal exercise capacity, 6-Minute Hall-Walk distance, ejection fraction and mitral regurgitation was also observed. In both groups, the degree of baseline mechanical asynchrony determined LV reverse remodeling to a similar extent. Similar results were observed in another study comparing 33 narrow complex patients with pre-existing LV dyssynchrony detected by tissue Doppler imaging to 33 wide complex patients after CRT.[81]

Like those with wide QRS complex patients, a properly designed randomized trial is needed to confirm the potential beneficial role of CRT in these narrow complex patients before adopting CRT into clinical practice. RethinQ was the first such study that enrolled 172 patients with narrow QRS complex who had echocardiographic evidence of LV mechanical dyssynchrony and a standard indication for an ICD.[82] Patients received the CRT device and were randomly assigned to the CRT group or to a control group (no CRT) for 6 months. The primary end point was the proportion of patients with an increase in peak oxygen consumption of at least 1.0 mL/kg of body weight per minute during cardiopulmonary exercise testing at 6 months. However, there was no statistical difference detected in the primary endpoint and other clinical or echocardiographic outcomes between the two groups. There are other ongoing clinical trials examining the role of CRT in narrow complex patients with various echo-determined mechanical dyssynchrony. However, CRT cannot be recommended to HF patients with QRS duration less than 120 ms at the present moment.

References

1. Yu CM, Hayes DL, Auricchio A. *Cardiac Resynchronization Therapy*. 2nd ed. Hoboken NJ: Wiley-Blackwell; 2008.
2. Baldasseroni S, Opasich C, Gorini M, et al. Left bundle-branch block is associated with increased 1-year sudden and total mortality rate in 5517 outpatients with congestive heart failure: a report from the Italian network on congestive heart failure. *Am Heart J*. 2002;143:398-405.
3. Epstein AE, DiMarco JP, Ellenbogen KA, et al. ACC/AHA/HRS 2008 Guidelines for Device-Based Therapy of Cardiac Rhythm Abnormalities: a report of the American College of Cardiology/American Heart Association Task Force on Practice Guidelines (Writing Committee to Revise the ACC/AHA/NASPE 2002 Guideline Update for Implantation of Cardiac Pacemakers and Antiarrhythmia Devices) developed in collaboration with the American Association for Thoracic Surgery and Society of Thoracic Surgeons. *J Am Coll Cardiol*. 2008;51:e1-e62.
4. Vardas PE, Auricchio A, Blanc JJ, et al. Guidelines for cardiac pacing and cardiac resynchronization therapy. The Task Force for Cardiac Pacing and Cardiac Resynchronization Therapy of the European Society of Cardiology. Developed in collaboration with the European Heart Rhythm Association. *Europace*. 2007;9:959-998.
5. Cazeau S, Ritter P, Bakdach S, et al. Four chamber pacing in dilated cardiomyopathy [see comments]. *Pacing Clin Electrophysiol*. 1994;17:1974-1979.
6. Cazeau S, Leclercq C, Lavergne T, et al. Effects of multisite biventricular pacing in patients with heart failure and intraventricular conduction delay. *N Engl J Med*. 2001;344:873-880.
7. Linde C, Leclercq C, Rex S, et al. Long-term benefits of biventricular pacing in congestive heart failure: results from the MUltisite STimulation in cardiomyopathy (MUSTIC) study. *J Am Coll Cardiol*. 2002;40:111-118.

8. Auricchio A, Stellbrink C, Sack S, et al. Long-term clinical effect of hemodynamically optimized cardiac resynchronization therapy in patients with heart failure and ventricular conduction delay. *J Am Coll Cardiol.* 2002;39:2026-2033.

9. Auricchio A, Stellbrink C, Butter C, et al. Clinical efficacy of cardiac resynchronization therapy using left ventricular pacing in heart failure patients stratified by severity of ventricular conduction delay. *J Am Coll Cardiol.* 2003;42:2109-2116.

10. Abraham WT, Fisher WG, Smith AL, et al. Cardiac resynchronization in chronic heart failure. *N Engl J Med.* 2002;346:1845-1853.

11. Young JB, Abraham WT, Smith AL, et al. Combined cardiac resynchronization and implantable cardioversion defibrillation in advanced chronic heart failure: the MIRACLE ICD Trial. *JAMA.* 2003;289:2685-2694.

12. Sastry PS. Occult fungal infection is the underlying pathogenic cause of atherogenesis. *Med Hypotheses.* 2004;63:671-674.

13. Lozano I, Bocchiardo M, Achtelik M, et al. Impact of biventricular pacing on mortality in a randomized crossover study of patients with heart failure and ventricular arrhythmias. *Pacing Clin Electrophysiol.* 2000;23:1711-1712.

14. Bristow MR, Saxon LA, Boehmer J, et al. Cardiac-resynchronization therapy with or without an implantable defibrillator in advanced chronic heart failure. *N Engl J Med.* 2004;350:2140-2150.

15. Cleland JG, Daubert JC, Erdmann E, et al. The effect of cardiac resynchronization on morbidity and mortality in heart failure. *N Engl J Med.* 2005;352:1539-1549.

16. McAlister FA, Ezekowitz JA, Wiebe N, et al. Systematic review: cardiac resynchronization in patients with symptomatic heart failure. *Ann Intern Med.* 2004;141:381-390.

17. Freemantle N, Tharmanathan P, Calvert MJ, Abraham WT, Ghosh J, Cleland JG. Cardiac resynchronisation for patients with heart failure due to left ventricular systolic dysfunction – a systematic review and meta-analysis. *Eur J Heart Fail.* 2006;8:433-440.

18. Bradley DJ, Bradley EA, Baughman KL, et al. Cardiac resynchronization and death from progressive heart failure: a meta-analysis of randomized controlled trials. *JAMA.* 2003;289:730-740.

19. Yu CM, Chau E, Sanderson JE, et al. Tissue Doppler echocardiographic evidence of reverse remodeling and improved synchronicity by simultaneously delaying regional contraction after biventricular pacing therapy in heart failure. *Circulation.* 2002;105:438-445.

20. Yu CM, Fang F, Zhang Q, et al. Improvement of atrial function and atrial reverse remodeling after cardiac resynchronization therapy for heart failure. *J Am Coll Cardiol.* 2007;50:778-785.

21. Bleeker GB, Schalij MJ, Nihoyannopoulos P, et al. Left ventricular dyssynchrony predicts right ventricular remodeling after cardiac resynchronization therapy. *J Am Coll Cardiol.* 2005; 46:2264-2269.

22. Yu CM, Gorcsan J III, Bleeker GB, et al. Usefulness of tissue Doppler velocity and strain dyssynchrony for predicting left ventricular reverse remodeling response after cardiac resynchronization therapy. *Am J Cardiol.* 2007;100:1263-1270.

23. Saxon LA, De Marco T, Schafer J, Chatterjee K, Kumar UN, Foster E. Effects of long-term biventricular stimulation for resynchronization on echocardiographic measures of remodeling. *Circulation.* 2002;105:1304-1310.

24. Zhang Q, Fung JW, Auricchio A, et al. Differential change in left ventricular mass and regional wall thickness after cardiac resynchronization therapy for heart failure. *Eur Heart J.* 2006;27: 1423-1430.

25. Hesketh T, Ding QJ. Standard definition of child overweight and obesity worldwide. Young Chinese people in Hong Kong are not representative of those in China. *BMJ.* 2000;321:1158-1159.

26. Vanderheyden M, Mullens W, Delrue L, et al. Myocardial gene expression in heart failure patients treated with cardiac resynchronization therapy responders versus nonresponders. *J Am Coll Cardiol.* 2008;51:129-136.

27. Yu CM, Fung JW, Zhang Q, et al. Improvement of serum NT-ProBNP predicts improvement in cardiac function and favorable prognosis after cardiac resynchronization therapy for heart failure. *J Card Fail.* 2005;11:S42-S46.

28. Yu CM, Bleeker GB, Fung JW, et al. Left ventricular reverse remodeling but not clinical improvement predicts long-term survival after cardiac resynchronization therapy. *Circulation.* 2005;112:1580-1586.

29. Pitzalis MV, Iacoviello M, Romito R, et al. Cardiac resynchronization therapy tailored by echocardiographic evaluation of ventricular asynchrony. *J Am Coll Cardiol.* 2002;40:1615-1622.

30. Yu CM, Fung JWH, Lin H, Zhang Q, Sanderson JE, Lau CP. Predictors of left ventricular reverse remodeling after cardiac resynchronization therapy for heart failure secondary to idiopathic dilated or ischemic cardiomyopathy. *Am J Cardiol.* 2003;91:684-688.

31. Bax JJ, Marwick TH, Molhoek SG, et al. Left ventricular dyssynchrony predicts benefit of cardiac resynchronization therapy in patients with end-stage heart failure before pacemaker implantation. *Am J Cardiol.* 2003;92:1238-1240.

32. Yu CM, Fung JW, Zhang Q, et al. Tissue Doppler imaging is superior to strain rate imaging and postsystolic shortening on the prediction of reverse remodeling in both ischemic and nonischemic heart failure after cardiac resynchronization therapy. *Circulation.* 2004;110:66-73.

33. Suffoletto MS, Dohi K, Cannesson M, Saba S, Gorcsan J III. Novel speckle-tracking radial strain from routine black-and-white echocardiographic images to quantify dyssynchrony and predict response to cardiac resynchronization therapy. *Circulation.* 2006;113:960-968.

34. Hugl B, Bruns HJ, Unterberg-Buchwald C, et al. Atrial fibrillation burden during the post-implant period after CRT using device-based diagnostics. *J Cardiovasc Electrophysiol.* 2006;17:813-817.

35. Yannopoulos D, Lurie KG, Sakaguchi S, et al. Reduced atrial tachyarrhythmia susceptibility after upgrade of conventional implanted pulse generator to cardiac resynchronization therapy in patients with heart failure. *J Am Coll Cardiol.* 2007;50:1246-1251.

36. Fung JW, Yu CM, Chan JY, et al. Effects of cardiac resynchronization therapy on incidence of atrial fibrillation in patients with poor left ventricular systolic function. *Am J Cardiol.* 2005;96:728-731.

37. Fung JW, Yip GW, Zhang Q, et al. Improvement of left atrial function is associated with lower incidence of atrial fibrillation and mortality after cardiac resynchronization therapy. *Heart Rhythm.* 2008;5:780-786.

38. Cleland JG, Daubert JC, Erdmann E, et al. Longer-term effects of cardiac resynchronization therapy on mortality in heart failure [the CArdiac REsynchronization-Heart Failure (CARE-HF) trial extension phase]. *Eur Heart J.* 2006;27:1928-1932.

39. Adamson PB, Smith AL, Abraham WT, et al. Continuous autonomic assessment in patients with symptomatic heart failure: prognostic value of heart rate variability measured by an implanted cardiac resynchronization device. *Circulation.* 2004;110:2389-2394.

40. Wang L, Lahtinen S, Lentz L, et al. Feasibility of using an implantable system to measure thoracic congestion in an ambulatory chronic heart failure canine model. *Pacing Clin Electrophysiol.* 2005;28:404-411.

41. Yu CM, Wang L, Chau E, et al. Intrathoracic impedance monitoring in patients with heart failure: correlation with fluid status and feasibility of early warning preceding hospitalization. *Circulation.* 2005;112:841-848.

42. Vollmann D, Nagele H, Schauerte P, et al. Clinical utility of intrathoracic impedance monitoring to alert patients with an implanted device of deteriorating chronic heart failure. *Eur Heart J.* 2007;9:716-722

43. Cowie MR, Conraads V, Tavazzi L, Yu CM; on behalf of SENSE-HF Investigators. Rationale and design of a prospective trial to assess the sensitivity and positive predictive value of implantable intrathoracic impedance monitoring (Optivol) in the prediction of heart failure hospitalizations: The SENSE-HF Study. *J Card Fail.* 2009;15:394-400.

44. La Rovere MT, Bigger JT Jr, Marcus FI, Mortara A, Schwartz PJ. Baroreflex sensitivity and heart-rate variability in prediction of total cardiac mortality after myocardial infarction. ATRAMI (autonomic tone and reflexes after myocardial infarction) investigators. *Lancet.* 1998;351:478-484.

45. Adamson PB, Kleckner KJ, VanHout WL, Srinivasan S, Abraham WT. Cardiac resynchronization therapy improves heart rate variability in patients with symptomatic heart failure. *Circulation.* 2003;108:266-269.

46. Bourge RC, Abraham WT, Adamson PB, et al. Randomized controlled trial of an implantable continuous hemodynamic monitor in patients with advanced heart failure: the COMPASS-HF study. *J Am Coll Cardiol.* 2008;51:1073-1079.

47. Walsh JT, Charlesworth A, Andrews R, Hawkins M, Cowley AJ. Relation of daily activity levels in patients with chronic heart failure to long-term prognosis. *Am J Cardiol.* 1997;79: 1364-1369.

48. Braunschweig F, Mortensen PT, Gras D, et al. Monitoring of physical activity and heart rate variability in patients with chronic heart failure using cardiac resynchronization devices. *Am J Cardiol.* 2005;95:1104-1107.

49. Maisel WH, Stevenson LW. Atrial fibrillation in heart failure: epidemiology, pathophysiology, and rationale for therapy. *Am J Cardiol.* 2003;91:2D-8D.

50. Hoppe UC, Casares JM, Eiskjaer H, et al. Effect of cardiac resynchronization on the incidence of atrial fibrillation in patients with severe heart failure. *Circulation.* 2006;114:18-25.

51. Kies P, Leclercq C, Bleeker GB, et al. Cardiac resynchronisation therapy in chronic atrial fibrillation: impact on left atrial size and reversal to sinus rhythm. *Heart.* 2006;92:490-494.

52. Molhoek SG, Bax JJ, Bleeker GB, et al. Comparison of response to cardiac resynchronization therapy in patients with sinus rhythm versus chronic atrial fibrillation. *Am J Cardiol.* 2004; 94: 1506-1509.

53. Delnoy PP, Ottervanger JP, Luttikhuis HO, et al. Comparison of usefulness of cardiac resyn-chronization therapy in patients with atrial fibrillation and heart failure versus patients with sinus rhythm and heart failure. *Am J Cardiol.* 2007;99:1252-1257.

54. Leclercq C, Victor F, Alonso C, Pavin D, Revault dG, Bansard JY, Mabo P, Daubert C. Comparative effects of permanent biventricular pacing for refractory heart failure in patients with stable sinus rhythm or chronic atrial fibrillation. *Am J Cardiol.* 2000;85:1154-1156, A9.

55. Gasparini M, Auricchio A, Regoli F, et al. Four-year efficacy of cardiac resynchronization ther-apy on exercise tolerance and disease progression the importance of performing atrioventricular junction ablation in patients with atrial fibrillation. *J Am Coll Cardiol.* 2006;48:734-743.

56. Khadjooi K, Foley PW, Chalil S, et al. Long-term effects of cardiac resynchronisation therapy in patients with atrial fibrillation. *Heart.* 2008;94:879-883.

57. Upadhyay GA, Choudhry NK, Auricchio A, Ruskin J, Singh JP. Cardiac resynchronization in patients with atrial fibrillation: a meta-analysis of prospective cohort studies. *J Am Coll Cardiol.* 2008;52:1239-1246.

58. Fung JW, Yip GW, Yu CM. Does atrial fibrillation preclude biventricular pacing? *Heart.* 2008; 94:826-827.

59. Gasparini M, Auricchio A, Metra M, et al. Long-term survival in patients undergoing cardiac resynchronization therapy: the importance of performing atrio-ventricular junction ablation in patients with permanent atrial fibrillation. *Eur Heart J.* 2008;29:1644-1652.

60. Koplan BA, Kaplan AJ, Weiner S, Jones PW, Seth M, Christman SA. Heart failure decompen-sation and all-cause mortality in relation to percent biventricular pacing in patients with heart failure: is a goal of 100% biventricular pacing necessary? *J Am Coll Cardiol.* 2009;53: 355-360.

61. Fung JW, Chan JY, Kum LC, et al. Suboptimal medical therapy in patients with systolic heart failure is associated with less improvement by cardiac resynchronization therapy. *Int J Cardiol.* 2007;115:214-219.

62. Abraham WT, Young JB, Leon AR, et al. Effects of cardiac resynchronization on disease progression in patients with left ventricular systolic dysfunction, an indication for an implant-able cardioverter-defibrillator, and mildly symptomatic chronic heart failure. *Circulation.* 2004;110:2864-2868.

63. Linde C, Abraham WT, Gold MR, St John SM, Ghio S, Daubert C. Randomized trial of car-diac resynchronization in mildly symptomatic heart failure patients and in asymptomatic patients with left ventricular dysfunction and previous heart failure symptoms. *J Am Coll Cardiol.* 2008;52:1834-1843.

64. Fung JW, Zhang Q, Yip GW, Chan JY, Chan HC, Yu CM. Effect of cardiac resynchronization therapy in patients with moderate left ventricular systolic dysfunction and wide qrs complex: a prospective study. *J Cardiovasc Electrophysiol.* 2006;17:1288-1292.

65. Sweeney MO, Hellkamp AS. Heart failure during cardiac pacing. *Circulation.* 2006;113: 2082-2088.

66. Leon AR, Greenberg JM, Kanuru N, et al. Cardiac resynchronization in patients with congestive heart failure and chronic atrial fibrillation: effect of upgrading to biventricular pacing after chronic right ventricular pacing. *J Am Coll Cardiol.* 2002;39:1258-1263.

67. Wilkoff BL, Cook JR, Epstein AE, et al. Dual-chamber pacing or ventricular backup pacing in patients with an implantable defibrillator: the Dual Chamber and VVI Implantable Defibrillator (DAVID) Trial. *JAMA.* 2002;288:3115-3123.

68. Kindermann M, Hennen B, Jung J, Geisel J, Bohm M, Frohlig G. Biventricular versus conventional right ventricular stimulation for patients with standard pacing indication and left ventricular dysfunction: the Homburg Biventricular Pacing Evaluation (HOBIPACE). *J Am Coll Cardiol.* 2006;47:1927-1937.

69. Doshi RN, Daoud EG, Fellows C, et al. Left ventricular-based cardiac stimulation post AV nodal ablation evaluation (the PAVE study). *J Cardiovasc Electrophysiol.* 2005;16:1160-1165.

70. Frias PA, Corvera JS, Schmarkey L, Strieper M, Campbell RM, Vinten-Johansen J. Evaluation of myocardial performance with conventional single-site ventricular pacing and biventricular pacing in a canine model of atrioventricular block. *J Cardiovasc Electrophysiol.* 2003;14:996-1000.

71. Cojoc A, Reeves JG, Schmarkey L, et al. Effects of single-site versus biventricular epicardial pacing on myocardial performance in an immature animal model of atrioventricular block. *J Cardiovasc Electrophysiol.* 2006;17:884-889.

72. Lieberman R, Padeletti L, Schreuder J, et al. Ventricular pacing lead location alters systemic hemodynamics and left ventricular function in patients with and without reduced ejection fraction. *J Am Coll Cardiol.* 2006;48:1634-1641.

73. Fung JW, Chan JY, Omar R, et al. The Pacing to Avoid Cardiac Enlargement (PACE) trial: clinical background, rationale, design, and implementation. *J Cardiovasc Electrophysiol.* 2007;18:735-739.

74. Yu CM, Lin H, Zhang Q, Sanderson JE. High prevalence of left ventricular systolic and diastolic asynchrony in patients with congestive heart failure and normal QRS duration. *Heart.* 2003;89:54-60.

75. Bleeker GB, Schalij MJ, Molhoek SG, et al. Relationship between QRS duration and left ventricular dyssynchrony in patients with end-stage heart failure. *J Cardiovasc Electrophysiol.* 2004;15:544-549.

76. Ghio S, Constantin C, Klersy C, et al. Interventricular and intraventricular dyssynchrony are common in heart failure patients, regardless of QRS duration. *Eur Heart J.* 2004;25:571-578.

77. Mor-Avi V, Vignon P, Bales AC, Spencer KT, Lang RM. Acoustic quantification indexes of left ventricular size and function: effects of signal averaging. *J Am Soc Echocardiogr.* 1998;11: 792-802.

78. Achilli A, Sassara M, Ficili S, et al. Long-term effectiveness of cardiac resynchronization therapy in patients with refractory heart failure and "narrow" QRS. *J Am Coll Cardiol.* 2003;42:2117-2124.

79. Turner MS, Bleasdale RA, Vinereanu D, et al. Electrical and mechanical components of dyssynchrony in heart failure patients with normal QRS duration and left bundle-branch block: impact of left and biventricular pacing. *Circulation.* 2004;109:2544-2549.

80. Yu CM, Chan YS, Zhang Q, et al. Benefits of cardiac resynchronization therapy for heart failure patients with narrow QRS complexes and coexisting systolic asynchrony by echocardiography. *J Am Coll Cardiol.* 2006;48:2251-2257.

81. Bleeker GB, Holman ER, Steendijk P, et al. Cardiac resynchronization therapy in patients with a narrow QRS complex. *J Am Coll Cardiol.* 2006;48:2243-2250.

82. Beshai JF, Grimm RA, Nagueh SF, et al. Cardiac-resynchronization therapy in heart failure with narrow QRS complexes. *N Engl J Med.* 2007;357:2461-2471.

19.1
Introduction

The last three decades have seen major advances in the pharmacological treatment of patients with heart failure. ACE inhibitors, beta blockers, Spironolactone and ARB's have all been shown to improve symptoms, and prolong life, by a reduction in the risk of sudden cardiac death (SCD) and the risk of death due to progressive heart failure. These treatments constitute what is termed optimal medical treatment. Nevertheless, despite optimal medical treatment patients with heart failure remain at increased risk of SCD and death due to progressive heart failure. In addition, many patients remain symptomatic in NYHA Classes II, III or even IV.

Device therapy for patients with heart failure seeks to build on the therapeutic benefits of optimal medical therapy to improve prognosis and symptoms. The implantable cardio-defibrillator (ICD) is a sophisticated pacemaker, which provides antitachycardia pacing if VT occurs with a backup defibrillator capability if antitacycardia pacing is unsuccessful or for the occurrence of VF. ICD's also provide backup pacing in the event of asystole or extreme bradycardia. They are easily implanted but are relatively expensive, thereby limiting their use in many countries. The biventricular pacemaker is another sophisticated pacemaker that is available for the treatment of patients with heart failure. This device has, in addition to the standard right atrial and right ventricular leads, a left ventricular lead to pace the left ventricle. This lead is usually inserted retrogradely through the coronary sinus but can be sited epicardially via a minithorocotomy. The rationale for biventricular pacing is to restore cardiac synchrony, hence the term cardiac resynchronization therapy (CRT). In some patients with heart failure (especially those with the poorest left ventricular function), the left ventricle is globular in appearance and tends to wobble rather than contract in a coordinated fashion. More detailed analysis of this wobbling appearance reveals that different regions of the ventricle are contracting and relaxing out of phase with each other, sometimes by as much as 180°, further reducing stroke volume. CRT, by pacing the septum

A. Owen
Princess of wales Hospital, Bridgend, U.K.
e-mail: Andrew.owen@abm-tr.wales.nhs.uk

(right ventricular lead) and the left ventricular lateral wall (left ventricular lead) seeks to restore synchrony and improve left ventricular function. In addition, for patients in sinus rhythm, atrial contraction can be timed to optimize ventricular filling. CRT devices are relatively inexpensive, but require substantial expertise to implant. Devices are also available that combine ICD and CRT capabilities, known as CRTD.

19.2
The Implantable Cardiodefibrillator (ICD)

Secondary prevention – Secondary prevention refers to the treatment of patients who have experienced the condition to be treated. Patients resuscitated from VT or VF arrest are at high risk of subsequent SCD and would seem ideal candidates to benefit from an ICD. Three trials have evaluated the efficacy of an ICD in this situation. All compared an ICD to amiodarone (the standard empirical treatment for such patients in the 1990's).

The AVID Trial[1] recruited patients who had survived a VF arrest (55%) or who had had symptomatic sustained VT. The mean age of patients was 65 years with a mean LV EF of 32%. The trial was stopped early after a mean follow up of 18 months because of overwhelming evidence of ICD efficacy in terms of all cause mortality. This result however may have been confounded by an imbalance in the use of beta blockers between the two groups: 42% in the ICD group and 16.5% in the amiodarone group at baseline. This is a ratio of 2.6:1, which increased during follow up to 3.9:1 at 24 months.

The CASH trial[2] solely recruited survivors of VF arrest. The mean age was 58 years and mean LV EF was 46%. Follow up continued until the end of the trial. There was a non significant reduction in all cause mortality with an ICD. Beta blocker use was precluded by trial design.

The CIDS trial[3] recruited survivors of VF arrest (50%), patients with symptomatic VT or patients with syncope (and inducible VT at EP testing). The mean age was 46 years and the mean LV EF was 34%. Follow up continued until the planned end of the trial. There was a non significant reduction in all cause mortality. In this trial, there was also an imbalance in the use of beta blockers: 53% in the ICD arm compared to 23% in the amiodarone arm.

In view of the inconclusive nature of these results, a meta analysis was undertaken.[4] An analysis using individual patient data was undertaken (no details of the methods used was provided) which suggested a benefit in favor of the ICD with a hazard ratio of 0.73 (95% CI, 0.60–0.87), $p < 0.001$ for all cause mortality. Subgroup analysis suggested that this benefit may have been confined to patients with a LV EF <35%. In the combined data set, there was still an imbalance in the use of beta blockers with 42% of patients in the ICD group prescribed beta blockers as to compared to 19% in the amiodarone group at baseline. A test for interaction between beta blocker use and treatment allocation was not significant ($p = 0.095$). No analysis adjusting for beta blocker use was presented. The presence of prior myocardial infarction or indeed ischemic heart disease generally, was not an inclusion criterion in any of the studies. In the combined dataset, however, 69% of patients had a history of prior myocardial infarction and only 12% had no evidence of ischaemic heart disease. The preponderance of prior myocardial infarction presumably reflects the prevalence of the etiology of SCD. Tests for interactions between a history of prior myocardial infarction, dilated cardiomyopathy (DCM) etiology and treatment allocation were not significant. Thus, it is not possible to conclude that patients with DCM or without a history of prior myocardial infarction do not benefit from ICD treatment. The authors estimated that, after 6 years of ICD treatment, the use of an ICD would prolong life by approximately 4 months for the entire cohort. For the subset of patients with an LV EF <35%, the extra life gained is similar (estimated from the survival curve[5]).

A fixed effects meta analysis using summary statistics was also presented for mortality, which yielded a hazard ratio of 0.72 (95% CI, 0.6–0.87), $p=0.006$. The test for heterogeneity was not significant, $p=0.3$. The authors justified a fixed effects model on the basis of a non significant test for heterogeneity and the similarity of the included trials. The heterogeneity test however has low power when few studies are included;[6] thus, a non significant test is not reliable evidence for the absence of heterogeneity. In addition, although the three studies were similar in many respects, there were some notable differences. CASH[2] only included VF survivors with no use of beta blockers. In the two other studies, beta blockers were allowed (in fact encouraged) but there was an unfortunate imbalance in their use in favor of the ICD arms. Thus, a random effects analysis may have been more appropriate.

In summary, the use of an ICD for the secondary prevention of SCD offers only a very modest prolongation of life (4 months after 6 years of treatment) and even this may be an overestimate because of the imbalance in the use of beta blockers in favor of the ICD. This modest benefit should be balanced against the discomfort and distress of inappropriate shocks (which may be as frequent as 30% of all shocks[7]). In addition shocks (whether appropriate or inappropriate) have a transient adverse effect on quality of life.[8] Current American College of Cardiology/ American Heart Association (ACC/AHA) guidelines give a Class I level of evidence A recommendation for the secondary prevention of SCD with an ICD, irrespective of LV EF[9] and irrespective of etiology, whereas current European Society of Cardiology (ESC) guidelines have a requirement for LV EF <40% and are ambiguous in relation to patients with DCM.[10] Both guidelines stipulate that patients should have a reasonable expectation of surviving at least 1 year with a good functional status. The CIDS[3] trial was the only trial examining secondary prevention of SCD with an ICD that had an exclusion criterion of this kind, and this was more specific: a non arrhythmic medical condition making 1 year survival unlikely. This would seem to be more appropriate than the wording used in the guidelines.

Primary prevention – Primary prevention of SCD refers to treatment of patients at increased risk of SCD, but who have not experienced a life threatening event. The efficacy of an ICD for the primary prevention of SCD has been evaluated in three landmark trials: MADIT II[11,12] (prior myocardial infarction), DEFINITE[13] (nonischaemic etiology, i.e., DCM) and SCD-HeFT[14] (no restrictions on etiology).

MADIT II[11] recruited patients with a prior myocardial infarction 1 month or more before entry and a LV EF <30%. A history of heart failure was not required but patients in NYHA Class IV were excluded. Patients were randomized to standard medical therapy or to standard medical therapy and an ICD. The study was therefore not blinded. Patients randomized to the ICD arm had a commercially available device inserted that was tested during implantation and was programmed according to the discretion of the local physician. The trial was stopped early after a median follow up of 20 months because of unequivocal efficacy of the ICD over medical treatment. The mean age was 65 years, the mean LV EF was 23% and approximately 65% had symptomatic heart failure (25% were in NYHA Class III). Patients in NYHA Class IV were excluded. The median time from myocardial infarction to randomization was 5 years, with only 12% of patients within 6 months. The use of beta blockers was reasonable at 75% in both groups. The hazard ratio for mortality was 0.69 (95% CI, 0.51–0.93), $p=0.016$ in favor of the ICD, i.e., a 31% relative risk reduction. Subgroup analysis did not reveal any interactions with treatment allocation, in particular with respect to age (a third of patients were over 70 years old), NYHA Class (split between I and II or greater) and QRS duration. The extra life gained as a result of the ICD however was modest at about 2 months after 3 years of treatment (estimated from the Kaplan–Meier plot[5]). A subsequent post hoc analysis has suggested that the benefit of an ICD is greatest for patients in whom the myocardial infarction was more distant, and in this analysis, no benefit accrued to patients within 18 months of a myocardial infarction.[12]

The DEFINITE trial[13] recruited patients with a history of symptomatic heart failure (patients in NYHA Class IV excluded) who had a nonischaemic etiology, a LV EF less than or equal to 35% and frequent ventricular ectopy (>10 beats per hour on 24 h holter monitoring or non sustained VT at more than 120/min). Randomization was to usual care or usual care plus ICD. The ICD was programmed to back up VVI pacing at 40/min. The mean age was 58 years, mean LV EF=21%. Both groups were medically well treated. After a mean follow up of 29 months the trial was terminated as planned. The hazard ratio for mortality in favor of the ICD was 0.65 (95% CI, 0.4–1.06), $p=0.08$. Subgroup analysis did not reveal any significant interactions with treatment allocation, in particular with, age (one-third of patients were >65 years), NYHA Class, LV EF or QRS duration.

The SCD-HeFT trial[14] recruited patients with NYHA Class II or III heart failure with a LV EF less than or equal to 35%. Patients were randomized to placebo, amiodarone or ICD (single lead, no testing at implantation and programmed to shock only). The median follow up was 45.5 months, 70% of patients were in NYHA Class II, 52% had ischaemic heart disease and the median age was 60 years. ICD therapy was associated with a decreased risk of death as compared to placebo (HR=0.77 (97.5% CI, 0.62–0.96), $p=0.007$). ICD treatment prolonged life for both IDCM and NIDCM by approximately 3 months after 5 years of treatment (estimated from the Kaplan–Meier plot[5]). Amiodarone therapy was associated with a similar risk of death as placebo (HR=1.06 (97.5% CI, 0.86–1.3), $p=0.53$). Subgroup analysis did not reveal any interaction between either amiodarone or ICD therapy and the cause of the heart failure. There was however a significant interaction between amiodarone therapy and NYHA Class, $p=0.004$. For patients in NYHA Class III, amiodarone therapy was associated with an increased risk of death compared with placebo (HR=1.44 (97.5% CI, 1.05–1.97)). There was no excess risk for patients in NYHA Class II. The interaction between ICD therapy and NYHA class was also significant, $p<0.001$. For patients in NYHA Class II, there was a reduced risk of death compared with placebo (HR=0.54 (97.5% CI, 0.4–0.74)). There was no apparent reduction in risk of death for patients in NYHA Class III.

The DINAMIT trial[15] evaluated the use of an ICD in patients with a recent (within a month) myocardial infarction and LV EF <35%. Over 80% had NYHA Class II or III heart failure. No benefit of the ICD over placebo was observed (HR=1.08 (95% CI, 0.76–1.55) $p=0.66$).

These trials provide the evidence base to inform the management of patients with heart failure in clinical practice. On the basis of MADIT II,[11] patients with NYHA Class I, II or III heart failure who have LV EF less than or equal to 35% and a remote myocardial infarction (more than 1 month) would gain a modest extension of life from an ICD. When applying clinical trial results to clinical practice, however, it is important to appreciate the type of patients actually recruited rather than relying on the inclusion criteria. In MADITT II,[11] although at least 1 month post myocardial infarction was an inclusion criterion, very few patients were actually recruited who had had a myocardial infarction within several months of the event. Thus we cannot draw any conclusions as to the efficacy of an ICD for this small group. Further, the lack of benefit of an ICD within the first month post infacrtion[15] and the MADITT II post hoc analysis[12] suggest that an ICD is unlikely to be of benefit until many months (possibly at least a year) post infarct. The SCD-HeFT trial[14] extends this result to patients with heart failure and ischaemic heart disease generally (no requirement for a prior myocardial infarction) but again only a modest extension of life is seen with an ICD. This trial raised the possibility that patients with NYHA III Class heart failure may not benefit from an ICD. In MADIT II,[11] the subgroup NYHA Class analysis was split between Class I and higher Classes, and there was no published subgroup analysis between Classes II and III as was provided in SCD-HeFT.[14] An unpublished personal communication cited in this paper[14] has indicated that both Class II and Class III patients benefited from an ICD in MADIT II.[11] Thus the available (published) evidence for the efficacy of an ICD in patients with NYHA Class III heart failure is less convincing than that for NYHA Class II patients. The ICDs were programmed differently in these two trials. There are currently no randomized trials to inform us how best to program an ICD for optimum function. We do not know whether the inclusion of complex antitachy-cardia pacing algorhythms offers any advantage (or even harm) compared to a simple shock only approach. The minimum VVI pacing rate is another issue that has not been addressed. Current ACC/AHA[9] and ESC[10] guidelines give a class I level of evidence A indication for NYHA Class II or III heart failure patients with LV EF <35% and with a history of prior myocardial infarction (at least 40 days post infarction) for treatment with an ICD. In addition the ACC/AHA guidelines[9] also include patients with NYHA Class I heart failure, a reflection of the patient population of MADITT II.[11] An ICD is not recom-mended for patients with heart failure within 1 month of a myocardial infarction. No recommendations are given for patients with extensive ischaemic heart disease but with-out a history of myocardial infarction.

For patients with heart failure due to DCM (i.e., no significant coronary artery disease) the value of an ICD is less clear. The DEFINITE trial[13] strongly suggested benefit, but did not reach the traditional standard of evidence required ($p < 0.05$). The SCD- HeFT trial[14] provides further evidence of the efficacy of an ICD in DCM, (HR=0.73 (97.5%CI, 0.50–1.07), $p = 0.06$) but this is from a subgroup analysis albeit prespecified. A meta-analysis[16] of ICD trials in DCM heart failure has been undertaken, which suggested benefit of an ICD. This analysis however has some important weaknesses. The arm of the COMPANION trial comparing CRTD with placebo[17] was included with the unsustainable assumption that CRTD is no better than ICD alone. The AMIOVIRT trial that compared ICD to amio-darone[18] was included with the assumption that placebo and amiodarone are interchange-able. Finally, a fixed effects model was assumed because the test for heterogeneity was not significant. This is a flawed assumption as this test has poor power when small numbers of trials are included.[6] A random effects meta analysis death from any cause including only trials that compare an ICD to control is given in the figure. The uncertainty over the benefit of an ICD for DCM NYHA Class II or III heart failure is reflected in the ACC/AHA[9] and ESC guidelines[10] with a Class I, level of evidence B recommendation.

These trials did not require electrophysiology testing or ventricular rhythm disturbances on holter ECG monitoring (DEFINITE[13] did require some ECG evidence of ventricular rhythm disturbance) as entry criteria. Thus, for primary prevention all that is required is the presence of NYHA Class II or III heart failure with a LV EF less than or equal to 35%.

A problem that arises in clinical practice that has not been addressed in clinical trials is how to manage the patient with an ICD who experiences frequent appropriate shocks; this has been found to be a marker of a worse prognosis compared to the case of patients who receive no shocks.[19] Such patients are often treated empirically with amiodarone to try and suppress ventricular rhythm disturbances that may provoke an ICD to discharge. There is no trial evidence to support this treatment strategy. Amiodarone may be associated with an increased risk of death in NYHA Class III heart failure. Dronedarone (a Class III antidysrhythmic agent based on the amiodarone molecule) has been found to increase the risk of death in patients with severe heart failure (NYHA class III or IV).[20] Thus, this empirical approach should only be considered as a last resort once all evidence based treatment has been exhausted, e.g., full dose treatment with beta blockers and ACE inhibitors.

19.3
Cardiac Resynchronization Therapy (CRT)

The efficacy of CRT was initially studied in small, short term studies MUSTIC,[21] PATHCHF[22] and MIRACLE[23] which clearly demonstrated improved exercise tolerance and quality of life. There were concerns however that this symptomatic improvement may be at the expense of an increase in mortality due to possible proarrhythmic effects of CRT. Larger studies were therefore undertaken to determine the effect of CRT on mortality.

The COMPANION trial[17] was the first to report. This trial recruited patients in NYHA Class III or IV heart failure, LV EF less than or equal to 35%, QRS duration > 120 ms, PR interval >150 ms. Patients were also required to be in sinus rhythm and have had an admission to hospital for heart failure within the previous 12 months. Patients were randomized to medical treatment, CRT or CRTD in a 1:2:2 ratio. The trial was terminated when the target of 1,000 events had occurred. Also, at this time, the predetermined boundaries for the termination of the trial for the primary end point of all cause mortality or hospital admission had been crossed for both device groups, in comparison to the medically treated group. The mean age was 67 years, 85% were in NYHA Class III, the mean LV EF was 22%, mean QRS duration was 160 ms (70% LBBB) and approximately 50% had an ischaemic etiology. The 12 month primary endpoint (death or hospital admission for heart failure) event rates for both device groups were reported and were significantly reduced compared to the medical group. The secondary endpoint of all cause mortality for the entire study period was reduced for both CRTD and CRT with hazard ratios of 0.64 (95%

CI, 0.48–0.86), $p=0.003$ and 0.76 (95% CI, 0.58–1.01), $p=0.06$ respectively. Quality of life was improved in both device groups. At 3 months, there was a net improvement of 15 points on the Minnesota living with heart failure questionnaire. Device therapy was associated with over 50% of patients having an improved NYHA Class compared to 24% in the medical group at 3 months. No comparisons between the two device groups were given but the event rates appeared to be very similar. Subgroup analyses did not reveal any interactions with treatment allocation, in particular for age group, LV EF, NYHA Class, heart failure etiology or QRS duration. There did however appear to be a trend for increasing benefit for longer QRS duration, but this was not quantified. The extra life gained for both devices was modest at approximately 1–2 months after 2 years of treatment (extra life estimated from the Kaplan–Meier curves[5]). Exercise distance (6-minute walk test) and symptoms were improved with both devices. This trial indicates that both CRT and CRTD are efficacious for patients with a QRS duration >120 ms in NYHA Classes III or IV and a LV EF less than or equal to 35%.

The CARE-HF trial[24] recruited patients in NYHA Classes III and IV heart failure with a LV EF less than or equal to 35% and a QRS duration >120 ms. Patients were required to be in sinus rhythm. Patients were randomized to CRT or optimum medical treatment. The mean age was 66 years, median LV EF was 25%, median QRS duration was 160 ms (75% >152 ms), only 7% were in NYHA Class IV and approximately 40% had an ischaemic etiology. CRT reduced mortality compared to medical therapy, hazard ratio 0.64 (95% CI, 0.48–0.85), $p<0.002$. Quality of life was improved with CRT. The Minnesota living with heart failure score improved by 10 points at 90 days and LV EF by 7 points at 18 months. Interactions with treatment allocation were not reported for subgroups, but important subgroups (heart failure etiology, age, NYHA class) all seemed to benefit. The extra life gained after 3 years of treatment was modest as approximately 2 months (estimated from the Kaplan–Meier plot[5]). Eight months of further follow up was subsequently reported.[25] The benefits previously reported were maintained. Further analysis of the cause of death revealed that CRT significantly reduced both the risk of SCD and the risk of death due to progressive heart failure. This trial supports the finding of COMPANION[17] that CRT improves symptoms and prolongs life. Although CRT has only a modest effect in prolonging life (similar to an ICD), unlike an ICD, CRT can have a dramatic effect in improving symptoms.

On the basis of these trials, the ACC/AHA[9] and ESC[10] guidelines give a Class I level of evidence A recommendation for CRT in patients with NYHA Class III or IV heart failure with LV EF less than or equal to 35% and QRS duration >120 ms, and in sinus rhythm.

19.4
Combined Resynchronization and Defibrillation Devices (CRTD)

There are two patient groups to be considered here: patients who have a secondary indication for an ICD (i.e., have sustained a cardiac arrest or experienced sustained VT) and patients in whom an ICD is indicated for primary prevention.

For secondary prevention the addition of CRT to ICD was addressed in three trials: MIRACLE-ICD,[26] CONTAK-CD[27] and MIRACLE-ICD II.[28] MIRACLE-ICD[26] recruited patients who had a secondary prevention indication for an ICD and were in NYHA Class III or IV, LV EF less than or equal to 35% and QRS duration >130 ms. Patients not in sinus rhythm were excluded. The trial compared CRTD with ICD alone. The trial was limited to 6 month follow up. No mortality benefit was observed with CRTD compared to ICD but improvements in quality of life and exercise distance were observed.

The CONTAK-CD[27] trial recruited patients who had a "conventional indication" for an ICD. At the time the trial was commenced (1998), this would have predominantly been for secondary prevention. Patients were also required to be in NYHA Class II, III or IV, have LV EF less than or equal to 35% and QRS duration >120 ms, and be in sinus rhythm. The trial design was changed from crossover to parallel during the course of the study making interpretation of the results difficult. Maximum follow up was for 6 months. Randomization was undertaken after implantation of the device (all patients had a CRTD device with CRT deactivated in those randomized to ICD). No mortality benefit was observed with CRTD compared to ICD. Improvements in quality of life peak VO_2, 6-minute walk test and NYHA Class were observed for patients in NYHA classes III and IV but not for those patients in Class II with CRT compared to ICD only. The MIRACLE-ICD II[28] recruited patients in NYHA Class II heart failure, LV EF less than or equal to 35%, QRS duration >130 ms and a Class I indication for an ICD. No meaningful benefits were observed with CRTD compared to ICD alone.

None of these three studies was designed to look at long term prognosis, but rather focused on short term (6 month) effects on symptoms. They suggest that for patients with a secondary indication for an ICD the addition of CRT improves symptoms and exercise distance for patients in NYHA Classes III and IV but not for patients in NYHA Class II heart failure. Whether the addition of CRT to an ICD in this patient population improves survival remains unknown. ACC/AHA[9] and ESC[10] guidelines do not give specific recommendations for this patient group. For patients in NYHA Class II, the evidence would suggest an ICD alone would be the appropriate treatment. For patients in NYHA Class III, the addition of CRT to ICD would be reasonable to improve symptoms, but CRT alone should be considered (see below).

The more commonly encountered problem is the management of patients with NYHA Class III heart failure, LVEF less than or equal to 35% and QRS duration >120 ms, and in sinus rhythm, who thus have an indication for an ICD and CRT. The question of whether adding an ICD to CRT is of value was addressed in the CAMPANION study[17] (summarized in the CRT section above). The combined device was demonstrated to be superior to no device. This was obviously going to be the case, unless by some bizarre interaction one device adversely affected the other. The combined device was not demonstrated to be superior to CRT either in terms of survival or symptoms. Unfortunately, the trial was discontinued before any benefit (if one exists) became apparent. A Bayesian network meta analysis[29] reaffirmed the superiority of CRTD and CRT over no device in terms of survival but did not demonstrate a benefit of CRTD over CRT. It was concluded that CRTD was probably superior to CRT, but conclusive evidence was lacking. It would seem improbable for CRTD to be able to improve quality of life or exercise distance over that achieved with CRT. Any mortality benefit is likely to be very small, certainly less than the 2 months extra life after 3 years treatment achieved with CRT in the CARE-HF trial.[24] Improvements of this order would not have been apparent from COMPANION.[17]

There have been no trials addressing the question of whether the addition of CRT to ICD in primary prevention is of any benefit. From the beneficial effects of this combination on symptoms in secondary prevention of SCD, it would seem likely that some symptomatic improvement could be expected for CRTD over ICD alone. Given that CRT improves LV EF and reduces the risk of both SCD and death due to progressive heart failure,[24, 25] it could be speculated that CRTD may improve survival over ICD alone.

Current ACC/AHA[9] and ESC[10] guidelines give a Class I, level of evidence A recommendation for CRTD and CRT in this patient group, based on the efficacy of these therapies over no device. The guidelines do not give any guidance on which of these devices to use. Given the substantial additional cost of CRTD, the implausibility of it being able to improve symptoms and the likely minimal extension to life, it would seem reasonable to implant CRT in this patient group unless there are particular reasons to include a defibrillator capability. This approach would be consistent with the uncertainty over the efficacy of an ICD for patients with NYHA Class III heart failure. Further, there will be some patients in whom CRT improves the LV EF to more than 35%, making the provision of an ICD inappropriate. In view of the lack of evidence, this would be a level of evidence C recommendation.

A related problem that occasionally occurs is what is the most appropriate device to implant in a patient who has previously had an ICD implanted for primary or secondary prevention and who becomes eligible for CRT, for example a patient previously in NYHA Class II who moves into Class III and who also satisfies the other criteria for CRT. To be consistent with the above suggestion the ICD should be explanted and replaced with a CRT device.

The efficacy of an ICD in patients with NYHA class IV heart failure has not been studied directly. The COMPANION trial[17] included a small proportion of patients in this group, but this trial did not compare ICD treatment alone to medical treatment. Consequently, the ACC/AHA[9] and ESC[10] guidelines do not recommend the use of an ICD in patients with NYHA Class IV heart failure.

19.5
Nonresponders to CRT

In clinical practice, the majority of patients treated with CRT are much improved, sometimes substantially so. There is, however, a group of patients in whom symptoms do not appear to be improved. Such patients have been described as "nonresponders." Nonresponders are generally felt to constitute 20–30% of the CRT population.[30] In clinical practice, where there is no control group and no blinding, lack of improvement may result from the benefit of CRT being less than the patient's expectation. Alternatively, a coincidental worsening of heart failure (despite CRT) or coincidental noncardiac conditions may be responsible for deterioration in symptoms. We therefore need to look at the randomized controlled trials for more solid evidence of the nonresponder concept. What constitutes a nonresponder has not been defined. The concept has arisen after the major trials reported and consequently is not specifically addressed.

In MUSTIC,[21] a blinded cross-over trial, 85% of patients preferred CRT, 4% preferred no CRT and 10% had no preference. Thus, we might infer that in this trial nonresponders constituted 15% of the total. In the MIRACLE trial,[23] a 6-month blinded parallel design CRT study, 20% of CRT patients felt no better or worse, compared to 43% in the no CRT group. This would suggest 20% of nonresponders. Note, however, that 57% of patients appeared to "respond" to no CRT, hence the importance of a blinded control group. This study also evaluated changes in NYHA Class. In the CRT group, 32% did not improve their NYHA class compared to 63% in the control group. In the COMPANION trial[17] (a nonblinded trial), 39% of the CRT group did not improve their NYHA Class compared to 62% in the control group. Thus, 38% of the control group did improve their NYHA Class, which as the trial was not blinded, was clearly not a placebo effect. These data remind us that patients with heart failure will improve and deteriorate spontaneously making it difficult to determine who is a true nonresponder and what is an apparent nonresponse due to a spontaneous deterioration in heart failure status coinciding with the post CRT implant period. Irrespective of how a nonresponse is defined, the question arises as to when it should be assessed in the post implant period. The beneficial effect of reducing or abolishing left ventricular dysynchrony with CRT can take some months to be fully realized. This sort of time period is necessary for left ventricular remodeling to occur with an associated improvement in LV EF and cardiac output. Further, for the patients to benefit fully from this improvement in left ventricular function, they would need to increase their physical activity to regain some degree of physical fitness, usually measured as peak VO_2. Typically, only very modest improvements of peak VO_2 are seen with CRT.[22] If assessment is delayed for too long, the natural history of worsening symptoms would start to annul the beneficial effects of CRT. In addition, deaths would start to confound the findings when groups are being assessed, as in clinical trials. Three to six months would therefore seem to be an optimum time to assess response. The use of NYHA Class changes is a very crude method to examine changes in symptoms. Patients may have important changes in symptoms and yet remain in the same NYHA Class.

Given the difficulties in determining if an individual has responded to CRT, we need to examine more closely what pathophysiology CRT is aimed at addressing, i.e., dysynchrony. All CRT trails have used a long QRS duration (>120 ms) as a surrogate for mechanical dysynchrony. Unfortunately this simple measure is not a necessary or sufficient condition for the presence of mechanical dysynchrony. In clinical practice, we see patients with a QRS duration of 120 ms or more who do not have mechanical dysynchrony. Applying CRT in such patients clearly cannot improve symptoms and can, on occasions, actually induce dysynchrony, which may translate into a deterioration of symptoms and possibly a worse prognosis. This is one group of patients who cannot respond to CRT. A second group of patients who are not likely to respond are those who do have mechanical dysynchrony, but in whom CRT does not achieve any meaningful improvement.

To apply these principles in clinical practice, all patients in whom CRT is being considered (i.e., are eligible according to current criteria) should have a detailed echocardiographic assessment to identify if dysynchrony is present, and if so its nature. Following implantation, a follow up echocardiographic assessment should be made to ensure it has resulted in improvement.

Many echocardiography measurements have been proposed as predictors of whether patients will respond to CRT. The PROSPECT study[31] examined 12 such measurements as predictors of response at 6 months. Two definitions of response were used, a 15% reduction in left ventricular end systolic volume and heart failure CSS (a combination of mortality, heart failure admissions and patient symptoms). None of the echocardiographic measurements was sufficiently reliable for the investigators to recommend them for general use in clinical practice. The tissue Doppler measurements were particularly disappointing, which is not surprising, given its poor temporal resolution. The study had a number of limitations. It did not assess the most fundamental marker of dysynchrony i.e., a prolonged isovolumic relaxation time (IVRT). A prolonged IVRT is a direct result of dysynchrony. When some regions of the left ventricle have delayed and/or prolonged contraction compared to others, relaxation of these regions is delayed resulting in a decrease in the rate of left ventricular pressure decline and a delay in the onset of filling. To be effective, CRT must reduce IVRT. Clearly, if IVRT is not prolonged, CRT is unlikely to be effective. Patients with a prolonged IVRT that is not reduced by CRT are also unlikely to benefit. This might arise, for example when the left ventricular lead is not sited at a site of delayed onset of contraction (the left ventricular lead is typically sited where the operator can achieve a good position rather than where it needs to be to achieve maximum benefit). The PROSPECT study[31] also did not address atrioventricular delay and its effect on response. Finally, the definition of response may not have been appropriate. Patients may have improved symptoms without a 15% reduction in left ventricular end systolic volume. Similarly, patients could be symptomatically improved and yet die within 6 months of implantation: CRT does not prevent death; it prolongs life by a few months.

How then should dysynchrony be assessed? For many patients, it is obvious from the 2-D echocardiogram. The quantification of dysynchrony is more difficult, with no set of measurements having been shown in multicentre trials to be of value. A prolonged IVRT is a global indication of dysynchrony (or on occasions generally delayed relaxation with no dysynchrony). The individual regional variations in left ventricular function that give rise to this can be assessed with M-mode, tissue Doppler or speckle tracking. However it is measured, it is most important to ensure that CRT has not worsened the situation.

Patients, in whom no dysynchrony is present, present a difficult management problem. Should they undergo CRT device implantation with the associated morbidity and even mortality, when they are unlikely to benefit? Conversely, is it right not to implant a CRT device in severely symptomatic patients (NYHA Class III and IV) when they fulfill current criteria for CRT? These are difficult judgements which need to be made on an individual patient basis in conjunction with the patient's wishes. It is most important to ensure that the patient is on optimal medical treatment. In particular, high dose ACE inhibitors can, by unloading the left ventricle, unmask previously unapparent dysynchrony,[32] thereby providing physiological evidence to support the use of CRT. When high dose ACE inhibitors have no effect, another option is to implant an ICD only. The remaining two options are to continue with medical therapy alone or to implant a CRT device on a "try it and see" basis. When dysynchrony is created or worsened with CRT (despite attempts at optimization, see below) deactivation of the device should be considered.

19.6
Patients in Atrial Fibrillation

Atrial fibrillation is common in real world patients with heart failure; a prevalence of up to 50% has been reported.[33] The clinical trials evaluating CRT have excluded patients with atrial fibrillation; consequently, we have no trial evidence to inform whether CRT is effective in this patient group. The ACC/AHA[9] and ESC[10] guidelines give a IIa level of evidence B recommendation for CRT in patients with atrial fibrillation who have NYHA Class III or IV heart failure, a LV EF less than or equal to 35% and QRS duration >120 ms. It is not clear how a level of evidence B can be advocated in the absence of trial evidence. Patient management therefore has to be on the basis of empirical principles. The inadequacy of evidence to support CRT in patients with atrial fibrillation means there is no compelling reason to use this treatment. A pragmatic approach would be to only use CRT when there is clear echocardiographic evidence of dysynchrony. Patients with heart failure and atrial fibrillation often have an inappropriate ventricular rate response, despite full dose beta blocker use and if necessary digoxin. It should be noted however that digoxin use appears to be associated with an increased risk of death in women with heart failure and sinus rhythm.[34] It should therefore be used with extreme caution (if at all) in women with heart failure and atrial fibrillation. For CRT to be effective, it is essential that biventricular pacing is not inhibited by an inappropriate ventricular response to atrial fibrillation. The intrinsic ventricular rate should be less than 70/min and ideally <60/min to ensure continuous biventricular pacing. Once a device is implanted, it is particularly important to interrogate it to ensure that biventricular pacing occurs on exercise. If the ventricular rate cannot be controlled with full dose beta blocker treatment, two options are available: 1) Increase the pacing rate above the intrinsic ventricular rate; this seems counter intuitive given that the beneficial effects of beta blockers are at least partly due to suppressing a tachycardia. 2) Ablate the AV node. This solves the problem, but there is at present no trial evidence to support this approach. The ESC[10] guidelines give a class IIb level of evidence B for this approach. The alternative to these approaches is to accept intermittent suppression of ventricular pacing, but clearly CRT cannot be effective if it is suppressed. Catheter ablation of atrial fibrillation appears to be feasible in patients with heart failure,[35] but trial evidence of its efficacy is lacking. The same principles apply when a patient with a CRT device develops atrial fibrillation.

19.7
Patients with Heart Failure and a Traditional Indication for Right Ventricular Pacing

The DAVID trial[36] examined, in patients with a LV EF less than or equal to 40% and a standard indication for an ICD, whether DDDR pacing at 70/min was superior to VVI at 40/min. The trial was discontinued early when it became apparent that DDDR pacing at

70/min was deleterious with an increased risk of death or hospital admission with heart failure. This trial result has been interpreted as indicating that long periods of right ventricular pacing are deleterious for patients with a reduced LV EF, probably because of creation or worsening of dysynchrony. An alternative explanation is simply that pacing such patients at 70 beats/min is deleterious relative to pacing at 40/min. These findings are reflected in the ACC/AHA[9] and ESC[10] guidelines with a Class IIb, level of evidence C recommendation that patients with LV EF less than or equal to 35% with NYHA Class I or II symptoms undergoing implantation of a permanent pacemaker and/or an ICD with anticipated frequent ventricular pacing should be considered for CRT.

Patients with a previously implanted right ventricular pacemaker receiving frequent ventricular pacing present an analogous problem that is not addressed in the guidelines. There is no trial evidence on how to manage these patients. It would seem reasonable however, to upgrade these patients to CRT if dysynchrony is apparent on echocardiography provided LV EF is less than or equal to 35% and they have at least NYHA Class II symptoms.

19.8
Optimization of CRT

Optimization of CRT refers to changing the pacing parameters to improve symptoms and or prognosis. No randomized controlled trials have been undertaken to demonstrate how best to do this. The atrioventricular (AV) delay can be adjusted to optimize ventricular filling, usually left ventricular filling. A prolonged PR interval often results in presystolic AV valve regurgitation, which tends to raise atrial pressure and is an ineffective use of time during the cardiac cycle. Reducing the AV delay can abolish this. If the AV delay is too short however, it will limit the filling resulting from atrial systole by the premature onset of ventricular systole. An AV delay of around 100 ms is usually a reasonable compromise. The intraventricular (VV) can be adjusted to minimize dysynchrony. In the COMPANION trial,[17] the AV delay was adjusted according to ECG measurements without apparent reference to echocardiographic information. No information was provided on the VV delay. In the CARE-HF trial,[24] the AV delay was adjusted to achieve maximum separation of the e and a filling periods (presumably of the left ventricle).[37] The VV delay was set to zero. Thus the trials do not give any information on how (if at all) the VV delay should be varied and nor do the ACC/AHA[9] or ESC[10] guidelines. It is important to note that a VV delay of zero achieved the beneficial effects of CRT observed in CARE-HF.[24] Therefore, changing the VV delay from zero should be undertaken with great caution. If it is decided to change the VV delay, this can be done (usually by trial and error) to optimize LV stroke distance, minimize the contraction delay between septum and posterior wall or between septum and lateral wall or minimize IVRT. None of these targets for optimization, however, has been demonstrated in multicentre controlled trials to be of any value. At present, in the absence of information from controlled trials it would seem wise only to adjust the VV delay in particular individual circumstances.

19.9
Summary

Device therapy for heart failure is now part of routine clinical practice and is incorporated into contemporary guidelines, whereas only 10 years ago it was an experimental concept undergoing clinical trials. CRT has the capability to dramatically improve patient symptoms but has only a modest effect in extending life. A minority of patients appear to gain less, if any, benefit from CRT. How best to define this group and what their management should be remains to be determined. The ICD is effective at terminating potentially life threatening rhythm disturbances, but rather disappointingly has only a modest effect in prolonging life, similar to that achieved with CRT. The combination of ICD with CRT has not been shown to offer any additional benefit to that of CRT alone. Any additional benefits are likely to be very limited and are unlikely to be of any practical importance.

The implantation peri-procedural mortality has not been well reported. In the COMPANION trial,[17] it was between 0.5 and 0.8%. With device implantation becoming more widespread, it is important to ensure that implantation mortality does not rise. With improving techniques and better equipment, a peri-procedural mortality of <1% should easily be achieved.

In many countries the cost of devices, particularly ICDs may limit their use. Local judgements will have to be made as to what constitutes "value for money" or "cost effectiveness."

References

1. The antiarrhythmics versus implantable defibrillators (AVID) investigators. A comparison of antiarrhythmic-drug therapy with implantable defibrillators in patients resuscitated from near-fatal ventricular arrhythmias. *N Engl J Med*. 1997;337:1576-1583.
2. Kuck KH, Cappato R, Siebels J, Rüppel R. Defibrillators in patients resuscitated from cardiac arrest: The Cardiac Randomized Comparison of Antiarrhythmic Drug Therapy With Implantable Arrest Study Hamburg (CASH). *Circulation*. 2000;102:748-754.
3. Connolly SJ, Gent M, Roberts RS, et al. Canadian Implantable Defibrillator Study (CIDS): a randomized trial of the implantable cardioverter defibrillator against amiodarone. *Circulation*. 2000;101:1297-1302.
4. Connolly AP, Hallstrom R, Cappato EB, et al.; on behalf of the investigators of the AVID, CASH and CIDS studies. Meta-analysis of the implantable cardioverter defibrillator secondary prevention trials. *Eur Heart J*. 2000;21:2071-2078.
5. Owen A. How should the efficacy of novel treatments be assessed in survival trials? *Int J Cardiol*. 2007;120:297-300.
6. Higgins JPT, Thompson SG. Quantifying heterogeneity in a meta-analysis. *Statist Med*. 2002;21:1539-1558.
7. Daubert JP, Zareba DS, Cannom DS, et al.; for the MADIT II Investigators. Inappropriate implantable cardioverter-defibrillator shocks in MADIT II: frequency, mechanisms, predictors, and survival impact. *J Am Coll Cardiol*. 2008;51:1357-1365.
8. Mark DB, Anstrom KJ, Sun JL, et al.; for the Sudden Cardiac Death in Heart Failure Trial Investigators. Quality of life with defibrillator therapy or amiodarone in heart failure. *N Engl J Med*. 2008;359:999-1008.

9. ACC/AHA/HRS 2008 Guidelines for Device-Based Therapy of Cardiac Rhythm Abnormalities: Executive Summary: A Report of the American College of Cardiology/American Heart Association Task Force on Practice Guidelines (Writing Committee to Revise the ACC/AHA/ NASPE 2002 Guideline Update for Implantation of Cardiac Pacemakers and Antiarrhythmia Devices): Developed in Collaboration With the American Association for Thoracic Surgery and Society of Thoracic Surgeons. *Circulation.* 2008;117:2820-2840.

10. ESC Guidelines for the diagnosis and treatment of acute and chronic heart failure 2008. The task force for the diagnosis and treatment of acute and chronic heart failure 2008 of the European Society of Cardiology. *Eur Heart J.* 2008;29;2388-2442.

11. Moss AJ, Zareba W, Jackson Hall W, et al.; for the multicentre automatic defibrillator implantation trial II investigators. Prophylactic implantation of a defibrillator in patients with myocardial infarction and reduced ejection fraction. *N Engl J Med.* 2002;346:877-883.

12. Wilber DJ, Zareba W, Hall J, et al. Time dependence of mortality risk and defibrillator benefit after myocardial infarction. *Circulation.* 2004;109:1082-1084.

13. Kadish A, Dyer A, Daubert JP, et al.; for the Defibrillators in Non-Ischemic Cardiomyopathy Treatment Evaluation (DEFINITE) Investigators. Prophylactic defibrillator implantation in patients with nonischemic dilated cardiomyopathy. *N Engl J Med.* 2004;350:2151-2158.

14. Bardy GH, Kerry LL, Daniel BM, et al.; for the Sudden Cardiac Death in Heart Failure Trial (SCD-HeFT) Investigators. Amiodarone or an implantable cardioverter–defibrillator for congestive heart failure. *N Engl J Med.* 2005;352:225-237.

15. Hohnloser SH, Kuck KH, Dorian P, et al.; on behalf of the DINAMIT Investigators. Prophylactic use of an implantable cardioverter–defibrillator after acute myocardial infarction. *N Engl J Med.* 2004;351:2481-4288.

16. Desai AS, Fang JC, Maisel WH, et al. Implantable defibrillators for the prevention of mortality in patients with nonischemic cardiomyopathy: a meta-analysis of randomized controlled trials. *JAMA.* 2004;292(23):2874-2879.

17. Bristow MR, Saxon LA, Boehmer, J et al.; for the Comparison of Medical Therapy, Pacing, and Defibrillation in Heart Failure (COMPANION) Investigators. Cardiac-resynchronization therapy with or without an Implantable defibrillator in advanced chronic heart failure. *N Engl J Med.* 2004;350:2140-2150.

18. Strickberger SA, Hummel JD, Bartlett MC, et al. Amiodarone versus implantable cardioverter-defibrillator: randomized trial in patients with nonischemic dilated cardiomyopathy and asymptomatic nonsustained ventricular tachycardia – AMIOVIRT. *J Am Coll Cardiol.* 2003;41:1707-1712.

19. Poole JE, Johnson GW, Hellhamp AS, et al. Prognostic importance of defibrillator shocks in patients with heart failure. *N Engl J Med.* 2008;359:1009-1017.

20. Køber L, Torp-Pedersen C, McMurray JJV, et al.; for the Dronedarone Study Group. Increased mortality after dromedaries. Therapy for severe heart failure. *N Engl J Med.* 2008;358: 2678-2687.

21. Cazeau S, Leclercq C, Lavergne T, et al.; for the multisite stimulation in cardiomyopathies (MUSTIC) study investigators. Effects of multisite biventricular pacing in patients with heart failure and intraventricular conduction delay. *N Engl J Med.* 2001;344:873-880.

22. Auricchio A, Stellbrink C, Sack S, et al.; for the Pacing Therapies in Congestive Heart Failure (PATH-CHF) Study Group. Long-term clinical effect of hemodynamically optimized cardiac resynchronization therapy in patients with heart failure and ventricular conduction delay. *J Am Coll Cardiol.* 2002;39:2026-2033.

23. Abraham WT, Fisher WG, Smith AL, et al.; for the MIRACLE study group. Cardiac resynchronization in chronic heart failure. *N Engl J Med.* 2002;346:1845-1853.

24. Cleland JGF, Daubert J-C, Erdmann E, et al.; for the Cardiac Resynchronization – Heart Failure (CARE-HF) Study Investigators. The effect of cardiac resynchronization on morbidity and mortality in heart failure. *N Engl J Med.* 2005;352:1539-1549.

25. Cleland JGF, Daubert J-C, Erdmann E, et al.; on behalf of the CARE-HF Study Investigators. Longer-term effects of cardiac resynchronization therapy on mortality in heart failure (the Cardiac REsynchronization-Heart Failure (CARE-HF) trial extension phase). *Eur Heart J.* 2006;27:1928-1932.

26. Young JB, Abraham WT, Smith AL, et al. Combined cardiac resynchronization and implantable cardioversion defibrillation in advanced chronic heart failure: The MIRACLE ICD Trial. *JAMA.* 2003;289(20):2685-2694.

27. Higgins SL, Hummel JD, Imran K, et al. Cardiac resynchronization therapy for the treatment of heart failure in patients with intraventricular conduction delay and malignant ventricular tachyarrhythmias. *J Am Coll Cardiol.* 2003;42:1454-1459.

28. Abraham WT, Young JB, Leon AR, et al.; on behalf of the Multicenter InSync ICD II Study Group. Effects of cardiac resynchronization on disease progression in patients with left ventricular systolic dysfunction, an indication for an implantable cardioverter-defibrillator, and mildly symptomatic chronic heart failure. *Circulation.* 2004;110:2864-2868.

29. Lam S, Owen A. Combined resynchronization and defibrillation therapy in left ventricular dysfunction: bayesian network meta-analysis of randomized controlled trials. *BMJ.* 2007; 335:925-934.

30. Maisch B, Soler-Soler J, Hatle L, et al. *The ESC Textbook of Cardiovascular Medicine.* In: Camm AJ, Luscher TF, Serruys PW, eds. Oxford: Blackwell Publishing; 2006.

31. Chung ES, Leon AR, Tavazzi L, et al. Results of the predictors of response to CRT (PROSPECT) trial. *Circulation.* 2008;117:2608-2616.

32. Henein MY, Amadia A, O'Sullivan C, Coats A, Gibson D. ACE inhibitors unmask incoordinate diastolic wall motion in restrictive left ventricular disease. *Heart.* 1996;76:326-331.

33. Owen A, Cox S. Diagnosis of heart failure in elderly patients in primary care. *Eur J Heart Failure.* 2001;3:79-81.

34. Rathore SS, Yongfeiwang MPH, Krumholz HR. Sex-based differences in the effect of digoxin for the treatment of heart failure. *N Engl J Med.* 2002;347:1403-1411.

35. Hsu L-F, Jais P, Sanders P, et al. Catheter ablation for atrial fibrillation in congestive heart failure. *N Engl J Med.* 2004;351:2373-2383.

36. The DAVID Trial Investigators. Dual-chamber pacing or ventricular backup pacing in patients with an implantable defibrillator: the dual chamber and vvi implantable defibrillator (david) trial. *JAMA.* 2002;288(24):3115-3123.

37. Cleland JGF, Daubert JC, Erdmann E, et al.; on behalf of the CARE-HF study Steering Committee and Investigators. The CARE-HF study CArdiac REsynchronisation in Heart Failure study/rationale, design and end-points. *Eur J Heart Failure.* 2001;3:481-489.

The Role of Surgery in Heart Failure

20

John Pepper

20.1
Introduction

Surgery for patients in advanced heart failure aims to correct or repair many of the pathophysiological changes that occur in heart failure, which are not corrected by medical treatment alone. The surgical techniques performed today include revascularization of hibernating myocardium, ventricular restoration surgery, mitral valve repair, use of ventricular assist devices, and heart transplantation.

These procedures have not been exposed to the same degree of scrutiny as medical treatment to provide the level of evidence needed to become a standard part of heart failure management. Current guidelines for different forms of operation and the strength of the evidence supporting them are summarized in the Table 20.1. The most established operations for heart failure are coronary artery bypass grafting (CABG) and heart transplantation.[1,2]

20.2
Revascularization of Hibernating Myocardium

The aim of myocardial revascularization, whether by CABG or percutaneous coronary intervention, is: (1) to correct myocardial ischemia and hence prevent further adverse ventricular remodeling and myocardial infarction, and (2) to improve myocardial contractility in regions of hibernating myocardium that have been shown to be viable.

The determination of hibernating myocardium and viability can be made by stress echocardiography or by various nuclear imaging techniques such as PET, SPECT, or thallium or by cardiovascular magnetic resonance imaging with gadolinium enhancement. It has been reported that the improvement in left ventricular function after CABG is related to the number of viable segments present; at least eight viable segments should be present

J. Pepper
Department of Surgery, Royal Brompton Hospital, Sydney Street, London, UK
e-mail: j.pepper@rbht.nhs.uk

M.Y. Henein (ed.), *Heart Failure in Clinical Practice*,
DOI: 10.1007/978-1-84996-153-0_20, © Springer-Verlag London Limited 2010

Table 20.1 Surgery for heart failure

Treatment	Current guidelines	Level of evidence	Randomized trial
Revascularization for IC MLM disease or equivalent	I	B	No
Revascularization for IC M absent LM disease	IIA	B	In progress
SVR	IIB	C	Yes
Cardiac transplant	L	B	No
Destination LVAD	IIA	B	Yes
M V repair	IIB	C	In progress

ICM ischemic cardiomyopathy; *SVR* surgical ventricular remodeling[1,2]

to ensure an absolute improvement in ejection fraction of at least 5%.[3] Patients with viable, hibernating myocardium also have a lower operative mortality and better symptomatic improvement following CABG.[4-6]

Until recently, there were no randomized controlled trials comparing revascularization against medical treatment in patients with advanced ischemic heart failure. The early randomized trials of CABG versus medical treatment excluded patients with heart failure symptoms (NYHA class greater than II) and those with severe impairment of left ventricular function (ejection fraction less than 35% in the CASS study and less than 50% in the ECSS study).[7,8] Subgroup analysis of 160 trial patients who had an ejection fraction of less than 50% and three vessel coronary artery disease or proximal left main stem or proximal left anterior descending artery stenosis showed that the 10-year survival in those who had CABG was better compared to those who were treated with medication (79% vs. 61%, $p=0.01$). The survival advantage for CABG was present regardless of the severity of impairment of left ventricular function. This survival advantage with CABG in patients with impaired left ventricular function has been consistently reported in the other early randomized trials. However, it must be emphasized that most of these patients presented with angina and not heart failure. Only 4% of the trial patients had heart failure symptoms and only 7.2% had an ejection fraction less than 40%. In addition, advances in the medical treatment of advanced heart failure in the last decade have improved survival significantly. The results of these early randomized studies may therefore not be applicable in the present day in a patient with advanced ischemic heart failure that is, someone with NYHA class III and IV heart failure symptoms and an ejection fraction less than 30%.

Several more recent nonrandomized studies have reported that CABG in patients with advanced ischemic heart failure can be performed with an acceptable risk (operative mortality of 1.7–5.3%) and improves ejection fraction by up to 40% above the baseline value. The reported 5-year survival is 60–75%.[9-12] Unfortunately, complete data are not reported for many of these studies and the patient population is not uniform. Hibernation studies were performed preoperatively in some reports (10.11) but not in others.[9] In addition, only 23–43% of patients had heart failure symptoms preoperatively. Accurate reporting of ventricular function, heart failure symptoms and NYHA functional class at late follow up is absent from most studies. This is of importance as many of the benefits noted in the studies may not be sustained at late follow up. Recurrence of heart failure symptoms is reported in 53% of patients at 5 years by Luciani.[10] However, only 48% of patients in this study had hibernation studies preoperatively. More favorable results are reported by Lorusso's study[11] which performed hibernation studies in all patients (18% recurrence of heart failure symptoms at 4 years, 40% at 8 years). However, the same study reports that left ventricular function although improving significantly immediately postoperatively (ejection fraction $40\pm2\%$ compared to $28\pm9\%$, $p<0.01$), subsequently fell at late follow up and was only marginally better compared to preoperatively (ejection fraction $30\pm9\%$ compared with $28\pm9\%$). This decline in left ventricular function at late follow up is also reflected in the NYHA functional class (35% in NYHA class III and IV at 8 years compared to 24% immediately postoperatively).

There is some evidence that recurrence of heart failure symptoms after CABG for ischemic heart failure may be related to the severity of ventricular dilatation. Yamaguchi et al[13] reported a recurrence of heart failure following CABG in 69% of patients when the left ventricular end systolic volume index (LVESVI) was greater than 100 mL/m² compared to only 15% when the LVESVI was less than 100 mL/m² ($p<0.01$). Five year survival was also worse when LVESVI was greater than 100 mL/m² (53.5% vs. 85%; $p<0.01$).[13] Similarly, Louie et al[14] reported a failure of CABG in 27% of patients with ischemic cardiomyopathy undergoing CABG for heart failure symptoms, all of whom had a left ventricle which was significantly more dilated compared with those in whom CABG was successful (LV end diastolic diameter of 81 mm vs. 68 mm). In these patients, it may be necessary to perform some form of ventricular restoration surgery in addition to CABG.

In summary, there is a sound pathophysiological basis for revascularization of viable hibernating myocardium in patients with ischemic heart failure. Early randomized trials have shown the efficacy of CABG in patients with three vessel coronary artery disease or left main stem or proximal left anterior descending coronary artery disease and impaired ventricular function. However, most of the trial patients did not have advanced heart failure. In addition, significant advances have been made in the medical treatment of these patients since the trials. More recent nonrandomized studies have reported that CABG in patients with advanced ischemic heart failure can be performed with an acceptable risk and improves ejection fraction and NYHA functional class. There is concern, however, that these improvements may not be sustained in the long term and many of these patients have a recurrence of heart failure symptoms with deterioration in ventricular function within 5 years. Patient selection is important and those with severely dilated ventricles may do less well with CABG alone. A large, well designed randomized controlled trial is needed to confirm these observations. Of interest, is not only the influence of CABG on long term survival in patients with advanced ischemic heart failure, but also the impact of it on functional capacity, quality of life, heart function, and of crucial importance, whether any benefits are sustained in the long term. Other factors in patient selection may also be important such as the presence of good target coronary vessels for revascularization, complete revascularization, and absence of right heart failure or raised pulmonary artery pressures.[10,15] In cases where the left ventricle is significantly dilated e.g., above a LVESVI of 100 mL/m², some sort of ventricular restoration surgery may be necessary in addition to myocardial revascularisation.

20.3
Ventricular Restoration

The aim of ventricular restoration is to restore the size, shape and geometry of the dilated left ventricle towards normal. Restoration of ventricular size reverses many of the pathophysiological processes described earlier by decreasing ventricular wall stress.[16] This in turn enhances myocardial perfusion, decreases oxygen consumption, and enables improved contractility of myocytes. Restoration of ventricular shape and geometry towards a more elliptical structure also leads to greater efficiency of ventricular systole as previously described. Ventricular restoration is achieved by resection of myocardium and reconstructing the remaining ventricle into a more elliptical shape. Several different techniques for ventricular restoration can be used depending on the underlying cause of the cardiomyopathy.

20.3.1
Ischemic Cardiomyopathy

Ventricular restoration in ischemic cardiomyopathy, also referred to as surgical ventricular restoration (SVR), is largely done using the Dor procedure.[17] The modified linear closure technique described by Mickleborough is also sometimes used.[18] The Dor procedure was initially described in 1985 for the resection of left ventricular aneurysms and has recently been modified for use in ischemic cardiomyopathy. Both techniques involve the resection of the akinetic or dyskinetic anterior free wall of the left ventricle. Typically, these patients have had an anterior myocardial infarction with scarring and akinesia or dyskinesia of the left ventricle anterior free wall which may extend onto the septum. This segment of nonfunctional myocardium is resected. In the Dor procedure, an oval dacron patch is then placed which would also exclude the infarcted part of the septum from the rest of the ventricle. The size of the patch is tailored to the required size of the ventricle, and the shape of the patch is fashioned such that it helps restore the geometry of the left ventricle towards a more elliptical configuration. SVR adds about 20 min to the duration of an operation for CABG and has not been found to increase the operative risk.[19] CABG is always performed at the same time. The aim is to (1) recruit hibernating myocardium and hence enhance myocardial contractility, (2) resect nonfunctional akinetic or dyskinetic myocardium and hence improve the efficiency of ventricular contraction, and (3) restore the left ventricle to its normal size, shape and geometry with the benefits discussed previously.

There are no randomized controlled trials on SVR. Numerous nonrandomized studies have been reported.[20–23] These studies report a hospital mortality of 2.8–8.1%, an absolute improvement in ejection fraction of 10–13% above baseline (or a relative improvement of up to 40% above baseline), and an improvement in NYHA functional class. The benefits of SVR appear to be sustained. In the RESTORE study, 85% of patients were free of congestive heart failure symptoms at 18 months.[20] Similarly, Di Donato reported an event-free survival of 82.1% at 3 years.[21] Actuarial survival was 89.2% at 18 months in the RESTORE study and 74% at 3 years in Di Donato's study.

The results of these nonrandomized studies are encouraging. They suggest that SVR in these very sick patients can be performed with acceptable hospital mortality, and improves ejection fraction and functional capacity. The early results of up to 3 years suggest that the improvement in congestive heart failure symptoms is sustained. The 3 year actuarial survival also appears impressive considering the patient population. Clearly, patient selection is important. The ideal patient may be one who has had an anterior myocardial infarction with akinesia or dyskinesia of the LV anterior free wall, dilatation of the LV, good target coronary vessels which can be grafted, and viable hibernating myocardium. The results of SVR may not be as good in patients who have pathology outside of the LV such as right ventricular failure or raised pulmonary artery pressures.

Clearly, a randomized controlled trial comparing SVR against optimal medical therapy is needed to confirm the findings of these nonrandomized studies. Furthermore, SVR is almost always combined with CABG, which in itself may improve cardiac function and functional capacity. It is unclear how much of the apparent benefits shown in the VRS studies are due to VRS and how much is due to CABG. The National Institutes of Health in the United States is sponsoring a multicentre prospective randomized trial, the surgical treatment for ischemic heart failure (STICH) trial which is due to be reported late in 2009.[24] It has recruited patients with ischemic LV dysfunction with an EF less than 35%, CAD amenable to surgical revascularization, and NYHA class 2–4 heart failure at 50 centers. It is designed to examine two hypotheses. Firstly, patients who undergo CABG with intensive medical treatment have an improved long-term survival compared to medical treatment alone. Secondly, in patients with anterior LV dysfunction, SVR to a more normal LV size with coronary bypass grafting improves survival compared to CABG alone. The overall study design is to randomly assign patients, stratified by presence or absence of angina and by the presence or absence of a large akinetic territory, either to surgery or to continued medical treatment. Those with large akinetic areas were eligible to undergo SVR. Patients without angina were divided into two groups: 1,600 patients with SVR-ineligible anatomy and 600 patients who are SVR eligible. The SVR-ineligible group was randomly assigned to one of three arms: medical treatment, CABG alone, or CABG and SVR. Finally in a subgroup of 600 patients with angina, those with heart failure and a large area of akinesis were randomly assigned to conventional CABG alone or CABG and SVR.

The need for a randomised trial has been widely recognised and the design much discussed [24]. The Hypothesis 2 substudy of the Surgical Treatment for Ischemic Heart Failure (STICH) has recently been reported by Jones et al [25]. This substudy compared CABG alone with the combined procedure of CABG with surgical ventricular reconstruction. Eligible patients were required to have coronary artery disease amenable to CABG, a left ventricular ejection fraction of 35% or less, and a dominant anterior region of myocardial akinesia or dyskinesia that was amenable to surgical ventricular reconstucion. All patients received standard medical and device treatment for heart failure.

Thousand patients were recruited from 96 medical centres in 23 countries. The patients in the two study group were closely matched for demographic characteristics, co-morbidity, the proportion who were on heart failure drugs, the CCS angina class, the NYHA heart-failure class, coronary anatomy and the extent of anterior myocardial akinesia or dyskinesia. Both groups of patients were equally successful in improving the postoperative CC angina and NYHA heart-failure class. There was similar improvement in the 6-min walk

test and similar reductions in symptoms. As one would expect, there was a greater reduction in the end-systolic volume index with the combined procedure (16ml/M^2 of BSA), as
compared with CABG alone (5ml/M^2). Unfortunately these data were obtained from only
373 patients at baseline and at 4 months.

The primary outcome of the trial was a composite of death from any cause or hospitalization for cardiac causes. There was no difference in the occurrence of the primary outcome between the CABG group (59%) and the combined procedure group (58%). The
30-day surgical rates of death for CABG alone (5%) and for the combined procedure (6%)
were similar and low overall, and no difference in the rate of death from any cause was
observed in a mean follow-up period of 48 months.

On the basis of this trial, Eisen,[26] in an editorial stated that the routine use of surgical
ventricular reconstruction in addition to CABG cannot be justified. There may be specific
subgroups of patients who might benefit from the combined procedure, but such an effect
is not apparent so far in the results of the STICH trial and may be difficult to detect, given
the heterogeneity of the study population.

There were several major problems with the conduct of this trial [27]. Myocardial viability
was only assessed in 20% of the patients. Therefore it is not clear whether the study was
examining the treatment of scar tissue or hibernating myocardium. The conduct of the
surgery also raises questions. 501 SVR procedures were performed in 127 sites over 5
years which results in an average of 0.7 SVR operations per site per year. Were the steps
taken to assure eligibility of the surgeon and the unit actually effective? The ESVI was
only reduced by 19% in STICH which compares unfavourably with a 36% reduction in the
RESTORE study. In 41% of patients undergoing the Dor procedure in STICH, a Dacron
patch was not used whereas in the RESTORE studies all patients received a patch. This
raises the question of whether inadequate operative procedures were performed in a large
proportion of the patients randomized to the Dor procedure.

20.3.2
Dilated Cardiomyopathy

Ventricular restoration in dilated cardiomyopathy can be achieved using partial left ventriculectomy (PLV), also called the Batista operation. This operation was first described by
Batista in 1996[28] and involves resection of segments of the lateral wall of the LV between
the papillary muscles, from the apex of the heart to the mitral annulus. The principle behind
PLV is similar to that of SVR (used in ischemic cardiomyopathy) in that they both aim to
reduce ventricular wall stress by reducing LV size. A key difference, however, is that functional myocardium is resected in PLV, whereas in SVR, nonviable, scarred, akinetic, myocardium is resected. The myocardium resected in SVR does not contribute at all towards
ventricular contractility. Rather, its presence impairs the efficiency of ventricular systole.
The myocardium resected in PLV, however, does contribute towards ventricular contractility and there is concern that excessive resection of such myocardium in an already com-
prised ventricle may actually impair LV function.

There are several studies reporting on PLV in dilated cardiomyopathy but only a few of
these are large enough to allow any meaningful interpretation of their results. There are,

unfortunately, no randomized controlled trials and even the biggest nonrandomized studies involved only about 60 patients.[29–31] The reported hospital mortality ranged from 3.2 to 31.5%. The studies demonstrate an initial improvement in ejection fraction and also NYHA functional class. However, these improvements do not appear to be sustained. In the Cleveland study,[29] more than half the patients were in NYHA class IV heart failure within 3 years and the 3-year event free survival was only 26% (events being defined as mortality, implantation of an LVAD, return to class IV heart failure or use of an implantable defibrillator).

The available evidence therefore does not support the widespread use of PLV in dilated cardiomyopathy. It carries a significant operative mortality and does not appear to improve long term symptom control, functional capacity or survival. Some smaller case series suggest that some patients may benefit from PLV but these groups of patients have yet to be clearly identified and until then, routine use of PLV in dilated cardiomyopathy cannot be recommended.

20.4
Mitral Valve Surgery

Mitral valve surgery is an option in advanced heart failure when significant mitral regurgitation is present. The mitral regurgitation in this situation is usually functional due to failure of mitral leaflet coaptation as a result of (1) dilatation of the left ventricle which pulls the subvalvular mitral apparatus and the papillary muscles apart, and (2) mitral annular dilatation. This tethering of the posterior wall of the LV tends to produce an assymetrical mitral annulus. As the disease progresses the entire annulus becomes dilated and the papillary muscles become widely splayed apart. It has been demonstrated that the presence of functional mitral regurgitation following myocardial function has an adverse effect on long term survival (62% at 5 years vs. 39%; $p < 0.001$) and is an independent predictor of adverse survival (RR 1.88; $p < 0.001$).[32] Furthermore, the severity of functional mitral regurgitation also determined long term survival. The 5 year survival of those with an effective regurgitant orifice area (ERO) of greater than 20 mm^2 was only 21% compared to 47% in those whose ERO was less than 20 mm^2 ($p < 0.001$, RR of death of 2.23, or 1.40 per 10 mm^2 ERO increase).[32] The SAVE study also reported that even mild mitral regurgitation had an adverse outcome on survival following myocardial infarction.[33]

The aim of mitral valve surgery in this situation is twofold: (1) to correct the mitral regurgitation and hence restore forward blood flow during LV systole; (2) to reduce the size of the dilated LV and reshape it from a spherical shape to a more normal elliptical shape. Both of these aims can be achieved by significantly reducing the size of the mitral annulus e.g., by the insertion of an undersized mitral annuloplasty ring. This procedure restores the zone of mitral leaflet coaptation and also reduces LV diameter significantly at its base. The ventricle is drawn together at its base, and the papillary muscles are pulled towards each other resulting in the long axis of the ventricle becoming more ellipsoid from base to apex.[34,35] As has been described earlier, ventricular wall stress is reduced when ventricular size is reduced. The LV also functions more efficiently when myofibrils are aligned in an oblique direction to the axis of the heart (as in a normal elliptically shaped heart) compared to when they are aligned in a horizontal direction to the axis of the heart (as in a dilated spherically shaped heart).

There are no randomized controlled trials of mitral valve surgery in advanced heart failure. The nonrandomized studies report an operative mortality of between 2.3 and 11%. All of the studies show a significant improvement in NYHA functional class and EF. In addition, Smolens[36] and Bolling[35] reported an improvement in cardiac output from 3.1 to 5.2 L/min at 22 months and a reduction in the sphericity of the LV from 0.82 to 0.74. Bishay[37] reported freedom from congestive heart failure symptoms of 88% at 1 year, 82% at 2 years, and 72% at 3 years. The reported actuarial survival is 73–90% at 1 year, 68–86% at 2 years, and 37–58% at 5 years.[36–39]

These non randomized studies suggest that mitral valve repair may be beneficial in advanced heart failure with significant mitral regurgitation. The operative mortality of 2.3–11% is acceptable in these very ill patients. The reported improvement in symptoms, functional capacity, and cardiac function, which appears to be sustained up to 3 years after operation, is encouraging. The reported actuarial survival of up to 58% at 5 years is also encouraging. Nevertheless, a randomized controlled trial comparing mitral valve surgery against optimal medical therapy in patients with advanced heart failure and significant mitral regurgitation is needed to confirm the findings of the nonrandomized studies. Patient selection may be important and those with associated significant right ventricular failure and irreversibly raised pulmonary artery pressures may not benefit from surgery to the left side of the heart.

20.4.1
Ventricular Restraint

The largest study in nonischemic cardiomyopathy took place in the Acorn Clinical Trial[40] which randomized 193 patients with significant heart failure and mitral regurgitation (88% nonischemic) to mitral repair alone vs. mitral repair with concomitant implantation of the CorCap cardiac support device (CSD). Mitral repair was associated with a progressive reduction in LV volumes over a 2-year period and there was improvement in quality of life measures, exercise performance and NYHA functional class. Reduction in LV dimensions was more pronounced in the CorCap-treated patients than in those treated with mitral repair alone. Both groups saw an early decrease in ejection fraction at 3 months followed by progressive improvement from 3 to 18 months after operation. Mann and colleagues[41] assessed the safety and efficacy of the device in 300 patients with heart failure. Of the 300 patients enrolled, 193 were randomized to mitral surgery alone or mitral surgery plus CSD. The 107 patients who did not need mitral surgery were randomized to medical treatment or medical treatment plus CSD. The primary end-point was a composite based on changes in clinical status, the need for major cardiac procedures for worsening heart failure, and a change in NYHA class. All patients had an LVEF of less than 35%, a LVEDD of 60 mm or greater, a 6-minute walk test of less than 450 m. The proportional odds ratio for the primary endpoint favored treatment with the CSD (1.73; 95% CI 1.07–2.79; $p=0.024$). When compared with the baseline, LVEF increased significantly at 12 months ($p=0.0009$) in the CSD-treated group compared with controls ($p=0.65$). But the changes in LVEF between groups were not significant ($p=0.45$). Therefore the CorCap CSD may have a role in preventing adverse remodeling after myocardial infarction. It requires an operation for its insertion but this could be through a small anterior thoracotomy.

A more recent development, the Paracor device, is currently being assessed in clinical trials in Europe and the United States. This is an elastic nitinol mesh that is designed to mechanically reinforce the heart to retard or hopefully halt the remodeling process. It can be deployed in a minimally invasive fashion. Klodell et al have reported their early results.[42] Fifty patients in NYHA ll or lll underwent the procedure which was well tolerated. At 6 months there was a significant improvement in the 6 minute walk ($+65.7$ M, $p=0.002$) and Minnesota Living with Heart Failure scores (-15.7, $p=0.002$). Long-term functional results are not yet available.

20.5
Left Ventricular Assist Devices

Left ventricular assist devices (LVADs) augment cardiac output in the failing heart by pumping blood from the left ventricle, through the LVAD, to the aorta. They have been used since the 1960s and were initially designed to provide short term mechanical circulatory support in patients with cardiogenic shock following cardiac surgery.[43] Since the 1980s, they have been used in patients awaiting heart transplantation who had decompensated chronic heart failure, so called "bridge-to-transplant." More recently, LVADs have been used in place of heart transplantation as permanent treatment in patients with advanced heart failure, so called "destination-therapy." The use of LVADs as a "bridge-to-recovery" is also being evaluated. In this case, reverse ventricular remodeling occurs while the heart is rested on an LVAD, and ventricular function recovers sufficiently for the LVADs to be explanted safely.

Engineering developments have enabled these pumps to be miniaturized to less than one third the mass and size of the first generation devices. This has made the task of insertion and removal considerably easier. As a result, such pumps are beginning to be used more often in the setting of acute cardiogenic shock. Results from anecdotal observations are encouraging but well defined trials have yet to be reported.

In the setting of chronic LV failure it is easy to underestimate the severity of right ventricular dysfunction. There is now a considerable experience with improving right ventricular function prior to implantation of a LVAD. In the event that these measures are insufficient a temporary RVAD can be inserted which can usually be removed within 14 days.

20.5.1
Bridge to Transplant

The use of LVADs as a bridge-to-transplant in patients with decompensated chronic heart failure is well established. It has been used in more than 4,000 patients worldwide. It is estimated that up to 20% of heart transplant recipients in the United States receive an

LVAD prior to transplantation.[44] The use of LVADs in these patients improves their cardiac output, NYHA functional class, and helps reverse any end-organ dysfunction e.g., renal and liver impairment. The physical condition of these patients improve significantly while on LVAD support and as many as 50% are well enough to be discharged home with an LVAD while waiting for a donor heart. The results of transplantation are improved in these patients who demonstrate a better survival at 1 year after transplantation compared to those who did not receive and LVAD (90% vs. 67%).[45,46]

The treatment of end-organ failure should be seen in perspective. Current figures for survival on hemodialysis for renal failure are 60% at 2 years, the use of the MARS charcoal filter in liver failure as a bridge to transplantation is associated with a 5-year survival of 66%, while LVAD bridge to heart transplantation is associated with a 5-year survival of 73%. The use of a LVAD can on occasion result in so great an improvement in the function of the native heart that the device can be removed and transplantation is no longer necessary. Recovery of hemodynamic and nutritional status with reversal of the metabolic and cellular abnormalities of heart failure improves survival after heart transplantation. This improvement results from reversal of cell deficiencies in the myocyte limiting contractile function. Abnormalities have been shown in the contractile proteins, the control of contraction, the provision of energy for contraction and expression of genes. Hypertrophied myocytes revert toward normal size, cell apoptosis and oncosis are reduced and calcium control by the sarcoplasmic reticulum is largely restored. Even the transcription of inhibitors of apoptosis is upregulated.

Overall, mechanical unloading by use of a LVAD leads to reversal of the adverse remodeling process, normalization of passive pressure–volume relationships and improved contractile response to increased heart rate and beta-agonists.

20.5.2
Bridge to Recovery

LVADs have long been used in postcardiotomy cardiogenic shock as a means to support the circulation until the heart recovers sufficiently following cardiac surgery. Approximately 30% of these patients survive to be discharged from hospital with good long term survival.[47,48] More recently, a small proportion of patients on long term LVAD support have been successfully weaned off LVAD support with reasonable left ventricular function and functional capacity.

The use of an LVAD decreases work load and ventricular wall stress. In most cases, the LVAD takes over the work of the left ventricle completely. The decrease in ventricular wall stress increases subendocardial perfusion, decreases oxygen consumption, and increases myocardial contractility.[49] Over time, reverse ventricular remodeling occurs. Zafeiridis et al[50] reported that after 75 days of LVAD support, cardiomyopathic hearts demonstrate a 28% reduction in myocyte volume, 20% reduction in cell length, 20% reduction in cell width, and 32% reduction in cell length-to-thickness ratio ($p < 0.05$), with a corresponding reduction in LV end diastolic diameter from 7.5 ± 0.5 to 5.5 ± 0.3 cm and LV mass from 347 ± 63 to 193 ± 23 g ($p < 0.05$). Several other studies have also reported a reduction in LV dimensions and improvement in cardiac function following long term LVAD support.[51–53]

The number of patients on long-term LVAD support who demonstrate sufficient myocardial function recovery for the LVAD to be explanted are small. The characteristics of these patients have yet to be fully identified. Patients with more acute onset heart failure e.g., those with viral myocarditis may demonstrate the greatest myocardial recovery while on LVAD support. The recovery in this instance is related more to resolution of the primary pathologic process rather than reverse ventricular remodeling. The results are less promising in patients with chronic heart failure. Only about 1–5% of such patients demonstrate recovery in ventricular function sufficient for the LVAD to be explanted.[54-57] Moreover, there is concern that this improvement in ventricular function may not be sustained after the LVAD is explanted. Hetzer[56] reported that 28 patients (out of 512 patients) showed myocardial recovery sufficient for the LVAD to be explanted. Of these, 16 continued to have normal heart function at a mean follow up of 2.6 years (range less than 1–5 years), while the remaining 12 either died or needed a heart transplant. The 16 patients who showed sustained recovery had a significantly shorter duration of heart failure prior to LVAD implantation compared to the 12 who had recurrence of heart failure (2 years vs. 9 years, $p<0.0002$). Similarly, Mancini (451) reported that five patients (out of 111 patients) had the LVAD explanted, but only one remained alive and well at 15 months without the need for another LVAD or heart transplantation. Frazier[55] meanwhile reported that 4 out of 5 patients who had the LVAD explanted were alive and well with follow- up extending up to 3 years in two of them.

Clearly, the numbers of patients showing sustained myocardial recovery following LVAD explantation is small and the predictors of such patients have not been fully identified at present. The duration of heart failure prior to LVAD implantation may be important as once significant myocyte loss and myocardial fibrosis occurs, ventricular remodeling may be irreversible.[56] It has been reported that patients who demonstrated significant myocardial recovery had a smaller LV end diastolic diameter (71 ± 2 mm vs. 81 ± 7 mm) and less myocardial fibrosis ($24\pm4\%$ vs. $34\pm2\%$) compared to those who showed no myocardial recovery.[58] There is also some evidence that the use of the beta agonist, clenbuterol, in combination with maximal heart failure drugs may augment myocardial recovery with an LVAD in a greater proportion of patients than has been reported hitherto.[57]

20.5.3
Destination Therapy

The efficacy of LVADs as permanent or destination therapy was demonstrated in the recently reported REMATCH trial.[58] The REMATCH study evaluated the HeartMate LVAD in patients with severe heart failure despite maximal medical treatment. Entry criteria were a need for intravenous inotropic therapy for symptomatic hypotension, decreasing renal function or worsening pulmonary edema together with LVEF less than 25% and peak oxygen consumption (MVO_2) less than 12 mL/kg/min. The investigating transplant centers had to overcome major ethical, logistic and economic hurdles in order to recruit 129 patients who were deemed unsuitable for transplantation and who were willing to be randomized. All cause mortality (the primary end-point) was 48% lower in the LVAD group ($p=0.09$ at 2 years, $p=0.001$ at 1 year). Median survival was 408 days in the LVAD group and only 150 days in the medically treated group. Few patients in the LVAD group survived for 2 years (23% vs. 8% in the medically treated group, $p<0.09$). Quality of life was limited by a 28% incidence of device infection at 3 months, a 42% incidence of bleeding at 6 months and a 35% probability of device failure at 2 years. Of the 68 patients who received a LVAD 10 had the device replaced. After REMATCH, 67 centers in the USA have started lifetime treatment programs. Clinical outcomes are now better than in REMATCH. The Health Care Advisory Board (USA) now predicts that LVADs will provide conventional treatment for advanced heart failure by 2010.

A recent Department of Health-commissioned study in the UK suggests that there is evidence that the odds of VAD survival is increasing with time ($p<0.04$).

The main concern with the use of LVADs is the high device-related morbidity associated with it. However, significant progress has been made since the REMATCH trial and the current newer generation of LVADs are safer, smaller, more efficient and more patient friendly. They are therefore likely to be associated with less morbidity compared with the LVADs used in the REMATCH trial. Currently, more than 60 centers in the United States have begun destination therapy programs with LVADs.

20.5.4
LVAD Development

In 1994 the devices and technology branch of the National Heart Lung and Blood Institute invited submissions for the development of innovative circulatory support systems as a long-term treatment for heart failure. The engineering strategy for these devices was to encompass a number of preferred characteristics. These were:

1. Small size and weight allowing the pump to be fully implantable.
2. Reduced blood contact surface area to decrease activation of the immune and coagulation systems.
3. A simple blood propulsion mechanism without prosthetic valves or the need for heparin.
4. A reliable operating system easily learned by the patient and safe in the community.

As a result of this initiative, new miniaturized centrifugal and axial flow devices have become available for clinical evaluation. These newer rotary pumps differ from the old larger pusher-plate pumps, by offering assistance to the ventricle rather than wholesale replacement. Thus with the rotary pump as a LVAD, the native LV continues to make a small but significant contribution to the cardiac output and thus the flow exhibits low pulsatility. These devices are preload and afterload sensitive. The overriding principle of controlling these pumps is to reach the desired flow with the lowest possible rotational speed, thus minimizing blood trauma and platelet activation. Careful afterload reduction is essential, together with close monitoring of antiplatelet therapy.

It is not yet clear whether the degree of ventricular unloading provided by these rotary pumps is sufficient to allow for recovery of LV and biventricular failure. The small observational studies available on these second generation rotary pumps suggest that the causes of mortality and morbidity are similar to the large pusher pumps but the frequency of complications is lower. Infection, bleeding and stroke remain the most significant problems, and there is an urgent need to understand the coagulopathy that can be problematic with the axial impellor pump.

In summary, LVADs have been shown to be efficacious as a bridge-to-transplantation and as destination therapy in advanced heart failure. The threshold level of heart failure beyond which patients will benefit from the insertion of an LVAD needs to be determined. Currently, LVADs are indicated in patients with advanced heart failure who cannot be weaned from inotropic support and who have a cardiac index of less than 2.0 L/min/m², a systolic blood pressure of less than 80 mmHg, and a pulmonary capillary wedge pressure of >20 mmHg.[1] As the technology improves and as LVADs get smaller, more efficient and safer, it is likely that this threshold level will change such that patients with less advanced heart failure may also benefit from a LVAD.

20.6
Heart Transplantation

Heart transplantation remains the most effective treatment for patients with end-stage heart failure. Although no randomized controlled trials are available, it appears to improve symptoms and survival. The reported survival following heart transplantation is 79–85% at 1 year, 75–80% at 3 years, and 69–75% at 5 years.[59] At the time of transplant, 41% of adult recipients were receiving intravenous inotropic support and 29% were on some type of mechanical circulatory support (22% on LVADs). The mean adult donor age is significantly higher for European centers than for North American centers (38.8 vs. 31.3 years) Approximately 20% of adult heart donors in Europe were aged 50 years or older, as compared to only 10% of adult heart donors in North America.

The shortage of donor hearts limits transplantation as a universal treatment for these patients. Only 95 heart transplants were performed in the UK in 2007/2008, a small increase on 2006/7 the figure for which was 88 (UKTSSA 2008). The contraindications to transplantation such as advanced age and other comorbidities further limit the use of heart transplantation in many patients. There is also morbidity associated with heart transplantation such as chronic rejection and complications from the use of immunosuppressive drugs. These include an increased incidence of renal failure and graft vascular disease.

It is generally accepted that heart transplantation should only be performed in patients with severe limitation of daily activities and with a peak oxygen consumption of less than 15 mL/kg/min unless there is significant refractory ischemia or arrhythmia not amenable to all other forms of treatment, both medical and surgical. The patients who show the greatest benefit from heart transplantation are those with refractory cardiogenic shock, dependence on inotropic or mechanical circulatory support or persistent NYHA class IV symptoms with a peak oxygen consumption less than 10 mL/kg/min.[1]

It is of concern that despite the ongoing stepwise improvement in early transplant survival, the overall slopes of the late post-transplant survival curves remain unchanged. It is becoming clear that a part of this lack of improvement is due to the fact that recent recipients and donors have more risk factors for later mortality than in previous eras. Nevertheless recent data demonstrates reduced incidence rates of coronary allograft vasculopathy and severe renal dysfunction in more recently transplanted patients. This would suggest that there has been a favorable impact of the recent immunosuppressive and management protocols on the natural history of cardiac allograft vasculopathy and the toxicity of the various drugs.

Despite all the limitations, heart transplantation remains the greatest success story for truly end-stage disease, with more than 50,000 patients now transplanted worldwide. The breadth of its impact far exceeds the actual recipients, because the lure of heart transplantation called attention to the newly defined population of advanced heart failure, whereas the restricted donor supply inspired the development of better heart failure management and of new strategies for replacement, such as mechanical cardiac devices.

References

1. Hunt SA, Baker DW, Chin MH, et al. ACC/AHA 2005 Guideline update for the Diagnosis and Management of Chronic Heart Failure in the Adult – Summary Article: A report of the American College of Cardiology/American Heart Association Task Force on Practice Guidelines (Writing Committee to update the 2001 Guidelines for the Evaluation and Management of Heart Failure): Developed in Collaboration with the American College of Chest Physicians and the International Society for heart an Lung transplantation: Endorsed by the Heart Rhythm Society. *Circulation.* 2005;112:1825-1852.
2. ACC.AHA 2004 Guidelines for coronary artey bypass graft surgery. *Circulation.* 2004;110: e340-e347.
3. Pagano D, Townend J, Horton R, et al. Coronary artery bypass grafting for ischaemic heart failure. The predictive value of quantitative PET for symptomatic and functional outcome. *J Thorac Cardiovasc Surg.* 1998;115:791-799.
4. Beller GA. Assessing prognosis by means of radionuclide perfusion imaging: what technique and which variables should be used. *J Am Coll Cardiol.* 1998;31:1286-1290.
5. Di Carli MF, Asgarzadie F, Schelbert HR, et al. Quantitative relation between myocardial viability and improvement in heart failure symptoms after revascularisation in patients with ischaemic cardiomyopathy. *Circulation.* 1995;92:3436-3444.
6. Maddahi J, Blitz A, Phelps M, Laks H. The use of positron emission tomography imaging in the management of patients with ischaemic cardiomyopathy. *Adv Card Surg.* 1996;7: 163-188.
7. CASS Principal Investigators. Coronary artery surgery study (CASS): a randomized trial of coronary artery bypass surgery. Survival data. *Circulation.* 1983;68:939-950.
8. European Coronary Surgery Study Group. Long-term results of prospective randomized study or coronary artery bypass surgery in stable angina pectoris. *Lancet.* 1982;2:1173-1180.
9. Trachiotis GD, Weintraub WS, Johnston TS, Jones EL, Guyton RA, Craver JM. Coronary artery bypass grafting in patients with advanced left ventricular dysfunction. *Ann Thorac Surg.* 1998;66:1632-1639.
10. Luciani GB, Montalbano G, Casali G, Mazzucco A. Predicting long-term functional results after myocardial revascularisation in ischaemic cardiomyopathy. *J Thorac Cardiovasc Surg.* 2000;120:478-489.
11. Lorusso R, La Canna G, Ceconi C, Borghetti V, Totaro P, et al. Long-term results of coronary artery bypass grafting procedure in the presence of left ventricular dysfunction and hibernating myocardium. *Eur J Cardiothorac Surg.* 2001;20:937-948.

12. Elefteriades JA, Tellides G, Samady H, et al. Coronary artery bypass for advanced left ventricular function. In: Roy Masters, ed. *Surgical Options for the Treatment of Heart Failure.* 1999:15-31.
13. Yamaguchi A, Ino T, Adachi H, et al. Left ventricular volume predicts postoperative course in patients with ischaemic cardiomyopathy. *Ann Thorac Surg.* 1997;65:434-438.
14. Louie HW, Laks H, Milgalter E, et al. Ischaemic cardiomyopathy. Criteria for coronary revascularisation and cardiac transplantation. *Circulation.* 1991;94(suppl III):III-290-III-295.
15. Jones EL, Weintraub WS. The importance of completeness of revascularisation during long-term follow up after coronary artery operations. *J Thorac Cardiovasc Surg.* 1996;112:227-237.
16. Schenk S, McCarthy PM, Starling RC, et al. Neurohormonal response to left ventricular reconstruction surgery in ischaemic cardiomyopathy. *J Thorac Cardiovasc Surg.* 2004;128:38-43.
17. Dor V, Kreitmann P, Jourdan J. Interest of "physiological" closure (circumferential plasty on contractive areas) of left ventricle after resection and endocardiectomy for aneurysm or akinetic zone comparison with classical technique about a series of 209 left ventricular resections. *J Cardiovasc Surg.* 1985;26:73.
18. Mickleborough LL, Carson S, Ivanov J. Repair of dyskinetic or akinetic left ventricular aneurysm: results obtained with a modified linear closure. *J Thorac Cardiovasc Surg.* 2001;121:675-682.
19. Maxey TS, Reece TB, Ellman PI, et al. Coronary artery bypass with ventricular restoration is superior to coronary artery bypass alone in patients with ischaemic cardiomyopathy. *J Thorac Cardiovasc Surg.* 2004;127:428-434.
20. Athanasuleas CL, Stanley AW Jr, Buckberg GD, Dor V, DiDonato M, Blackstone EH. Surgical anterior ventricular endocardial restoration (SAVER) in the dilated remodelled ventricle after anterior myocardial infarction. RESTORE group. Reconstructive Endoventricular Surgery, returning Torsion Original Radius Elliptical Shape to LV. *J Am Coll Cardiol.* 2001; 37(5):1210-1213.
21. Di Donato M, Toso A, Maioli M, Sabatier M, Stanley AWH, Dor V; RESTORE Group. Intermediate survival and predictors of death after ventricular restoration. *Sem Thorac Cardiovasc Surg.* 2001;13(4):468-475.
22. Mickleborough LL, Merchant N, Ivanov J, Rao V, Carson S. Left ventricular reconstruction: early and late results. *J Thorac Cardiovasc Surg.* 2004;128(1):27-37.
23. Suma H, Isomura T, Horii T, Hisatomi K. Left ventriculoplasty for ischemic cardiomyopathy. *Eur J Cardiothorac Surg.* 2001;20:319-323.
24. Velazquez EJ, Lee KL, O'Connor CM, et al. Rationale and design of the surgical treatment for ischemic heart failure (STICH) trial. *J Thorac Cardiovasc Surg.* 2007;134:1540-1547.
25. Jones RH, Velazquez EJ, Michler RE, et al. Coronary bypass surgery with or without surgical ventricular reconstruction. *N Engl J Med.* 2009;360:1705-1717.
26. Eisen HJ. Surgical ventricular reconstruction for heart failure. *N Engl J Med.* 2009;360:1781-1784.
27. Buckberg GD. Questions and answers about the STICH trial: a different perspective. *J Thorac Cardiovasc Surg.* 2005;130:245-249.
28. Batista RJV, Santos JLV, Takeshita N, et al. Partial left ventriculectomy to improve left ventricular function in end stage heart disease. *J Card Surg.* 1996;11:96-97.
29. Franco-Cereceda A, McCarthy PM, Blackstone EH, et al. Partial left ventriculectomy for dilated cardiomyopathy: is this an alternative to transplantation? *J Thorac Cardiovasc Surg.* 2001;121:879-892.
30. Moreira LFP, Stolf NAG, Higuchi ML, Bacal F, Bocchi EA, Oliveira SA. Current perspectives of partial left ventriculectomy in the treatment of dilated cardiomyopathy. *Eur J Cardiothorac Surg.* 2001;19:54-60.
31. Izzat MB, Kabbani SS, Suma H, Pandey K, Morishita K, Yim APC. Early experience with partial left ventriculectomy in the Asia-Pacific region. *Ann Thorac Surg.* 1999;67:1703-1707.

32. Grigioni F, Enriquez-Sarano M, Zehr KJ, Bailey KR, Tajik J, et al. Ischemic mitral regurgitation: long term outcome and prognostic implications with quantitative Doppler assessment. *Circulation*. 2001;103:1759-1764.

33. Lamas GA, Mitchell GF, Flaker GC, et al. Clinical significance of mitral regurgitation after acute myocardial infarction: survival and ventricular enlargement investigators. *Circulation*. 1997;96:827-833.

34. Bolling SF, Deeb M, Brunsting L, Bach DS. Early outcome of mitral valve reconstruction in patients with end stage cardiomyopathy. *J Thorac Cardiovasc Surg*. 1995;109:676-683.

35. Bolling SF, Pagani FD, Deeb GM, Bach DS. Intermediate term outcome of mitral reconstruction in cardiomyopathy. *J Thorac Cardiovasc Surg*. 1998;115:381-386.

36. Smolens IA, Pagani FD, Bolling SF. Mitral valve repair in heart failure. *Eur J Heart Failure*. 2000;2:365-371.

37. Bishay ES, McCarthy PM, Cosgrove DM, et al. Mitral valve surgery in patients with severe left ventricular dysfunction. *Eur J Cardiothorac Surg*. 2000;17:213-221.

38. Chen FY, Adams DH, Aranki SF, et al. Mitral valve repair in cardiomyopathy. *Circulation*. 1998;98(19S):124II-127II.

39. Calafiore AM, Gallina S, Mauro MD, et al. Mitral valve procedure in dilated cardiomyopathy: repair or replacement? *Ann Thorac Surg*. 2001;71:1146-1153.

40. Acker MA, Bolling S, Shemin R. Mitral valve surgery in heart failure: insights from the Acorn Clinical Trial. *J Thorac Cardiovasc Surg*. 2006;132:568-577.

41. Mann DL, Acker MA, Jessup M; Acorn Trial Principal Investigators and Study Coordinators. Clinical evaluation of the corcap cardiac support device in patients with dilated cardiomyopathy. *Ann Thorac Surg*. 2007;84:1226-1235.

42. Klodell CT, Aranda JM, McGiffin DC, et al. Worldwide surgical experience with the Paracor HeartNet cardiac restraint device. *J Thorac Cardiovasc Surg*. 2008;135:188-195.

43. DeBakey ME. Left ventricular bypass pump for left ventricular assistance. *Am J Cardiol*. 1971;27:3-11.

44. Frazier OH, Delgado RM. Mechanical circulatory support for advanced heart failure. *Circulation*. 2003;108:3064-3068.

45. Drews TN, Loebe M, Jurmann MJ, et al. Outpatients on mechanical circulatory support. *Ann Thorac Surg*. 2003;75:780-785.

46. Frazier OH, Rose EA, Macmanus Q, et al. Multicentre clinical evaluation of the Heartmate 1000 IP left ventricular assist device. *Ann Thorac Surg*. 1992;53:1080-1090.

47. Pennington DG, Bernhard WF, Golding LR, et al. Long-term follow up of postcardiotomy patients with profound cardiogenic shock treated with ventricular assist device. *Circulation*. 1985;72:216-226.

48. Pae WE, Miller CA, Matthews Y, Pierce WS. Ventricular assist devices for postcardiotomy cardiogenic shock. *J Thorac Cardiovasc Surg*. 1992;104:541-553.

49. Dipla K, Mattiello JA, Jeevanandam V, et al. Myocyte recovery after mechanical circulatory support in humans with end-stage heart failure. *Circulation*. 1998;97:2316-2322.

50. Zafeiridis A, Jeevanandam V, Houser SR, Margulies KB. Regression of cellular hypertrophy after left ventricular assist device support. *Circulation*. 1998;98(7):656-662.

51. Frazier OH, Benedict CR, Radovancevic B, et al. Improved left ventricular function after chronic left ventricular unloading. *Ann Thorac Surg*. 1996;62:675-681.

52. Levin HR, Oz MC, Chen JM, et al. Reversal of chronic ventricular dilatation in patients with end-stage cardiomyopathy by prolonged ventricular mechanical unloading. *Circulation*. 1995;91:2717-2720.

53. Nakatani S, McCarthy PM, Kottke-Marchant K, et al. Left ventricular echocardiographic and histologic changes: impact of chronic unloading by an implantable ventricular assist device. *J Am Coll Cardiol*. 1996;27:894-901.

54. Mancini DM, Beniaminovitz A, Levin H, et al. Low incidence of myocardial recovery after left ventricular assist device implantation in patients with chronic heart failure. *Circulation*. 1998;98:2383-2389.
55. Frazier OH, Myers TJ. Left ventricular assist system as a bridge to myocardial recovery. *Ann Thorac Surg*. 1999;68:734-741.
56. Hetzer R, Johannes M, Weng Y, et al. Bridging to recovery. *Ann Thorac Surg*. 2001;71: S109-S113.
57. Kumpati GS, McCarthy PM, Hoercher KJ. Left ventricular assist device bridge to recovery: a review of the current status. *Ann Thorac Surg*. 2001;71:S103-S108.
58. Muller J, Wallukat G, Weng YG, et al. Weaning from mechanical cardiac support in patients with idiopathic dilated cardiomyopathy. *Circulation*. 1997;96:542-549.
59. Birks EJ, Tansley PD, Hardy J, et al. Left ventricular assist device and drug therapy for the reversal of heart failure. *N Engl J Med*. 2006;355:1873-1884.
60. Rose EA, Gelijns A, Moskowitz AJ, et al. Long term use of a left ventricular assist device for end stage heart failure (REMATCH). *N Engl J Med*. 2001;345:1435-1443.
61. Taylor DO, Edwards LB, Aurora P, et al. Registry of the International Society for Heart and Lung Transplantation: twenty-fifth official adult heart transplant report – 2008. *J Heart Lung Transplant*. 2008;27:943-956.

Index

Printing: Ten Brink, Meppel, The Netherlands
Binding: Stürtz, Würzburg, Germany

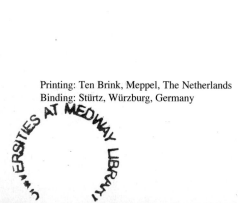